INFECTION
CONTROL

and Management of Hazardous
Materials for the Dental Team

INFECTION CONTROL

and Management of Hazardous
Materials for the Dental Team

Second Edition

Chris H. Miller, Ph.D.
Professor of Oral Microbiology
Director of Infection Control Research and Services
Associate Dean for Research and Graduate Education
Indiana University School of Dentistry
Indianapolis, Indiana

Charles John Palenik
Director of Sponsored Programs
Indiana University School of Dentistry
Indianapolis, Indiana

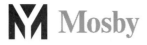 Mosby

St. Louis   Baltimore   Boston   Carlsbad   Chicago   Minneapolis   New York   Philadelphia   Portland
London   Milan   Sydney   Tokyo   Toronto

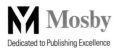

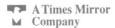

Publisher: John Schrefer
Editor: Penny Rudolph
Associate Developmental Editor: Kimberly Frare
Project Manager: Carol Sullivan Weis
Production Manager: Florence Achenbach
Designer: Jen Marmarinos

SECOND EDITION

Copyright © 1998 by Mosby, Inc.

Previous edition copyrighted 1994

Printed in the United States of America

Mosby
11830 Westline Industrial Drive
St. Louis, Missouri 64146

Library of Congress Cataloging in Publication Data
Miller, Chris H.
    Infection control and management of hazardous material for the
dental team / Chris H. Miller, Charles John Palenik. —2nd ed.
        p.   cm.
    Includes bibliographical references and index.
    ISBN 0-8151-5688-X
    1. Dental offices—Sanitation.   2. Cross infection—Prevention.
3. Dentistry—Safety measures.   4. Hazardous substances—Safety
measures.   I. Palenik, Charles John.   II. Title.
    [DNLM: 1. Infection Control, Dental—methods.   2. Waste
Management—methods.   3. Dental Waste.   4. Cross Infection—
prevention & control.   WU 29 M6467i 1998]
RK52.M46   1998
617.6′0028′9—dc21
DNLM/DLC
for Library of Congress   98–13526
                                                                  CIP

98 99 00 01 02 / 9 8 7 6 5 4 3 2 1

PREFACE to Second Edition

This second edition continues to emphasize the basic concepts of infectious disease spread upon which future developments can be based. It also emphasizes the actual practice of infection control by describing the specific procedures used and supplies and equipment needed for disease prevention and office safety. This edition continues to be a learning tool for all dental assisting, dental hygiene, and dental students and for established dental health care professionals developing or reorganizing their office safety programs.

Infection control in dentistry is continually being modified with the discovery of new information about infectious diseases and their causative agents. Occasionally a newly recognized disease appears, and sometimes known diseases change their patterns of occurrence, and these all influence disease prevention schemes. Thus this second edition is necessary to keep pace with recent developments and with new thinking on how to best practice infection control and office safety in light of a constantly changing pattern of diseases.

New features in this edition include three new chapters on emerging diseases, dental unit water asepsis, and fire prevention and emergency plans. Other new information appears on respiratory diseases, TB skin testing, prevention of TB in health care facilities, hepatitis C, and occupational exposures to HIV. New information on reactions to latex gloves also has been added along with procedures to be used during treatment of those with a latex allergy. The popular *Step-by-Step Procedures* in the first edition have been retained and expanded to facilitate training of students and the practicing dental team. Also, the clinical asepsis protocol in the first edition has been expanded into its own chapter to emphasize the importance of chairside infection control procedures. The chapter on managing the office safety program also includes a new 71-point checklist to help establish or reorganize the entire infection control program for the office. Other new information in this area includes a list of supplies and equipment needed to establish an instrument processing system and tips on how to design or reorganize an instrument processing area for the office.

We thank our colleagues who share their thoughts and expertise, allowing us to expand our thinking. We thank the front line dental professionals for their questions, concerns, and ideas that keep us informed about private practice environments. We thank the manufacturers and distributors of infection control products and equipment for their interests in developing new ways to attack infectious diseases. We thank the professional organizations in dentistry that provide forums for the discussion of disease prevention. We also thank our students who continue to challenge us to justify our statements, to develop meaningful approaches to learning, and to remain lifelong students ourselves.

Chris H. Miller
Charles John Palenik

PREFACE to First Edition

Controlling the spread of disease agents and maintaining office safety are two of the most rapidly expanding areas within and among all dental health-care professions. Significant regulatory actions by federal, state and local agencies recently have been issued for the protection of both patients and the dental team. These mandates have permanently changed how dental care is provided, and these changes must be reflected in the curricula offered in allied dental and dental education programs to assure proper training for everyone entering the dental health-care professions. Successful prevention of disease spread and proper management of hazardous materials require the interaction of the entire dental team. Allied dental personnel play key roles in organizing, managing, and maintaining these office safety programs. These responsibilities require an understanding of procedures used for infection control and office safety and also an understanding of basic concepts needed to respond to future changes in these rapidly evolving areas.

Therefore the purpose of this book is to provide basic concepts, specific step-by-step procedures, current regulatory mandates related to infection control, and the management of hazardous materials for the dental team. Although the book is written for students in allied dental health programs, it can be used to emphasize infection control procedures, hazardous materials management, and current regulatory mandates in undergraduate and graduate dental programs. The book also updates office safety procedures for practicing dentists, hygienists, and assistants.

Since prevention of disease spread is based in the discipline of microbiology, the book includes basic concepts in microbiology with descriptions of bacteria, viruses and fungi, how infectious diseases develop, oral microbial diseases and bloodborne disease agents. It also contains an explanation of how disease agents may be spread in dental environments and a description of regulations relating to office safety with approaches to compliance. Prevention of certain diseases is addressed in a chapter on available immunizations, and specific infection control procedures are presented in detail, including step-by-step procedures for the use of protective barriers, processing contaminated instruments, surface asepsis, aseptic techniques, laboratory and radiographic asepsis, and waste management. Management of hazardous materials and a description of the related regulations are described, as is an approach to manage an office safety program.

We thank our illustrator (Mark Dirlam), photographers (Michael Halloran and Alana Barra), and typist (Kim Tillman). We also thank our students and colleagues for their challenging questions and their desire to learn and to share information.

CHRIS H. MILLER
CHARLES JOHN PALENIK

CONTENTS

PART I   THE MICROBIAL WORLD

1   Scope of Microbiology and Infection Control   2

2   Characteristics of Microorganisms   5

3   Development of Infectious Diseases   23

4   Emerging Diseases   35

5   Oral Microbiology and Plaque-associated Diseases   43

PART II   INFECTION CONTROL

6   Bloodborne Pathogens   54

7   Oral and Respiratory Diseases   70

8   Infection Control Rationale and Regulations   83

9   Immunization   106

10   Protective Barriers   115

11   Instrument Processing   135

12   Surface and Equipment Asepsis   175

13   Dental Unit Water Asepsis   190

14   Aseptic Techniques   205

15   Laboratory and Radiographic Asepsis   210

16   Waste Management   222

17   A Clinical Asepsis Protocol   230

PART III   OFFICE SAFETY

18   Managing the Office Safety Program   236

19   Managing Chemicals Safely in the Office   247

20   Employee Fire Prevention and Emergency Plans   275

APPENDIXES

A   Infection Control and Hazardous Materials Management Resource List   280

B   CDC Infection Control Guidelines for Dentistry   283

C   CDC Guidelines for Prevention of Tuberculosis in Dental Settings   295

D   Office Safety and Asepsis Procedures (OSAP) Research Foundation   298

E   Exposure Incident Report   308

F   Chemicals Used for Infection Control   310

G   Infection Control Recommendations for the Dental Office and the Dental Laboratory   317

H   The OSHA Bloodborne Pathogens Standard   329

GLOSSARY   343

I
PART

THE MICROBIAL WORLD

Chapter 1

SCOPE OF MICROBIOLOGY AND INFECTION CONTROL

ROLE OF MICROORGANISMS IN INFECTION CONTROL

Microbiology is the study of small life forms, including bacteria, special fungi called molds and yeasts, protozoa, certain algae, and viruses. There are several subdisciplines within microbiology that concentrate on specific types of microorganisms, such as *bacteriology, mycology* (study of fungi), *protozoology,* and *virology,* or on the activities of selected microorganisms such as those important in the fields of medical microbiology, dental microbiology, food microbiology, industrial microbiology, and environmental (aquatic, soil, sewage, and space) microbiology. There are also very close relationships to the fields of immunology (study of the immune system) and biochemistry (the chemistry of life forms).

The field of infection control (controlling microbial contamination and infection) is deeply seated within the discipline of microbiology. In fact, microbiology had its beginnings as a science concerned with the control and identification of microorganisms in attempts to explain and prevent disease. An understanding of the physical and chemical properties of microorganisms, where microorganisms exist, how they grow, how they are influenced by the environment or special physical and chemical agents, and how they cause specific diseases of concern form the basis for killing microorganisms and understanding and preventing their spread from person to person. Also, a general knowledge of immunology and body defense mechanisms contributes to the understanding of disease prevention through immunization and through reliance on the body's natural barriers against infection.

DISCOVERY OF MICROORGANISMS AND INFECTION CONTROL PROCEDURES

Diseases were recognized long before their causative agents. The Italian physician, Girolamo Fracastorius, in 1546, is generally given the credit for being the first to recognize the existence of tiny living particles that cause "catching" (contagious) diseases by being spread by direct contact with humans and animals and by indirect contact with objects. Since microorganisms are too small to be seen with the naked eye, their actual existence was not established until Antoni van Leeuwenhoek first observed what he called "animalcules" (bacteria, yeasts, and protozoa) in 1667. The microorganisms became visible when he observed tooth scrapings and gutter water under a simple microscope.

The relationship of these "little animals" to disease was not established until "The Golden Age of Microbiology" in the mid- to late 1800s by researchers such as Louis Pasteur (France), Robert Koch (Germany), Ignaz Semmelweis (Vienna), Oliver Wendell

Holmes (USA), Lord Joseph Lister (England), and Willoby D. Miller (USA) who became known as the "Father of Oral Microbiology." By 1900, microorganisms known as bacteria had been described and recognized as the cause of numerous diseases such as anthrax, diphtheria, tuberculosis, cholera, tetanus, leprosy, epidemic meningitis, gonorrhea, brucellosis, pneumonia, abscesses, food poisoning, and dental caries.

The Golden Age of Microbiology also brought about the basis for disease prevention through use of *infection control procedures.* Semmelweis in Vienna and Holmes in the USA first recognized the importance of handwashing in preventing the spread of disease agents. The use of heat to destroy vegetative bacteria and resistant bacterial spores was recognized by Pasteur and John Tyndall. They used boiling water to kill bacteria, and the process known as *pasteurization* (destroying pathogens in milk by heating it to 63° C [145.4° F] for 30 minutes or to 72° C [161.6° F] for 15 seconds) is still used today. Lord Lister as a surgeon became concerned about postoperative infections and demonstrated that boiling instruments and washing his hands and surgical linens with phenol before surgery greatly reduced these complications. He also proposed that infections of open wounds were caused by microorganisms in the air, so he sprayed the air around his patients with phenol before surgery. These procedures were considered bold and outrageous at the time but they truly paved the way for sterile and aseptic techniques that are now practiced throughout the world.

The activities of the human body's immune defense mechanisms were recognized about four centuries ago when it was known that some individuals who recovered from a sickness did not get that disease a second time. Edward Jenner is credited with recognizing the concept of immunization when he realized in the 1790s that milkmaids who caught cowpox, a mild disease, were protected from the more serious disease of smallpox. He injected the fluid from cowpox pustules into a healthy boy and later injected the boy with fluid from human smallpox lesions. The boy did not get smallpox.

Pasteur became known as the "Father of Immunology" for his work in developing immunization techniques against chicken cholera, anthrax in cattle, and rabies in humans.

The viral diseases of polio, smallpox, and rabies had been described for centuries but a microbial cause for these and other diseases was not apparent until 1898 when Loeffler and Frosch demonstrated that an agent smaller than bacteria, and that could not be seen through the microscopes of the day, caused foot-and-mouth disease in animals. For the next 40 or so years, there was fierce scientific debate as to the nature of such small disease agents, that were named viruses, the latin word for poisons. Similar agents that infected bacteria were discovered in 1915 and in 1922 were named *bacteriophages* ("bacteria eaters"). Then in 1940 the electron microscope was developed, and Stanley at the Rockefeller Institute in Princeton, New Jersey, published the first pictures of a virus magnified 35,000 times its normal size. This tobacco mosaic disease virus was first erroneously described as a large protein molecule. Today we know that viruses contain nucleic acids (RNA or DNA), a few molecules of enzymes, structural proteins, and sometimes lipids. However, it is interesting to note that a recently discovered group of "unconventional viruses" (including agents causing Creutzfeldt Jakob disease and kuru in humans and scrapie in animals) are now called *prions,* a term that means "proteinaceous infectious particle," because they apparently lack RNA or DNA that is present in conventional viruses.

By 1943, viruses were described as the cause of smallpox, chickenpox, rabies, poliomyelitis, yellow fever, mumps, the common cold, hepatitis A, and influenza. Over the next 30 years, several other viruses were first isolated or seen through the electron microscope, including rubella virus, measles virus, Epstein-Barr virus, and other herpes viruses.

Microbe hunters similar to Pasteur and Koch have been active throughout the history of microbiology and infection control. Within the last 25 or so years new infectious diseases or the causative agents of recognized diseases have been discovered (see Chapter 4). Diseases will continue to emerge as new or renewed opportunities develop for microorganisms to associate with humans and cause diseases. These might result from closer interactions between the populations of the world and their unique diseases, changes in the disease-producing abilities of microorganisms, unknown factors that may enhance susceptibility of the body to microbial infections, lack of appreciation for maintenance of current vaccine programs and insect control projects, and enhanced complacency concerning the general cleanliness of objects we contact and personal hygiene.

IMPORTANT ACTIVITIES OF MICROORGANISMS

Microorganisms are actually more beneficial than harmful to mankind but we usually hear about or see only their harmful activities of causing diseases, spoiling food, occluding water lines, or destroying fabrics. Bacteria in the soil convert dead plants, animals, and insects into usable nutrients needed for survival of the live plants. Other soil microorganisms convert atmospheric nitrogen and carbon dioxide into forms that are required for growth by all plants. Bacteria also form the basis of modern sewage treatment by degrading the organic material in the sewage as it flows over or is mixed with bacterial masses in treatment plants. Also bacteria are cultured in large vats to make several products such as vinegar, vitamins, alcohol, organic acids, enzyme cleaners, drain openers, antibiotics, insecticides, and special chemicals used in biomedical research. Microorganisms are used in making rubber products, tobacco, and spices and are used also in processing leather. Some bacteria are used to help clean up oil spills in the oceans because they can degrade the components of crude oil. Special fungi called yeasts make bread dough rise and are used in beer production. Bacteria or fungi are used to pickle cucumbers, produce cultured dairy products such as yogurt and sour cream, and to make cheeses. Bacteria or yeasts are also used to synthesize special agents such as insulin, other hormones, and hepatitis B vaccines used to treat or prevent diseases.

Harmful activities of microorganisms usually result when they are someplace they should not be and when they grow out of control. Microorganisms do not really intend to harm or destroy things; they simply "wish" to survive and grow (increase their numbers). Unfortunately, their growth results in the production of substances that may harm or change their habitat. If their habitat is the human body, disease may occur. If it is food, the food may spoil. If they accumulate in a water line, the water flow is stopped or reduced. Thus harmful activities of microorganisms are actually accidents resulting from their growth.

The first approach to preventing the harmful activities of microorganisms is to attempt to keep them in their proper place by preventing contamination (e.g., infection control or exposure control). If they get someplace where they should not be, they must be removed, killed, or kept from growing to harmful numbers (e.g., by cleaning, sterilization, disinfection, growth inhibition, immunization, or antimicrobial therapy).

SELECTED READINGS

Brock TD: *Milestones in microbiology,* Washington DC, 1975, American Society for Microbiology.

Gest H: *The world of microbes,* Menlo Park, California, 1987, Benjamin Cummings.

Chapter 2

CHARACTERISTICS OF MICROORGANISMS

There are four groups of microorganisms with varying degrees of importance in the field of dentistry and allied dental health. These are *bacteria, viruses, fungi,* and *protozoa.* Although each group has a different life-style and each group is composed of many different types, they all share two common characteristics: they are too small to be seen by the naked eye, and many members of each group can live on or in the human body, which may result in development of harmful infections.

BACTERIA

Bacterial Names and Differentiation

Bacteria are named like most other life forms, with a first name *(genus)* and a last name *(species).* Each genus is composed of one or more species, and some species may be further subdivided into types and strains. For example, the genus *Streptococcus* is composed of approximately 21 different species, and the oral species *S. mutans* is divided into eight subtypes (a-h).

Bacteria have different characteristics and activities that allow them to be distinguished from each other. These include cell morphology (size and shape), staining characteristics, colony characteristics (appearance during growth on agar media), metabolic properties, immunologic properties, and DNA characteristics.

All size and shape is determined by observation under a microscope that magnifies approximately 1,000 times normal size. Because bacteria are difficult to see even under a regular light microscope, procedures for staining the cells with special dyes were developed to aid visualization. A staining procedure developed by Dr. Christian Gram differentiates bacteria into one of two groups. Those that appear blue or purple are called *gram-positive,* and those that appear pink or red are called *gram-negative.* Gram–positive and gram-negative bacteria have other important differences, which will be described later. Other staining procedures also aid in identifying bacteria. For example, the Ziehl-Neelsen or Kinyoun acid-fast stain helps visualize acid-fast bacilli (AFB) and greatly aids in the identification of *Mycobacterium tuberculosis,* the causative agent of tuberculosis.

Another way to visualize bacteria is to place (inoculate) them onto the surface of a semisolid growth medium, called agar, contained in a covered dish, called a petri plate (described later). If the agar medium contains all the proper nutrients and is incubated at the proper temperature, each bacterium begins to multiply into a small mass of cells (a colony) that can be seen with the naked eye (Figure 2-1). Each visible colony contains hundreds of thousands of bacterial cells and frequently has an appearance (shape, color, size, consistency) different from those of another species. Thus colony morphology is one aspect used to differentiate bacteria.

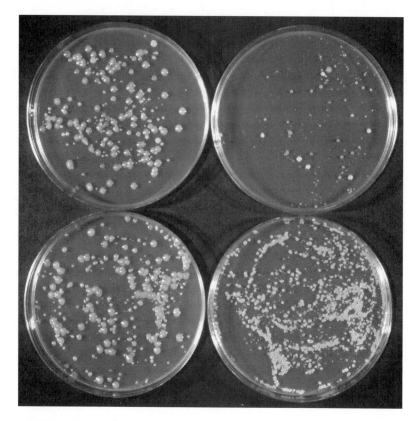

FIGURE 2-1   Colonies of different bacteria on an agar growth medium in petri plates. Colonies of different bacteria vary in size and appearance. Each plate contains a different number of colonies, and each colony contains thousands of cells.

Metabolism is the physical and chemical changes that occur during bacterial growth (multiplication or increase in numbers of cells). Different bacteria have different metabolic properties, which distinguishes one from another. Detecting these differences may involve performing many tests, such as, for example, determining the nutrients (e.g., sugars and amino acids) used for growth, the requirements for oxygen or carbon dioxide during growth, the waste materials (e.g., acids) produced during growth, and the *enzymes* (e.g., catalysts that chemically change a substance such as breaking down proteins into amino acids) made during growth.

Table 2-1 describes various macromolecules and their subunits to assist in understanding the characteristics of microorganisms. Bacteria having different chemical substances on their surfaces or that make different extracellular substances (substances that are released from the cell to the outside environment) cause the synthesis of different *antibodies* (special proteins in serum) when bacteria are placed into animals. These antibodies are part of the immune defense system of humans and lower animals and will be further explained in Chapter 3. Antibodies formed against one bacterium will usually bind only to that bacterium and not to others, and this binding can be visualized in the laboratory by a variety of techniques. Thus exposing an animal to a known bacterium, allowing the animal to

Table 2–1 Microbial Biochemicals

MACROMOLECULE	BASIC COMPOSITION	EXAMPLES OR OCCURRENCE
Protein	Amino acids (e.g., tryptophan, leucine)	Enzymes, viral capsid, cell walls, cytoplasmic membranes, flagella
Polysaccharide	Monosaccharides (e.g., glucose, fructose)	Capsules, storage granules, dextran
Lipid	Fatty acids, glycerol	Cytoplasmic membranes, viral envelopes
Nucleic acid	Adenine, guanine, cytosine, thymine, ribose	DNA, RNA
Glycoprotein	Polysaccharide, protein	Fimbriae, viral envelope
Lipoprotein	Lipid, protein	Cell wall
Lipopolysaccharide	Lipid, polysaccharide	Endotoxin

make antibodies to that bacterium, mixing the animal's serum with unknown bacteria in the laboratory, and looking for a visualized positive reaction can help determine the identity of the unknown bacteria.

All of the properties of bacteria are controlled by specific genes in their DNA. Thus because different bacteria have different properties, they also have different DNA. Several techniques can be used to detect these differences in DNA, and these techniques greatly aid in differentiating and identifying bacteria.

Cell Morphology and Structure
Size and Shape

Bacteria are single cells with one of three basic shapes. Spherical cells are called *cocci* (singular: *coccus*); rodshaped cells are called *bacilli* (singular: *bacillus*); curved or spiral cells are called *spirilla* (singular: *spirillum*). The cocci and bacilli may exist as single cells or they may exist in small clusters or in chains (Figure 2-2). The average diameter of a coccus is about one *micrometer* (μm). Common bacilli are about one μm wide and 5 to 10 μm long.

Spirilla are 0.2 to 1.0 μm wide and up to 30 μm long. A micrometer is one-millionth of a meter or one-thousandth of a millimeter, and a millimeter is the smallest division on a metric ruler. Approximately 25,000 cocci laid side by side would create a line just one inch long! In comparison, a human red blood cell is about 7 μm in diameter.

Structure

Although bacterial species differ in shape, size, and activity, their structure is similar. Understanding this structure helps explain their role in causing diseases, their resistance to methods of killing, and their activities that are beneficial to mankind. The structures of a representative bacterial cell are shown in Figure 2-3; the functions of these structures are listed in Table 2-2.

Cytoplasm. The *cytoplasm* is contained within the cytoplasmic membrane and is a viscous material consisting of water, enzymes and other proteins, carbohydrates, lipids, nu-

A

B

C

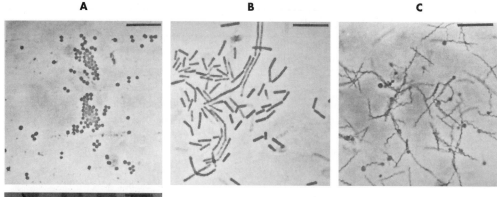

D

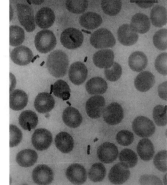

FIGURE 2-2   The common morphologies of prokaryotic cells as revealed by phase-contrast photomicrographs of unstained **(A)** *Staphylococcus aureus* (cocci), **(B)** *Bacillus subtilis* (rods), and **(C)** *Treponema denticola* (spirals) compared with **(D)** human red blood cells. *Bacillus subtilis* has been mixed with the red blood cells in **D** for size comparison. Bar = 10 μm. (From Slots J, Taubman MA: *Contemporary oral microbiology and immunology,* St. Louis, 1992, Mosby, p. 12.)

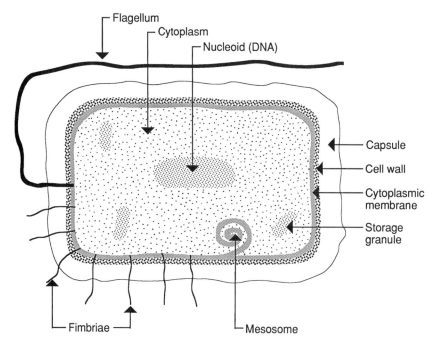

FIGURE 2-3   Diagram of a composite bacterial cell.

Table 2-2 Bacterial Structure and Function

STRUCTURE	FUNCTION/ACTIVITY
Cytoplasmic membrane	Transport of nutrients; energy metabolism; secretion of wastes; DNA synthesis; cell wall synthesis
Cell wall	Cell shape; protection from mechanical damage
Outer membrane of gram-negative bacteria	Contains endotoxin; transport of nutrients
Capsule	Protection from drying; antiphagocytic; attachment to surfaces
Flagella	Locomotion
Fimbriae (Pili)	Attachment to surfaces; transport of DNA between cells
Nucleoid	DNA controls cell activities
Endospore	Protection against adverse conditions

cleic acids, essential nutrients, oxygen, and waste products. Embedded in the cytoplasm is the bacterial *nucleoid,* consisting of a single long chromosome of DNA that contains most of the genes (approximately 2500) controlling cell activities. The nucleoid is usually diffused throughout the cytoplasm rather than well defined as in mammalian cells. Some bacteria also have extrachromosal DNA in small units in the cytoplasm, called plasmids. Plasmids frequently carry genes that express special activities such as resistance to chemical and physical agents and antibiotics.

The cytoplasm also contains submicroscopic particles called ribosomes that serve as physical sites for the synthesis of proteins from amino acids. Some bacteria may have granules in the cytoplasm that consist of stored substances such as starch, lipids, or iron.

Cytoplasmic Membrane.   The *cytoplasmic membrane* surrounds the cytoplasm and is composed of lipids and protein substances. Its structure is similar to that of mammalian cells, and its functions include regulating the entrance and exit of nutrient materials and waste products, maintaining proper pressure within the cell to keep it from "bursting," containing the enzymes responsible for synthesizing the outer cell wall, serving as the physical site for attachment and allocation of newly formed chromosomal DNA during cell division, controlling release of certain extracellular enzymes, and serving as the site of many metabolic reactions through which the cell gains energy for growth.

Mesosomes, present mostly in gram-positive bacteria, are inward foldings of the cytoplasmic membrane. This structure houses many hydrolytic enzymes that are released into the extracellular environment and break down macromolecules into their subunits that are taken into the cell as food.

Antimicrobial agents in many disinfectants, hand washing agents, and mouth rinses kill or inhibit the growth of bacteria by acting on the cytoplasmic membrane. Chlorhexidine gluconate, present in hand washing products and mouth rinses, is thought to affect the cell membrane and interfere with energy metabolism and uptake of nutrients.

Cell Wall.   The bacterial *cell wall* is a rigid structure that gives the cell its characteristic shape (coccus, rod, spirillum) and is not present in mammalian cells. It is a very complex structure in which its basic components *(peptidoglycan)* forms a very tight-knit "net" over the entire surface of the cell. Peptidoglycan (peptide: small protein; glycan: polysaccharide) consists of very long polysaccharide chains with short side-chains of peptides. The peptides of one polysaccharide chain are linked to the peptides of other polysaccharide chains, forming a large continuous macromolecule. Besides giving the cell its characteristic shape, the peptidoglycan also protects the cell from mechanical crushing. Gram-positive bacteria have several layers of peptidoglycan in their cell walls and are much more resistant to external physical forces than the gram-negative bacteria because the latter have only a very few layers of peptidoglycan.

The cell wall peptidoglycan is the site of action of several antimicrobial agents. *Lysozyme* is an enzyme present in saliva, tears, nasal secretions, and other body secretions and is present inside white blood cells (e.g., phagocytes, described later) that destroy bacteria. This enzyme lyses susceptible bacteria by breaking the bond between the subunits of the polysaccharide chain in peptidoglycan. The antibiotic penicillin and its many derivations act by preventing cross-linking of the peptidoglycan units as the cell wall is being synthesized during cell division. Other antibiotics such as vancomycin and the cephalosporins also prevent cell wall synthesis. The action of all of these antimicrobial agents results in "holes" forming in the peptidoglycan that cause a loss of the cytoplasm into the external environment (lysis) and cell death.

Outer Membrane.   Gram-negative (but not gram-positive) bacteria have an outer membrane just external to the cell wall. It covers the entire cell surface, and its basic structure and composition is like the cytoplasmic membrane. The outer membrane, however, contains a very important component called *endotoxin* that is composed of lipid, polysaccharide, and protein (lipopolysaccharide-protein complex). When endotoxin is released from bacteria present in the body (after cell death and lysis or in some instances during its synthesis), it can cause damage to nearby body cells and stimulate several reactions in the body, including fever, inflammation, bone destruction, hemorrhage, and vomiting. The action of endotoxin is thought to play a role in many infectious diseases, including periodontal diseases, dysentery, meningitis, typhoid fever, gonorrhea, and cholera.

Capsule.   Some gram-positive and gram-negative bacteria contain another structure called the *capsule.* It is also referred to as a slime layer or glycocalyx. The capsule covers the entire outer surface external to the cell wall in some gram-positive bacteria or external to the outer membrane in some gram-negative bacteria. It is produced by the cytoplasmic membrane and secreted through the cell wall and remains associated with the cell surface in the form of a gelatinous covering. Usually it consists of polysaccharide but in a few instances it may contain proteins. Some species may have large capsules, such as *Streptococcus pneumoniae* (the cause of lobar pneumonia and middle ear infections); others may have only a thin layer of capsular material, such as *Streptococcus mutans* (a cause of dental caries).

Capsules contain a large amount of water (hydrated) and may help bacteria survive in dry environments. The presence of a capsule also influences how bacteria interact with cells and other surfaces in the human body. Surface polysaccharides in the microcapsule of *S. mutans* are involved in sucrose-induced plaque formation on tooth surfaces (see Chapter 5). The presence of capsules also reduces the ability of white blood cells to surround, engulf, and destroy the bacterium through a process called *phagocytosis* (eating cells) and digestion (see Chapter 3). Thus, bacteria with capsules tend to escape these early body defense mechanisms against bacterial disease agents. Bacteria without capsules are more easily engulfed and destroyed.

Flagella.   Some bacteria have long, threadlike appendages called *flagella* (singular: *flagellum*). These protein structures are attached to the cytoplasmic membrane extending through the cell wall and, if present, the outer membrane and capsule. They have a whip-like motion and allow the bacterium to move through fluids and be motile. The number of flagella per bacterial cell may range from one to many, exhibiting different arrangements over the cell surface.

Fimbriae and pili.   These structures are hairlike protein appendages projecting from the cytoplasmic membrane into the external environment. They are much shorter than flagella and have two major functions. Sex pili, found mainly on gram-negative bacteria, serve as a tube through which DNA can be passed directly from a donor cell to a recipient cell during a process called conjugation. This process permits properties expressed by the DNA genes of one cell to be transferred to and expressed by another cell. *Fimbriae,* also called *pili,* serve as mechanisms by which cells can attach to other cells or environmental surfaces. The fimbriae act as a bridge between the cell and other surfaces. Attachment fimbriae provide a very important virulence property. Almost all bacteria that cause harmful infections on or through mucous membranes must first attach to the epithelial cells of the mucous membrane or they will be washed away by secretions of the body. Attachment fimbriae provide the mechanisms of attachment in such diseases as "strep throat," scarlet fever, gonorrhea, and diphtheria and cause some bacteria to attach to each other during the formation of dental plaque.

Endospores.   Some bacteria have developed a defense mechanism against death caused by adverse environmental conditions. When available nutrients become depleted, cells of *Bacillus* and *Clostridium* form a large internal structure that contains the DNA and other substances surrounded by several coats of protein. This dense, thick-walled structure is called a *spore* or *endospore* and is one of the most resistant forms of life against heat, drying, and chemicals (Figure 2-4). Once formed, the spore can remain dormant for years and then, when exposed to the proper nutrients and other growth requirements, it can germinate into an actively dividing (vegetative) cell. Only one endospore forms within a bacterial cell and it germinates into only one vegetative bacterial cell. This is in contrast to fungal spores in which several spores may form a single cell. Bacterial spores are particularly important in the field of infection control because of their high resistance to heat and antimicrobial chemicals. Spores of *Bacillus stearothermophilus* and *Bacillus subtilis* are used to biologically monitor the use and functioning of heat or ethylene oxide gas sterilizers (see Chapter 11). Also, spores of *B. subtilis* and *Clostridium sporogenes* are used to test the antimicrobial effectiveness of liquid sterilants used at room temperature.

Growth and Control

Bacterial growth is defined as an increase in cell numbers; it is also referred to as multiplication. The cells divide by a process called *binary fission,* in which each cell divides into two daughter cells (Figure 2-5). In the next generation, each of these daughter cells divides into two similar cells, and this continues until the environmental conditions no longer support growth because of a lack of nutrients, a buildup of toxic products, or changes in pH, temperature, and availability of oxygen, or the application of physical or chemical agents that kill the bacteria.

Bacteria have a tremendous ability to multiply, and under optimal growth conditions

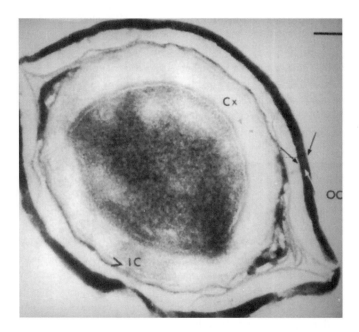

FIGURE 2-4   Thin-section of a *Bacillus megatherium* spore showing two spore coats (*IC,* inner coat; *OC,* outer coat). The germ cell wall of the spore coat is seen immediately underlying the thick cortex *(Cx).* Bar = 100 nm. (From Aaronson AI, Fitz-James P: *Bact Rev* 40:360-402, 1976.)

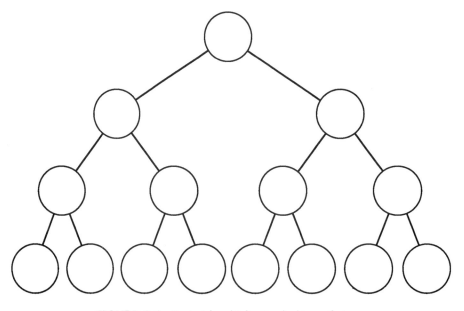

FIGURE 2-5   Bacterial multiplication by binary fission.

a population of some bacteria such as *Escherichia coli* can double in number (go from one generation to the next) in just 20 minutes. If such growth continues for just 24 hours, one cell can multiply to a mass of cells that is equal to the size of Earth (more than 3 trillion billions of cells)! This of course can never happen because nutrients soon become depleted and growth stops. To be more realistic, 10 milliliters (mL) of an overnight broth culture of a bacterium seldom achieve a total population of more than 10 billion cells.

Growth Requirements

Bacteria are influenced by a variety of physical and chemical conditions of the environments in which they exist. Each bacterial species requires certain conditions for growth, and if those conditions do not exist at a given site, the bacterium will not be found at that site. Even subtle differences are important. For example, the differences in the physical and the chemical environments between the buccal surface of a tooth and a periodontal pocket just a few millimeters away are sufficient to result in important differences in the types and numbers of bacteria that are found at these two sites (see Chapter 5). The greater the differences among environmental sites, the greater the differences in the types and numbers of bacteria present. Thus the bacteria that survive and grow in the human body can be very different from those that survive in the oceans. Conversely, some bacterial species can survive and grow in widely different environments. There are five major chemical or physical conditions that influence growth of bacteria.

Temperature.   Bacteria can be divided into three groups based on the temperature required for optimum growth. *Thermophils* grow best at 56° C (132.8° F) with a range of 45° C to 70° C (113° F to 158° F). Such bacteria were found in the hot waters of the "Old Faithful" geyser in Yellowstone National Park. More importantly, the spore-forming, thermophilic bacterium, B. *stearothermophilus,* was selected many years ago to test the use and functioning of heat sterilizers because of its resistance to heat. *Mesophils* grow at temperatures ranging from 22° C to 45° C (71.6° F to 113° F) with optimal growth at body temperature, 37° C (98.6° F). Most of the bacteria that grow and survive in the human body, including those that cause infectious diseases (such as dental caries, periodontal diseases, tuberculosis, bacterial pneumonia, tetanus, and many others) are mesophils. *Psychrophils* grow between temperatures of 1° C and 22° C (33.8° F and 71.6° F), with optimal growth at the typical refrigerator temperature, 7° C (44.6° F). The bacteria present in the oceans, as well as many of those that spoil food stored in a refrigerator, are psychrophils. Refrigeration has long been used to maintain the freshness of food or extend the storage life of many items that may be contaminated with microorganisms. It slows down or prevents the growth of many bacteria and molds but refrigeration cannot be considered a means of killing microorganisms. If psychrophils are present, they will continue to grow at normal rates at these low temperatures. If fresh pasteurized milk or high-quality hamburger is purchased at the food market and stored unopened in the refrigerator, it will eventually spoil because microorganisms, some of which may be psychrophils, will grow, using the nutrients in the milk or meat, and will produce physical and chemical changes associated with food spoilage.

Thus if an item or solution becomes contaminated with microorganisms, placing it in the refrigerator or freezer cannot be relied on to kill the microorganisms to make it "safe" for use.

Acidity.   pH is a measure of acidity, and the pH scale ranges from 0 (high acid) to 14 (high alkalinity). Values from 0 to 7 are acidic and values from 7 to 14 are basic or alkaline in nature. The neutral pH of 7 indicates an equal amount of acid and base or no acid or base present. Examples of acidic solutions are stomach acid (pH 1.5) and orange juice (pH 2.9). Examples of basic or alkaline solutions are household ammonia cleaners (pH 11.9) and human blood (about pH 7.4). Pure water has a pH of 7.0.

Most bacteria that survive in the human body grow over a pH range of approximately 5.5 to 8.5, with optimal growth at pH 7.0. Bacteria that produce acids during growth are called *acidogenic;* those that survive and grow in an acidic environment (usually below pH 5.5) are called *aciduric.* Acidogenic and aciduric bacteria are important in the initiation and progression of dental caries, as described in Chapter 4.

Nutrients.   Bacteria, like mammalian cells, must synthesize all of the macromolecules of protein, polysaccharides, lipids, and nucleic acids (DNA and RNA) needed to grow. These macromolecules are synthesized from the building blocks of amino acids, monosaccharides, fatty acids, and purines/pyrimidines, respectively. Bacteria also must use a variety of smaller molecules such as vitamins and inorganic substances (e.g., sodium, potassium, iron, chlorine, manganese, magnesium, sulfur, phosphorus, calcium, and trace elements). If a bacterium cannot synthesize a given building block such as an amino acid or a vitamin such as niacin, these substances must be available from the environment for the bacterium to survive and grow. Just as we require "eight essential vitamins," bacteria also require nutrients for growth.

Different bacteria have different nutritional requirements. For example, *S. mutans* may require six amino acids, five vitamins, all four purines and pyrimidines, and other small molecules plus an energy source, nitrogen, oxygen, inorganic salts, and trace elements from its environment. Conversely, some types of *E.coli* need only carbon dioxide, a nitrogen source, and trace elements and from this meager "diet" can synthesize all of the macromolecules needed for growth.

Many organic nutrients available for growth may not be in a form that can be used by the bacteria. For example, amino acids are the building blocks for proteins, and many bacteria require certain amino acids to synthesize their own proteins needed for growth. In many instances, proteins rather than the amino acid building blocks are present in the environment but the entire protein molecules are too large to get into bacterial cells. Thus many bacteria make extracellular *proteases,* which are enzymes released into the environment that break down proteins into amino acids that can enter the cell. Bacteria also may produce extracellular enzymes that degrade polysaccharides into monosaccharides or lipids into fatty acids, which then can be taken into the cell and be used for growth.

Unfortunately, when these extracellular bacterial enzymes are produced in the human body during a bacterial infection, they may degrade proteins, polysaccharides, or lipids that are important components of body cells, causing damage to these cells. This is one of the mechanisms by which bacteria cause disease.

Oxygen Metabolism.   Bacteria are divided into four groups based on their requirement for oxygen:

Obligate aerobes require the presence of oxygen at concentrations of approximately 20% and cannot grow at low oxygen concentrations
Microaerophiles can tolerate only low concentrations of oxygen at no more than 4%
Obligate anaerobes cannot tolerate oxygen and grow only in its absence
Facultative anaerobes can grow in the presence or absence of oxygen

Almost all bacteria (regardless of their growth requirement for oxygen) have enzymes that produce toxic substances (e.g., superoxide and hydrogen peroxide) from oxygen that can kill the bacteria. These toxic substances also are produced by white blood cells and help these cells kill bacteria after phagocytosis (see Chapter 3). Some bacteria that produce these toxic substances in the presence of oxygen have mechanisms to remove them to prevent death. One mechanism involves the enzyme *superoxide dismutase* that converts superoxide to hydrogen peroxide and molecular oxygen. Hydrogen peroxide is converted to water and oxygen by the enzyme *catalase.*

Obligate aerobes, microaerophiles, and facultative anaerobes, all of which can grow in the presence of oxygen, have superoxide dismutase and catalase to detoxify the oxygen metabolites. Obligate anaerobes do not have these enzymes and therefore cannot tolerate the presence of oxygen. Approximately 99% of the bacteria that live in the mouth are either obligate anaerobes or facultative anaerobes.

Water. All life forms require water to dissolve nutrients and to permit nutrient entrance or transport into cells. Also, the water molecule is required in several enzymatic reactions to break down (e.g., hydrolyze) certain substances.

Culturing Bacteria

All of the nutritional and physical growth requirements must be met to culture (grow) bacteria in the laboratory. Culture media in the form of a liquid (broth medium) or in a semisolid form (agar medium) provide the nutrients. Agar is a polysaccharide from seaweed that is liquid at boiling temperatures and turns semisolid when it cools to room temperature. Agar is added to a solution of nutrients, brought to a boil, sterilized, and poured into covered dishes (petri plates) or into tubes to cool and solidify. Samples of bacteria are then placed into sterilized broth media or onto the surface of sterile agar media and incubated under the appropriate atmospheric conditions (anaerobically: without air; aerobically: in air) at the proper temperature.

If bacteria grow in the broth culture, the broth becomes turbid (cloudy). If bacteria grow on the surface of agar media, visible colonies of bacteria (see Figure 2-1) appear that may be well separated from each other, or if a large number of bacteria were originally placed on the agar, a confluent solid mass of growth (lawn) may appear all over the surface.

An agar medium is primarily used to physically separate bacterial cells from each other to obtain a *pure culture* (growth of only one type of bacterium). Most samples taken from the human body or from nature that are cultured for the presence of bacteria contain many different species. When the sample is spread or streaked (inoculated) over the surface of an agar medium, individual cells or small groups of cells, called *colony-forming units* (CFU), are deposited at different sites on the surface. As the agar plate is incubated, each cell or CFU begins to multiply into a pure colony (clone). Thus all of the cells in the colony are derived from the cells or CFU originally deposited at that site and exist as a pure culture that can be picked off the agar medium and kept separate from all other bacteria. Occasionally, more than one type of bacterial cell can be deposited next to another on the agar surface during inoculation and both will grow into a mixed, rather than a pure, colony. Such colonies must be picked off and restreaked on a fresh agar plate to separate the types into pure colonies.

Agar plates also provide a means to quantitate the number, or CFU, of bacterial cells present in a sample. Each single colony that develops on the agar plate after incubation represents one CFU present in the original sample.

Most bacteria can survive and grow separately from other cells, if the environment is appropriate. There are special bacteria that can grow only while inside other living cells. Their general structures and mechanisms for growth are the same as the free-living bacteria but they lack some of the metabolic machinery necessary to exist separately. Thus they use the machinery of other cells to grow. Examples of these special bacteria are members of the genera *Rickettsia,* which can cause diseases such as Rocky Mountain spotted fever, typhus, and ehrlichiosis, and *Chlamydia,* which can cause sexually transmitted diseases, pneumonia, and trachoma (disease of the eye).

Metabolic Activities

Metabolism is the sum total of chemical reactions that occur in the cell. It involves the uptake of nutrients into the cell, converting them to substances needed by the cells for survival and multiplication and release of waste products (Figure 2-6). Metabolism includes two phases: *catabolism,* or the breakdown of nutrients to smaller or more easily usable molecules, and *anabolism,* or the synthesis of new molecules. Catabolism provides the building blocks or carbon skeletons and the energy needed for anabolism. Anabolism provides the macromolecules needed to make cell components, such as cell walls, DNA, cytoplasmic membranes, fimbriae, flagella, cytoplasmic granules, and capsules. Both catabolic and anabolic reactions require biologic catalysts called enzymes.

Enzymes.   Metabolism occurs through the action of enzymes, which are catalysts made of protein. Catalysts speed up chemical reactions and are used over and over because they are not changed during the reaction. Action of some enzymes requires small molecules such as magnesium or calcium, called cofactors; other enzymes require organic molecules such as vitamins, called coenzymes. An enzyme (E) molecule binds to a specific molecule referred to as the substrate (S), and it binds to the part of the substrate molecules

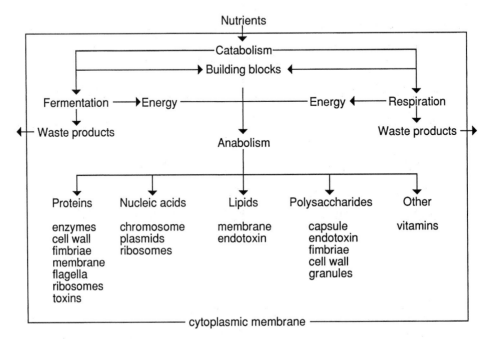

FIGURE 2-6 General bacterial metabolism. Nutrients are taken into the cell and processed through catabolic reactions that generate the building blocks and energy needed to synthesize macromolecules through anabolic reactions. Waste products generated exit the cell.

that will be changed. This binding causes the breaking of chemical bonds or the formation of new chemical bonds in the substrate molecule, changing the substrate to a new substance called the product (P). This reaction is written as:

$$E + S \rightarrow ES \rightarrow E + P$$

There are approximately 1000 different enzymes in a bacterial cell, and their names all end with the suffix -ase (e.g., protease, hydrolase). Some enzymes break down extracellular substrates into subunits (products) that can be then taken into the cell and used for growth. Other enzyme reactions may change one small molecule into another small molecule. In the example given, *pyruvic acid* (produced in the cells from the metabolism of sugar) is changed into *lactic acid* by the enzyme *lactate dehydrogenase* (LDH). Lactic acid produced by streptococci and lactobacilli in dental plaque leaves the cell as a waste product and can cause demineralization of the tooth surface, producing dental caries (see Chapter 5.)

$$
\begin{array}{ccc}
\text{O} & & \text{O} \\
\parallel & & \parallel \\
\text{C-OH} & & \text{C-OH} \\
| & & | \\
\text{C=O} & \rightarrow & \text{H-C-OH} \\
| & & | \\
\text{H-C-H} & & \text{H-C-H} \\
| & & | \\
\text{H} & & \text{H}
\end{array}
$$

Pyruvic acid   Lactic acid

Catabolism.   Bacterial multiplication requires the synthesis of new cell components, and these anabolic reactions require energy. Catabolism provides some of the building blocks for the macromolecules and the energy needed to drive anabolism. All bacteria require nutrients that can serve as sources of energy, and the energy is released from the nutrients as they are processed through catabolic reactions. Two major catabolic pathways that generate energy in bacteria are *fermentation* and *respiration*. The pathway used depends on the types of enzymes and metabolic machinery present in the bacterial cell.

Energy Production.   A common energy source for many bacteria is glucose. After glucose is transported into the cells, it is processed through one of two major catabolic pathways known as fermentation or respiration (described later). These are the reactions associated with the release of energy from the glucose but the energy cannot be used to drive anabolic reactions unless it is transferred to special molecules such as adenosine triphosphate (ATP). The ATP then participates in the energy-requiring anabolic reactions such as the synthesis of polysaccharides from monosaccharides.

Fermentation.   Fermentation is an anaerobic process that usually involves the breakdown of sugars (called glycolysis) with end products of organic acids or alcohols. During fermentation of sugars, hydrogen atoms (also referred to as electrons) are released from the sugar breakdown products. These electrons then bind to organic molecules, changing their structure. In respiration, these electrons bind to oxygen or inorganic substances (as described later). During the fermentation of glucose, pyruvic acid usually accepts the released electrons, changing to lactic acid as a final end product. This is the metabolic path-way that is responsible for dental caries formation, and it is active in caries-conducive oral bacteria such as *S. mutans* and *Lactobacillus* spp. The metabolic machinery present in these oral bacteria give the cells only one metabolic choice, the generation of building blocks and energy for anabolism through the fermentation of sugar to mainly lactic acid. Other bacteria may produce other products from fermentation, depending on the species and the nutrients available.

Respiration.   Respiration of sugars by infectious bacteria also involves glycolysis to pyruvic acid as described for fermentation. The electrons released from the sugar break-down products, however, are transferred to oxygen in aerobic respiration through a series of molecular processes called the electron transport chain. The pyruvic acid, rather than being changed to an end product lactic acid as in fermentation, is further processed through a series of reactions that yield considerably more energy in the form of ATP.

Controlling Growth

Controlling the growth of bacteria is accomplished by preventing their multiplication or by killing them. Such control is important to prevent damage they may cause by growing where they should not be (e.g., in our bodies, on food, in drinking water).

Preventing Growth.   Preventing growth can be achieved by changing or eliminat-ing a physical or nutritional requirement for growth or by using a chemical agent that in-terferes with cell division. Agents or conditions that prevent bacterial growth without killing them are called *bacteriostatic*.

Storing items in the refrigerator stops or slows down bacterial growth unless they are psychrophils. Freezing bacteria stops their growth and, because of formation of ice crys-tals inside the cell, can rupture the cell membrane. Some cells commonly survive, however, and may begin to grow when thawed.

Eliminating the availability of oxygen prevents the growth of aerobes. Adding oxygen prevents growth of anaerobes. Changing the pH beyond optimal values stops growth ex-cept for bacteria that can survive extreme pH values, such as aciduric bacteria in the mouth. Treating bacterial diseases with *antibiotics* can result in inhibiting growth or in killing the cells, depending on the bacterium and the antibiotic used. Antibiotics are chemicals that interfere with some metabolic activity of the bacterium but usually do not affect the metabolic activity of our body cells. This is referred to as selective toxicity. For example, penicillins prevent the formation of the cell wall in certain bacteria, which pre-vents their growth and usually kills the bacterium. Penicillins do not affect the growth of our body cells because our cells do not have cell walls.

Killing Bacteria.   Killing bacteria is accomplished by physical or chemical means and is a very important aspect of disease prevention and infection control. Agents or con-ditions that kill microorganisms rather than just prevent their growth are called *bactericidal, virucidal,* or *fungicidal* agents or conditions. Probably the most sure way to kill bacteria (or any other type of microorganism) in the shortest amount of time is to expose them to high temperatures such as those achieved in a steam, dry heat, or unsaturated chemical va-por sterilizer (see Chapter 11). The heat may destroy proteins, break down DNA and RNA, or cause structural damage to the cell membrane.

Several chemicals can kill bacteria and other microorganisms, and the type of chemi-cal used is frequently determined by location of the microorganisms to be killed. Strong chemicals cannot be used to kill microorganisms on or in the body, whereas inanimate objects, such as operatory surfaces, can withstand treatment by such agents. Chemicals kill microorganisms by several mechanisms, depending on the properties of the chemical.

VIRUSES

Viruses cause many different diseases and can infect humans, lower animals, plants, fungi, bacteria, algae, and protozoa. Viruses are important in dentistry because they can cause:

Specific oral diseases
Diseases elsewhere in the body that may result in lesions occurring in the mouth
Bloodborne diseases, such as acquired immunodeficiency syndrome (AIDS) and hepatitis B
Other types of diseases that may be transmitted in the dental office without use of proper infection control procedures

Structure

Human viruses are smaller than bacteria, ranging from 0.02 to 0.3 μm. They may have many different shapes but their general structure consists of a *nucleic acid core* (DNA or RNA) surrounded by a protein coat called a *capsid*. Some viruses also have an outer structure of lipids, proteins, and polysaccharides called the *envelope* (Figure 2-7).

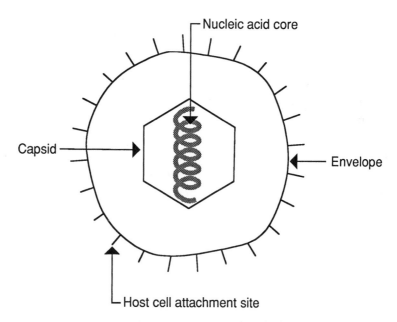

FIGURE 2-7   Diagram of a representative virus. The shape of the nucleocapsid (capsid + nucleic acid core) varies. Some viruses do not have an envelope and the host cell attachment sites are located on the capsid.

Life Cycle

Unlike most bacteria, viruses are not free-living in that they do not have the metabolic machinery to synthesize new protein coats and nucleic acids. They must use both the nutrients and the metabolic machinery of living cells to multiply (replicate themselves). Thus, viruses, like the special bacteria *Rickettsiae* and *Chlamydiae,* are called obligate intracellular parasites. Their life cycle is summarized in Table 2-3.

To replicate after entering the body, a virus must first adsorb to a surface of a living cell. This attachment is specific for each type of virus and the virus attaches to certain host cells through special receptors on the capsid or on the envelope. After adsorption, the virus is taken into the cell, and the capsid is removed to release the nucleic acid and a few molecules of enzymes that help initiate replication. At this point in the life cycle, the nucleic acid of the virus (depending on the virus involved) may induce the *lytic cycle, a persistent infection,* or *cell transformation*.

Lytic Cycle

In the lytic cycle, the nucleic acid takes over the metabolic machinery of the cell and directs it to produce more virus particles inside the cell. The macromolecules of the host cell are broken down to provide the nutrients needed to synthesize new virus capsids and virus nucleic acids. These then are assembled into new virus particles that are released when the host cell lyses. Each infected host cell may produce thousands of new viruses, each of which can infect a new host cell to produce more viruses. Some viruses are released slowly from their host cells by budding through the host cell cytoplasmic membrane, acquiring a portion of the cell membrane as their envelope.

Persistent Infections

A persistent virus infection may be latent, chronic, or slow. A latent persistent infection may occur if the nucleic acid of the virus is incorporated into the DNA of the host cell chromosomes. This incorporated viral nucleic acid is replicated along with the host cell chromosomes during normal cell division and is carried to each newly formed host cell. The viral nucleic acid may be reactivated later to induce a lytic cycle. This type of latent

---

Table 2-3   Life Cycle of a Virus

STEP	ACTIVITY
Adsorption	Virus particle attaches to host cell surface
Penetration	Virus enters host cell
Uncoating	Capsid is degraded to release nucleic acid
Replication*	Host cell machinery used to synthesize new viral nucleic acid and protein capsid
Assembly	Capsid assembled around nucleic acid
Release	Viral particle migrates to cytoplasmic membrane for budding or the host cell lyses to release all internal contents

*Some viruses will incorporate their nucleic acid into the host cell chromosomal DNA, resulting in (1) delay of the viral replication through the lytic cycle or (2) changing of host cell properties through transformation without host cell lysis.

persistent infection is caused by herpesviruses such as herpes simplex, which causes cold sores. A chronic persistent infection such as hepatitis B is caused by lysis of the infected cells but the symptoms are often unrecognized. Slow persistent infections are those in which the virus replicates very slowly, causing recognizable damage only after several years.

Host Cell Transformation

Some viruses infect host cells and cause changes in the properties of cells without causing lysis of the cell. These new properties may result in uncontrolled cell growth such as the formation of certain tumors like warts caused by the human papilloma virus.

Controlling Virus Replication

Viruses cause diseases by killing or changing the cells of our body. Artificially controlling the growth of viruses inside the body with chemicals is impossible in most cases. Antimicrobial chemicals (including antibiotics) act by inhibiting the metabolic machinery of the microorganisms. Because viruses use the metabolic machinery of the host cell to replicate, such chemicals would cause damage to the host cells. Thus because most virus diseases cannot be treated, the approach is to prevent them from occurring through immunization or infection control procedures.

Viruses can be killed when outside of the body by exposure to heat or chemicals as described for bacteria.

FUNGI

Fungi include mushrooms, molds, and yeasts, with certain members of the latter two types capable of causing diseases in humans. Such diseases may involve the lungs or other organs or tissues (e.g., histoplasmosis, coccidiodomycosis, blastomycosis, cryptococcosis, and phycomycoses), or the skin (e.g., athlete's foot, ringworm, candidiasis) and infections of the nails, scalp, and hair. In dentistry, the most important fungal infection is *oral candidiasis* (e.g., thrush, denture stomatitis). This is caused by the fungus *Candida albicans,* which may exist as a yeast cell or as a filamentous fungus (mold). This organism also may cause skin infections, vaginal infections, or widespread infection in the body.

Candida albicans occurs as a member of the normal oral microbiota in approximately 30% of adults. It is an opportunistic pathogen in that it usually causes harmful infections only when given a special opportunity resulting from depressed body defenses, immature body defenses as in the newborn, changes in the body's physiology, trauma to tissues (e.g., poor-fitting dentures), debilitating systemic diseases, and long-term antibacterial therapy.

Oral infections with *C. albicans* are usually easily treated with topical antifungal agents, and the yeast cells can be killed outside the body by exposure to heat and certain chemicals as described for bacteria and viruses.

SELECTED READINGS

Boyd RF, Hoerl BG: *Basic medical microbiology,* ed 4, Boston, 1991, Little, Brown.
Emmons CW, Binford CH, Utz JP, Kwong-Chung KJ: *Medical mycology,* ed 3, Philadelphia, 1989, Lea & Febiger.

Moat AG: *Microbial physiology,* New York, 1988, Wiley.

Rodgers HJ: *Bacterial cell structure. Aspects of microbiology,* Washington DC, 1983, American Society for Microbiology.

Voke WA, Gebhardt BM, Hammarskjold M-L, Kadner RJ: *Essentials of medical microbiology,* Philadelphia, 1996, Lippincott-Raven.

Chapter 3

DEVELOPMENT OF INFECTIOUS DISEASES

There are several causes of diseases in the body. Some are associated with microorganisms but others result from a malfunctioning of an organ (e.g., hyperthyroidism, diabetes), a nutritional deficiency (e.g., rickets, scurvy), an allergic reaction (e.g., hayfever, asthma, poison ivy), and abnormal growth of cells (e.g., cancer, tumors).

An *infectious disease* occurs when a microorganism in the body multiplies and causes damage to the tissues. The microorganisms that cause infectious diseases are called *pathogens.*

There are two types of infectious diseases: *endogenous* and *exogenous.* These terms refer to the source of the microorganism. Endogenous diseases are caused by microorganisms that are normally present on or in the body without causing harm but something happens that allows them to express their disease-producing potential. Examples of oral endogenous infectious diseases caused by members of the normal oral flora are *dental caries, pulpitis, periodontal diseases,* and *cervicofacial actinomycosis.* The causative agents of these diseases are called *opportunistic pathogens.* They cause diseases only when given a special opportunity to enter deeper tissues of the body or to accumulate to levels that can harm the body.

An exogenous disease is caused by microorganisms that are not normally present on or in the body but contaminate the body from the outside. Most infectious diseases are exogenous diseases (e.g., hepatitis B, "strep throat," acquired immunodeficiency syndrome [AIDS], measles, chickenpox, the common cold, influenza).

Some exogenous microorganisms can also cause disease without entering and multiplying in the body. These are called *toxigenic diseases* and occur after eating food in which microorganisms have multiplied and produced *toxins,* or poisons (e.g., *Staphylococcus* food poisoning, botulism).

STEPS IN DISEASE DEVELOPMENT

The steps for development of exogenous infectious diseases are listed in Box 3-1. Exogenous infectious diseases develop through six basic steps, each of which may be slightly modified, depending on the specific microorganism involved and the related environmental conditions. The basic steps are described below as related to disease development in a dental office environment. Prevention of disease development occurs by interfering with one of the basic steps as described in the Infection Control section, Chapters 6 through 15.

Source of the Microorganism

The major sources of disease agents in the dental office are the mouths of the patients. Although microorganisms can be present almost anywhere in the office (surfaces, dust, water,

---

Box 3-1   Steps in the Development of an Infectious Disease

Source of microorganism
Escape of microorganism from the source
Spread of microorganism to a new person
Entry of microorganism into the person
Infection (survival and growth of microorganism)
Damage to the body

From Miller CH and Cottone JC: *Dental Clin North Am* 37:1-20, 1993.

air, and the dental team), microorganisms of greatest concern are in the mouths of patients. These microorganisms are more fully described in Chapter 5 and include those that may be present in saliva, respiratory secretions, and blood that may escape from the mouth during dental care. Pathogenic microorganisms also may be harbored by members of the dental team but the chances for the spread of these agents in the office is much lower than those involving patient microorganisms. Nevertheless, spread of microorganisms from the dental team to patients is an important concern that is described in Chapter 7.

Although the patient's mouth is in general the most important source of pathogens in the dental office, it is not possible to accurately detect which patients may indeed be harboring these pathogens. Therefore, to successfully prevent the spread of pathogens in the office, infection control procedures must be applied during the care of **all** patients using the concept of **universal precautions** (the consideration of all patients to be infected with pathogenic microorganisms). The importance of universal precautions is based on an understanding of *asymptomatic carriers* of disease agents and an analysis of the four stages of the infectious disease process in the body as related to spread of disease agents to others.

Asymptomatic Carrier

Persons who have disease agents on or in their bodies but have no recognizable symptoms of the diseases are called asymptomatic carriers. These persons are probably the most important source for spread of disease agents because they may spread pathogens to others and may not even be aware that they are infected. Also, the dental team will not be aware of the potentially infectious nature of patients because carrier patients may look normal, with no recognizable symptoms.

An asymptomatic carrier state may occur at different stages during an infectious disease.

Stages of an Infectious Disease

There are four stages during an infectious disease: *incubation, prodromal, acute,* and *convalescent.* Pathogens may be spread to others during each of these stages.

Incubation Stage.   The incubation stage of an infectious disease is the period from the initial entrance of the infectious agent into the body to the time when the first symptoms of the disease appear. During this time, the disease agent is simply surviving in the body or is multiplying and producing harmful products that ultimately damage the body. This incubation period may range from a few hours to years, depending on the disease-producing potential of the microorganism, the number of microorganisms that enter the body, and the resistance of the body to the microorganism. All infectious diseases have an incubation stage, because we seldom, if ever, are exposed to a sufficient number of microorganisms to cause immediate symptoms. The entering microorganisms must multiply to sufficient numbers that overwhelm local or body-wide defense systems before enough damage occurs to result in a recognizable symptom (e.g., fever, swelling, skin discoloration, ulceration, pain, bleeding, watery eyes, "running nose," etc.). The length of the incubation stage varies. For influenza, it is usually 2 to 3 days, whereas that for hepatitis B is usually several weeks. For some of the rare "slow virus" infections, it may be 50 or 60 years. Persons infected with the human immunodeficiency virus (HIV-1) may be free of recognizable symptoms for 10 years or longer after the virus initially enters the body.

Prodromal Stage.   Prodromal means "running before," and this stage of a disease involves the appearance of early symptoms. The microorganism multiplies to numbers just large enough to cause the first symptoms commonly called *malaise* (not feeling well). These symptoms may include slight fever, headache, and upset stomach.

Acute Stage.   The acute stage is when the symptoms of the disease are maximal and the person is obviously ill. Although this person certainly has a potential to spread disease agents, they may not be the most important source in the dental office. The acutely ill are not likely to come to the dental office for care except in an emergency. Their presence in the office also may depend on the severity of their symptoms and the nature of the disease.

Convalescent Stage.   The convalescent stage of a disease is the recovery phase. The number of microorganisms may be declining or the harmful microbial products are being rapidly destroyed as the body defenses successfully combat the disease. Nevertheless, infectious agents are present and may be spread during this stage. Although the patient is aware of the disease, the declining symptoms may not be recognizable by others.

Some people may never fully recover from an infectious disease. The symptoms may occur over a long period or may occur intermittently. The chronic ("long-term") stages may occur in diseases such as hepatitis B and tuberculosis, in which the disease agent may be retained in the body for long periods. As more fully described in Chapter 5, some people may be infected with the hepatitis B virus and not experience any symptoms until 25 or more years later, with development of severe liver damage. Yet the virus was present in their bodies all of this time and may have been spread to others.

Normal Patient

A normal patient in this context is one who has no infectious diseases and is not a carrier of obvious pathogens. Normal and asymptomatic patients appear the same with no recognizable symptoms, however. This substantiates universal precautions because one cannot always differentiate between normal patients and those capable of spreading harmful microorganisms.

Even normal patients have opportunistic pathogens in their mouths, as more fully described in Chapter 5.

Escape from the Source

Step 2 in the development of an infectious disease is the escape of microorganisms from the source. Microorganisms escape from the mouth during natural mechanisms such as coughing, sneezing, and talking. This is indeed how respiratory diseases such as the com-

Table 3-1   Modes of Disease Transmission

MODE	EXAMPLE
Direct contact	Contact with microorganisms at the source such as in the patient's mouth
Indirect contact	Contact with items contaminated with a patient's microorganisms such as surfaces, hands, contaminated sharps
Droplet infection	Contact with sprays, splashes, aerosols, or spatter containing microorganisms

mon cold, measles, chickenpox, and influenza are normally spread. Providing dental care results in several artificial mechanisms by which microorganisms can escape from the patient's mouth.

Anything that is removed from a patient's mouth is contaminated (hands, instruments, handpieces, x-ray film, cotton products, needles, teeth, saliva, tissue, appliances, temporaries, etc.). In addition, microorganisms can escape from the mouth in spatter droplets and aerosol particles generated by use of the handpiece, ultrasonic scaler, and air/water syringe. Spatter droplets are the larger droplets that may contain several microorganisms and can hit the skin, eyes, nostrils, lips, and mouth of the dental team. These droplets settle rapidly from the air and can contaminate nearby surfaces. Aerosol particles are mostly invisible but contain a few microorganisms that may be inhaled or remain airborne for some time, depending on their size and on the air currents in the office.

Spread of Microorganisms to Another Person

Microorganisms that have escaped from a patient's mouth may be spread to others by three basic modes of disease transmission: *direct contact, indirect contact,* and *droplet infection* (Table 3-1).

Direct Contact

Touching soft tissue or teeth in the patient's mouth results in direct contact with microorganisms with immediate spread from the source. This gives microorganisms an opportunity to penetrate the body through small breaks or cuts in the skin and around the fingernails of ungloved hands.

Indirect Contact

A second mode of spread called indirect contact can result from injuries with contaminated sharps (e.g., needlesticks) and contact with contaminated instruments, equipment, surfaces, and hands. These items and tissues can carry a variety of pathogens, usually because of the presence of blood, saliva, or other secretions from a previous patient.

Droplet Infection

A third mode of spread is droplet infection. This mode encompasses aerosols and spatter, as mentioned earlier. Spatter generated during care may contact unprotected broken skin

---

Table 3-2   Routes of Entry of Microorganisms into the Body

ROUTES	EXAMPLES
Inhalation	Breathing aerosol particles generated from use of prophylaxis angle
Ingestion	Swallowing droplets of saliva/blood spattered into the mouth
Mucous membranes	Droplets of saliva/blood spattered into the eyes, nose, or mouth
Breaks in the skin	Directly touching microorganisms or being spattered with saliva/blood onto skin with cuts or abrasions; punctures with contaminated sharps

---

or mucous membranes of the eyes, noses, and mouths of members of the dental team. This delivers microorganisms directly to the body. Smaller aerosol particles also may be spread through the air, providing a potential for inhalation of the microorganisms.

Entry into a New Person

Microorganisms that are spread to a new person frequently cause no damage unless they actually enter the body. There are four basic routes of entry, which have been mentioned earlier (Table 3-2). Microorganisms at the surface of the skin can enter through small cuts or abrasions that are often unnoticed. Injuries with contaminated sharp items cause direct penetration through the skin into the body. Also, microorganisms in spatter or aerosols may contact and enter the body through mucous membranes of the eye, nose and mouth, or they may be inhaled. Ingestion is another route of entry.

Infection

Infection is the multiplication and survival of microorganisms on or in the body. An infection does not always indicate disease but disease seldom results without infection (exception, toxigenic diseases). Our bodies are constantly infected, with large numbers of bacteria multiplying and surviving in our mouths, intestines, and skin on a normal basis.

Damage to the Body

As mentioned earlier, infecting microorganisms usually must multiply to a harmful level for disease to occur. Thus, a harmful infection is the final step in development of an infectious disease. The final two steps of infection and damage are very complex and involve a battle between the infecting microorganism and the body's defenses, as described in the next section.

HOST-MICROORGANISM INTERACTIONS

Microorganisms present on or in the body multiply if the conditions are appropriate. Bacteria and fungi take in available nutrients, metabolize, multiply, and produce extracellular products that may damage the body. Viruses invade appropriate host cells, replicate, and damage the host cell during the process. The body attempts to restrict microbial invasion and multiplication and to counteract harmful microbial products. The result of these interactions is health or disease.

Pathogenic Properties of Microorganisms

Pathogenic properties of microorganisms are properties that facilitate development of disease and are categorized into those that enhance infection, interfere with host defenses, and cause direct damage to the body (Table 3-3).

Enhance Infection

Properties that enhance the initial survival and multiplication of microorganisms in the body are the surface fimbriae on bacteria and host cell attachment sites on viral envelopes or capsids. These allow the microorganism to attach to host cells or other surfaces; for viruses, this attachment is required before multiplication.

Attachment to host surfaces is also necessary for infection by many bacteria, especially if they are to establish themselves on mucosal surfaces such as in the mouth. Bacteria that do not attach to or are not mechanically trapped in oral sites are washed off surfaces and swallowed. The accumulation of dental plaque is an example of the result of bacterial attachment to host surfaces, in this case leading to dental caries. Other examples of diseases requiring initial attachment by bacteria are streptococcal pharyngitis, genitourinary gonorrhea, gonococcal pharyngitis, conjunctivitis, *Salmonella* gastroenteritis, and shigellosis.

Bacteria that attach to specific body sites must be able to multiply in the environment of that site to become established and eventually cause damage. Thus their nutritional requirements must be compatible with the specific host site. This is another reason why only specific bacteria can survive at and damage specific sites in the body. For example, lactobacilli and many strains of *Streptococcus mutans* can survive in an environment high in acid (they are aciduric), such as within a carious lesion. Thus, although many other oral bacteria cannot multiply under these conditions, these aciduric species continue to thrive in the lesion and contribute to the progression of caries.

Interfere with Host Defenses

Many microorganisms are pathogenic because they interfere with host defense mechanisms. Bacteria with capsules, such as *Streptococcus pneumoniae* that causes lobar pneumonia, resist phagocytic engulfment, and others, such as *Mycobacterium tuberculosis* that causes tuberculosis, may be engulfed but resist phagocytic digestion. Such bacteria gain a foothold during infection because they evade destruction by phagocytes, one of the early lines of defense. The same is true for bacteria such as *Actinobacillus actinomycetemcomitans,* an important periodontopathogen, that produces a toxin (leukocidin) that kills certain phagocytes. Other microorganisms interfere with the latter stages of host defense, cell-mediated and antibody-mediated immunity. For example, HIV-1 can destroy certain T-lymphocytes that are involved in regulating the immune response. Also, some streptococci can produce protease enzymes that destroy antibody molecules.

Table 3-3 Pathogenic Activities and Properties of Microorganisms

ACTIVITY	PROPERTY	EXAMPLE
Enhances infection	Attaches to host cells	
	bacterial fimbriae	*Streptococcus pyogenes*
	bacterial surface polymers	*Streptococcus mutans*
	viral envelope or capsid	All viruses
	Multiplies at body site	
	utilizes available nutrients	Most pathogens
	resists acids	*Lactobacillus acidophilus*
Interferes with host defense	Destroys phagocytes	
	leukocidin	*Actinobacillus actinomycetemcomitans*
	exotoxin A	
	Inhibits phagocyte attraction	*Pseudomonas aeruginosa*
	extracellular products	*Capnocytophaga* sp.
	Avoids phagocyte engulfment	
	bacterial capsule	*Streptococcus pneumoniae*
	bacterial fimbriae	*Streptococcus pyogenes*
	Resists phagocytic digestion	
	resistant bacterial surfaces	*Mycobacterium tuberculosis*
	products inhibit killing	*Legionella pneumophila*
	Suppresses or avoids immune system	
	kills lymphocytes	Human immunodeficiency virus
	changes surface antigens	Influenza viruses
	destroys antibodies	*Streptococcus sanguis*
	avoids contact with antibodies	Herpes simplex viruses
Damages cells or tissues	Produces histolytic enzymes	
	collagenase	*Porphyromonas gingivalis*
	hyaluronidase	*Staphylococcus aureus*
	Contains endotoxin	Gram-negative bacteria
	Produces exotoxins	
	tetanus toxin	*Clostridium tetani*
	botulinum toxin	*Clostridium botulinum*
	enterotoxins	*Staphylococcus aureus*
	Produces cytotoxic chemicals	
	hydrogen sulfide	*Fusobacterium nucleatum*
	ammonia	*Bacteroides* sp.
	acids	*Streptococcus mutans*
	Induces damage by the immune system	
	causes persistent, localized infections	Periodontopathogens
	causes chronic infections	Hepatitis B virus

Direct Damage to the Body

As bacteria or fungi multiply in the body, they produce extracellular enzymes that can degrade macromolecules. If these macromolecules are parts of host cell surfaces or are tissue components, this process can kill cells or damage the tissue. Examples of such *histolytic enzymes* are collagenase produced by the bacterial species of *Porphyromonas, Bacteroides,* and *Clostridium;* hyaluronidase produced by some streptococci; and a variety of proteolytic enzymes produced by many bacteria.

Bacteria also produce waste products, many of which are *cytotoxic* such as ammonia, acids, and hydrogen sulfide, or cause demineralization of enamel and dentin, such as lactic and other organic acids. Gram-negative bacteria contain endotoxin that when released affects phagocytes and blood platelets and can induce an inflammatory response. Other bacteria may produce exotoxins that interfere with cell or body functions, such as food poisoning toxins and tetanus toxins.

Viruses cause damage by killing or interfering with the normal functions of the host cells they invade, and all types of microorganisms contain or produce substances that stimulate an inflammatory response or an immune response. These host responses are protective but if continually stimulated over time by persistence of the microorganism these responses may produce more damage than protection. One example is the damage that occurs in periodontal disease with the long-term presence of plaque and its antigens in periodontal pockets.

Host Defense Mechanisms

Host defense against harmful infections are grouped into two categories: *innate* (defenses that are always active) and *acquired* (defenses that must be stimulated to become active).

Innate Host Defenses

Innate host defenses consist of four groups of properties or activities of the body that guard against infection by contaminating microorganisms (Table 3-4). Although these defenses are quite formidable, they do not prevent all diseases.

Physical Barriers.   The unbroken skin serves as an excellent barrier and prevents microorganisms from penetration to deeper tissues where multiplication and spread to other body sites may occur. The mucous membranes of the eyes, nose, mouth, respiratory tree, vagina, and intestinal tract also provide resistance to penetration by microorganisms. The architecture of the skin with its many layers and the arrangement of cells of mucous membranes serve as the mechanisms that resist penetration.

Another physical barrier is the architecture of the respiratory tree that prevents particles of 5 μm and greater in size from reaching the alveoli (air sacks) of the lung. This restricts entrance of many microorganisms that may be present in large droplets or dust particles that are inhaled.

Mechanical Barriers.   Mechanical barriers include the cleansing action of secretions such as saliva and tears and excretions such as urine that wash away microorganisms present at these respective body sites. Innate protection of the respiratory tree also includes the secretion of "sticky" mucus that tends to trap inhaled particles that are then moved up and away from the lungs by the *ciliary escalator* (movement of the hairlike cilia on the surface of mucosal epithelial cells that moves the mucus toward the throat). The natural reflexes of coughing and sneezing also expel particles from the respiratory tree.

Table 3-4 Innate Host Defense Mechanisms

MECHANISM	EXAMPLES
Physical barriers	Skin
	Mucous membranes
	Architecture of respiratory tree
Mechanical barriers	Washing action of secretions and excretions
	Sticky nature of mucus
	Ciliary escalator
	Desquamation of skin and mucous membrane cells
	Coughing and sneezing
	Hair in the nose
Antimicrobial chemicals	Hydrochloric acid in stomach
	Organic acids on skin and in vagina
	Lysozyme
	Phagocytic killing systems
	Interferon
	Complement fragments
	Microbial products
Cellular barriers	Phagocytes

Adapted from Miller CH and Cottone JC: *Dental Clin North Am* 37:1-20, 1993.

Another mechanical barrier involves the desquamation (shedding) of skin cells and mucous membrane cells. As these outer surface cells are lost, microorganisms attached to these cells also are removed from the body.

Antimicrobial Chemicals. A variety of antimicrobial chemicals are present in the body that kill or inhibit the multiplication of microorganisms. Hydrochloric acid in the stomach and organic acids on the skin and in the vagina can prevent bacterial multiplication. The enzyme lysozyme that can lyse and kill some bacteria is present in saliva, tears, nasal secretions, intestinal secretions, colostrum, and inside phagocytes. Other antimicrobial mechanisms of phagocytes involve oxygen products, peroxidase, and lactoferrin. Many of our body cells produce a substance called *interferon* when the cells are infected with a virus. This interferon is released from infected cells and makes nearby cells resistant to virus replication.

A special group of proteins called the *complement system* is present in blood and tissue fluids and can participate in antimicrobial activities by working in concert with the immune response (it "complements" the immune system). The complement system may attract phagocytes to a site of infection, enhance phagocytosis of microorganisms, lyse certain gram-negative bacteria, and destroy the envelope of some viruses.

Cellular Barriers. As previously described, certain white blood cells such as *neutrophils* and *macrophages* can destroy microorganisms through the process of phagocytosis. These phagocytes first engulf ("swallow-up") microorganisms and then kill and digest them by enzymes that degrade the microbial structures. Phagocytes provide a very important defense system and are present throughout the body in connective tissue, tissue and lymphatic fluid, lymph nodes, blood, and many organs.

Acquired Immunity

If a microorganism invades the body, it usually activates a special host defense system directed specifically against that invading microorganism. After this system is activated, it attempts to prevent serious harm from that microorganism and may provide protection against subsequent invasion of the body by that same microorganism. *Immunity* is a state of being resistant to the harmful effects of a microorganism. This defense system is called acquired immunity because this system is always ready to respond to microbial infections but does not actually do so until after an infection has occurred. In contrast, the innate body defenses are always active, even before infection has occurred.

Activation of the Immune Response.   The immune response is activated by *antigens*. Examples of antigens are bacteria, viruses, fungi, protozoa, extracellular macromolecules produced by these microorganisms, and other macromolecules or cells that are normally not present in the body. During an infection, while the innate body defenses are trying to kill or limit the spread of the invading microorganism, the microorganism and its macromolecular products (antigens) are recognized as being foreign to the body. This recognition is accomplished by special macrophages distributed throughout the body that process antigens through phagocytosis and then interact with the cells of the immune system: B-lymphocytes and T-lymphocytes. This interaction causes these lymphocytes to multiply and yield large numbers of cells that can recognize the specific invading antigens. These lymphocytes then begin a series of activities that can destroy the microorganism or interfere with its pathogenic properties. These activities are grouped into two categories: cell-mediated response and antibody-mediated response.

Cell-mediated Response.   The activated T-lymphocytes develop into several different types of T-lymphocytes that can: (1) regulate the antibody-mediated response, (2) destroy virus-infected host cells in an attempt to stop further multiplication of the virus in the body, (3) produce chemicals called *lymphokines* that in general activate other types of cells (e.g., phagocytes) to be more active in killing the invading microorganism, and (4) destroy certain nonmicrobial cells in the body that have changed and become recognized as foreign to the body (e.g., cancer cells).

Antibody-mediated Response.   The activated B-lymphocytes develop into different types of B-lymphocytes that produce lymphokines (that act like those produced from T lymphocytes) and into plasma cells that produce antibodies. Antibodies are protein molecules that can bind to the specific antigens that originally stimulated their formation. When the antibodies bind to these antigens, the antigens (e.g., microorganisms or their harmful products) are destroyed, inactivated, or more easily removed from the body, depending on the nature of the antigen (Table 3-5).

Long-term Immunity

The initial immune response to an invading microorganism usually results in an increased number of lymphocytes that can respond to that microorganism if it attempts to invade the body again. During subsequent invasions, the body "remembers" that microorganism and, because of the large number of specific lymphocytes now present, can respond rapidly to destroy the microorganism before it can damage the body. Thus, once we have had an in-

Table 3-5   Protective Activities of Antibodies

ACTIVITY	EXAMPLES
Enhance phagocytosis to destroy microorganisms	Binding to the bacterial capsule eliminating its antiphagocytic activity
	Binding to a microorganism and attaching the microorganisms to the surface of a phagocyte that promotes engulfment
	Activating the complement system that in turn activates phagocytes
Interfere with microorganism attachment to host cells to prevent infection	Binding to bacterial fimbriae or to viral capsid and envelope before the microorganism attaches to host cells
	Binding to microorganism surfaces and causing several cells or viral particles to clump
Inactivate toxins to prevent damage to the body	Binding to bacterial leukocidin molecules, preventing damage to neutrophils
Inactivate histolytic enzymes to prevent damage to the body	Binding to the collagenase molecule, preventing destruction of collagen
Lysis of gram-negative bacteria or enveloped viruses	Binding to the surface of microorganisms activates the complement system that destroys the outer membrane or viral envelope
Lysis of virus-infected cells	Binding to virus-infected cells and attaching the cell to a macrophage that then kills the virus-infected cells

fectious disease, we frequently do not get that same disease again. There are notable exceptions, including dental caries, periodontal disease, and gonorrhea. Also, in some instances, different microorganisms can cause the same disease. For example, there are more than 100 viruses that can cause the common cold, and an immune response to one microorganism seldom protects against another.

Artificial Immunity

Artificial immunity involves being immunized or vaccinated against a specific disease. We are inoculated with an antigen (e.g., a dead microorganism, a weakened microorganism, the antigenic part of a microorganism, or an inactivated toxin) that will not cause disease or damage to the body but will stimulate the immune system. On receiving the vaccine, the body is deceived and, believing it is a real infection, mounts an immune response for protection. In most instances, this protection lasts for many years but in some cases booster inoculations are needed periodically to maintain protection. Disease for which vaccines are available in the United States, including hepatitis B, are described in Chapter 8.

Damage by the Immune System

Activation of the immune system by certain antigens can cause damage to the body. Approximately 10% of the population are allergic to substances that can directly serve as an antigen or are changed into antigens after they enter the body. The immune response to the antigen (in these cases called an *allergen*) results in damage to the body, usually occurring at the body site exposed to the allergen. For example, some people who breathe in pollens have antibody-mediated and allergic reactions in the nose and eyes, called *hayfever,* or in the respiratory tree, called *asthma*. Allergies to foods (e.g., chocolate) are usually expressed as *"hives"* on the skin. Allergy to a substance that is distributed throughout the body (e.g., penicillin inoculation) may result in a widespread reaction affecting the blood system, lungs, and heart, called *systemic anaphylactic shock*.

Cell-mediated allergic reactions also occur in some persons with chronic infections such as may occur in hepatitis B, syphilis, and tuberculosis. Oils from the poison ivy plant, nickel from jewelry, and chemicals in latex gloves also may cause cell-mediated allergic reactions, called *contact dermatitis*.

Skin testing is used to determine which specific allergens are causing problems. In many instances an allergic person "outgrows" the allergy but some remain allergic for life and must take special precautions to avoid contact with the allergens.

SELECTED READINGS

Miller CH: Microbial pathogenicity and innate host resistance. In Schuster GS, editor: *Oral microbiology and infectious diseases,* ed 2, Baltimore, 1983, Williams & Wilkins.

Miller CH, Cottone JC: The basic principles of infectious diseases as related to dental practice, *Dental Clin North Amer* 37:1-20, 1993.

Mims CA, Dimmock NJ, Nash A, Stephen J: *Mim's pathogenesis of infectious diseases,* ed 4, San Diego, 1995, Academic Press.

Schaechter M, Medoff G, Schlessinger D, editors: *Mechanisms of microbial diseases,* Baltimore, 1989, Williams & Wilkins.

Sigal LH, Yacov R, editors: *Immunology and inflammation-basic mechanisms and clinical consequences,* New York, 1994, McGraw-Hill.

Chapter 4

EMERGING DISEASES

Emerging diseases are new infectious diseases that haven't been recognized before or are known infectious diseases with changing patterns. Infectious diseases can be expected to continually emerge and the list in Table 4-1 will continue to grow as this happens. Diseases emerge because conditions change that bring microorganisms and humans together in new ways. These changing conditions can be grouped into five categories, as listed in Table 4-2.

ECOLOGICAL CHANGES

Ecological changes that result in disease emergence usually involve *zoonotic* diseases (diseases involving animals) or insect-borne diseases. Such changes involve bringing humans into close contact with animals or insect vectors, resulting in the spread of microorganisms from animals to humans. One example is the emergence of Korean hemorrhagic fever, a disease of humans involving high fever and internal bleeding, caused by the Hantaan virus from rodents. When rice fields are created, field mice flourish because of the new source of food. Harvesting the rice brings humans into close contact with these infected mice, resulting in spread of the virus.

Changing weather conditions in the Southwest United States, to a more mild and wet season in the summer of 1993, likely enhanced contact between humans and rodents carrying a previously unrecognized hantavirus now named Sin Nombre virus. The rodent population flourished and humans probably entered the wilds more frequently as a result of the favorable weather. This likely caused the initial cluster of 24 human cases of hantavirus pulmonary syndrome in this area. This syndrome produces symptoms of fever, muscle aches, nausea, vomiting, headache, and ultimately severe respiratory distress with death in about one-half of those infected. Although the initial outbreak occurred in the Four Corners region of the U.S. (New Mexico, Arizona, Colorado, Utah), over 150 cases have been confirmed in 30 states. The deer mouse (which is widely distributed in North America) is found to be the most common host for the Sin Nombre virus. Disease also is associated with cotton rats, rice rats, and the white-footed mouse.

Other rodent viruses cause human diseases, including the Machupo virus that causes Bolivian hemorrhagic fever, the Argentine hemorrhagic fever virus, and the Lassa fever virus. The exact mode of spread of microorganisms from rodents to humans is not always known but may involve contact with rodent feces or aerosolized urine.

Another ecological change resulted in disease emergence in 1987 along the Senegal river in Africa. Building dams in the river valley facilitated irrigation as planned but it also greatly increased the water breeding grounds for the mosquitoes that carry viruses. This caused the emergence of Rift Valley fever, a viral disease caused by a mosquito vec-

Table 4-1   Some Recently Recognized Disease/Microorganism Associations

YEAR*	MICROORGANISM	DISEASE
1970	Coxsackievirus	Hand-foot-mouth disease
1973	Rotavirus	Infantile diarrhea
1975	Parvovirus B19	Fifth disease; aplastic crises-chronic hemolytic anemia
1976†	Ebola virus	Ebola hemorrhagic fever
1977	*Cryptosporidium parvum*	Acute enterocolitis
1977	*Legionella pneumophila*	Legionnaires' disease
1977	Hantaan virus	Hemorrhagic fever with renal syndrome
1977	Hepatitis D virus	Hepatitis D (bloodborne)
1981	*Staphylococcus aureus*	Toxic shock syndrome associated with tampons
1982	*Escherichia coli,* O157:H7	Hemorrhagic colitis; hemolytic uremic syndrome
1983	HIV type 1	HIV disease; HIV infection and AIDS
1983	*Helicobacter pylori*	Gastric ulcers
1987	Hepatitis E virus	Hepatitis E (water/foodborne)
1988	Human herpesvirus 6	Roseola (actual disease known since 1910)
1989	Hepatitis C virus	Hepatitis C (bloodborne)
1989	*Ehrlichia chaffeensis*	Human ehrlichiosis
1990	Barmah forest virus	Polyarthritis in West Australia
1990	*Hemophilus influenzae*	Brazilian purpuric fever (new strain-*aegypticus*)
1991	Guanarito virus	Venezuelan hemorrhagic fever
1992	*Vibrio cholerae* O139	Epidemic cholera (new strain)
1992	*Bartonella henselae*	Cat-scratch disease
1993	Hantavirus	Hantavirus pulmonary syndrome
1994	Sabia virus	Brazilian hemorrhagic fever
1995	Hepatitis G virus	Hepatitis G
1995	Human herpesvirus 8	Associated with Kaposi's sarcoma

*Year microorganism was isolated, identified, or first associated with disease.
†Subsequent outbreaks have occurred in 1979 and in 1995.

tor that results in high fever and sometimes retinitis and, rarely, fulminant hepatitis with hemorrhage.

Lyme disease was initially recognized here in the U.S. in 1975 in a group of children who lived in Lyme, Connecticut. Lyme disease is caused by the bacterial spirochete *Borrelia burgdorferi* that is transmitted to humans through the bite of ticks. The disease results in a rash (associated with the tick bite) and starts with flu-like symptoms. Weeks later, the subject may develop cardiac or neurological problems, muscle aches and pains, or intermittent attacks of arthritis. The emergence of this disease was likely due to ecological changes in forests near populated sites that increased the population of the deer and the deer tick, the vector of Lyme disease in humans. Situations that enhance humans venturing near and into forests also contribute to this emergence and may involve campers, hunters, hikers, bird-watchers, and even golfers. Today there are about 10,000-14,000 cases

Table 4-2 Causes and Examples of Disease Emergence

CAUSE	DISEASE EXAMPLES
Ecological changes	Korean hemorrhagic fever
	Bolivian hemorrhagic fever
	Argentine hemorrhagic fever
	Lassa fever
	Hantavirus pulmonary syndrome
	Lyme disease
	Rift Valley fever
Changes in human demographics or behaviors	HIV disease
	Hepatitis B and C
	Tuberculosis
International travel and commerce	Cholera
	Encephalitis
Technology	*E. coli* hemolytic uremic syndrome
	Salmonella food poisoning
	HIV disease
	Hepatitis B and C
	Legionnaires' disease
Microbial changes	Influenza
	Infections with microbial changes
Breakdown in public health measures	Cryptosporidiosis
	Diphtheria

of Lyme disease reported annually throughout the U.S., with most cases occurring in the northeastern states.

CHANGES IN HUMAN DEMOGRAPHICS OR BEHAVIORS

Human population movements or changes in how humans associate with each other can create new conditions that favor disease spread. Movement and crowding of people into cities in poor countries results in numerous infectious disease problems such as the spread of dengue virus from mosquitoes breeding in open water containers, causing dengue hemorrhagic fever. This also leads to other mosquito-borne diseases such as yellow fever and several forms of viral encephalitis. The movement of HIV-infected persons from the villages of Africa to large cities introduced the infection to larger susceptible populations. The movement of over 500,000 starving Rawandans into Zaire in 1994 resulted in over 50,000 deaths in the refugee camps from cholera and *Shigella* dysentery.

Human demographics also play a role in disease spread in the U.S. Increased population densities, as may occur with the homeless or with institutionalized persons (e.g., prisoners), have contributed to the increase in the numbers of tuberculosis cases in the U.S. in recent years. Bringing children together in some day care centers has contributed to the spread of disease agents such as cytomegalovirus. Human behavior also influences disease spread and emergence. Unprotected sexual contacts among various populations and an increase in injection drug abuse facilitates the sharing of human body fluids among individuals. If the body fluids are infected with microorganisms, the microorganisms rapidly reach new hosts. These behaviors are the primary reasons for the emergence and spread of HIV disease and the continued occurrence of most cases of hepatitis B and C.

The behaviors of misuse and overuse of antibiotics lead to conditions that select for antibiotic-resistant strains of bacteria, for example, antibiotics prescribed when not necessary and antibiotics used for prevention of infections. Such practices have resulted in the emergence and occurrence of harmful infections by antibiotic-resistant strains that are much more difficult to treat. This is more fully described below under Microbial Changes.

INTERNATIONAL TRAVEL AND COMMERCE

In a few hours, or a few days at the most, just about anyone can travel just about anywhere. We carry our microorganisms with us when we travel and can easily spread them to others in far away lands. Also, microorganisms that contaminate water, foods, plants, animals, insects, and goods can be literally shipped throughout the world. A recent example of this is the emergence of cholera in South and Central America. Cholera is an intestinal bacterial disease spread by contaminated water or food and results in severe diarrhea and dehydration. A new strain of the cholera causative agent (*Vibrio cholerae* O139 Bengal) emerged in Southern Asia in 1992 where cholera is endemic. Within a year this new strain was detected in South and Central America, where, along with *V. cholerae* O1, it has caused over a million cases of cholera involving about 10,000 deaths. This is the first epidemic of cholera in South and Central America in this century. The exact mode of spread of strain O139 from Asia to South and Central America is not known but it is suggested that it involves the water on and in cargo ships. *Vibrio cholerae* has been isolated from the ballast, bilge, and sewage waters from cargo ships.

Evidence that *V. cholerae* O1, originally detected in Indonesia, has reached U.S. shores is that this strain was isolated from oysters and oyster-eating fish in Mobile Bay, Alabama, in 1992. However, there has not been an associated epidemic or even a large outbreak of cholera in the U.S. During the period when a million cases of cholera developed in South and Central America (1991 to 1994), only 158 cases were reported in the U.S. This difference likely involves better import controls and sanitation in the U.S.

Another example of shipping industry involvement in disease emergence is viral encephalitis spread by the Asian tiger mosquito. Encephalitis involves infection of the central nervous system that may cause fever, headache, vomiting, nausea, lethargy, paralysis, or convulsions. Tiger mosquitoes were originally found in Asia but they now have been detected (along with the encephalitis) in the U.S., Brazil, and Africa. Apparently these mosquitoes were transported from Asia in water that collected in used automobile tires on the decks of cargo ships. Since coming to the U.S. in 1982, the Asian tiger mosquito has established itself in at least 21 states and is involved in causing Eastern equine encephalomyelitis.

An interesting incident involving foreign commerce occurred in Reston, Virginia, in 1989. Monkeys from the Philippines were shipped to an animal care facility in Reston. The monkeys were infected with an Ebola-like virus that caused a hemorrhagic fever, and the virus was spread to other monkeys in the facility. It was feared that this deadly virus might escape the facility and cause an epidemic in humans. Fortunately, the Reston virus was different from the African strains of the Ebola virus (see below) and did not cause disease in humans.

TECHNOLOGY

Technology advancements involving the development of new devices and processes are important to many aspects of life. However, sometimes this new technology creates new ways to bring microorganisms and humans together. For example, mass food processing combines large amounts of raw materials for widespread distribution. Unfortunately, a small amount of contaminated raw material can taint a large amount of processed food. This is apparently what happened in 1993 when a pathogenic strain of *Escherichia coli* (O157:H7) contaminated meat used to make hamburger for a fast food chain. The *E. coli* was distributed to restaurants over a four state area in the Northwest U.S., infecting about 700 people and causing two deaths. Another important point is that undercooking of the meat allowed the *E. coli* to survive and cause problems. This strain of *E. coli* was first recognized in 1983 and causes hemorrhagic colitis involving bloody diarrhea and abdominal cramps. A life-threatening complication called hemolytic uremic syndrome (HUS) may develop and this was the cause of the two deaths in the 1993 outbreak. HUS involves malfunction of the kidneys and lysis of red blood cells. Fifteen additional outbreaks with the O157:H7 strain were reported in 1993, resulting in a total of 60 outbreaks now reported in the U.S. Most outbreaks were the result of consumption of contaminated, undercooked ground beef; others involved contaminated fruits, yogurt, water, and dried salami.

In 1994 about 4,000 cases of *Salmonella* food poisoning occurred over 36 states because of contamination of a batch of ice cream mix processed by a large food company. The mix was prepared and pasteurized (heated to 161° F for 15 seconds to kill disease-producing bacteria) and transported to the packaging and distribution plant. Unfortunately, the mix was transported in a truck that had just previously been used to transport raw eggs. Eggs are the leading source of *Salmonella* food poisoning in the U.S. Apparently the truck had not been properly disinfected before transporting the ice cream mix, which was not re-pasteurized before freezing, packaging, and distribution.

The life-saving technology of concentrating special blood products to administer to hemophiliacs and others is very important. Unfortunately, it also created a very efficient way to transmit bloodborne viruses (e.g., HIV and hepatitis B and C viruses) to those who receive these blood products. Blood transfusion with contaminated blood presents a similar mode of spread. As of June 1997, 4,567 cases of AIDS has occurred in those with hemophilia or other coagulation disorders, and 8,075 cases of AIDS has occurred in transfusion recipients. Today, blood can be tested for the presence of HIV and hepatitis B and no longer serves as a significant mode of spread for these agents.

The development of water-handling devices has certainly made our lives easier but it has led to new sites that harbor potential pathogens. For example, Legionnaires' disease (a pneumonia caused by the bacterium *Legionella pneumophila*, see Chapter 7) was first recognized in 1976 among attendees at an American Legion convention in Philadelphia. A few hundred staying at a particular hotel became contaminated with *L. pneumophila* either through the hotel water system or the air-conditioning system and became ill. Since then it is known that *L. pneumophila* exists in our natural waters and tends to accumulate on surfaces of water-handling devices (e.g., cooling fins of air-conditioning units, in humidifiers, grocery store vegetable sprayer nozzles, shower heads, therapeutic whirlpools, dental unit waterlines). Inhalation of contaminated water aerosols or aspiration of oral fluids colonized with this opportunistic bacterium may lead to disease, mainly if a person is compromised and particularly susceptible to respiratory diseases.

MICROBIAL CHANGES

Most mutations in the microbial world are probably lethal because the change destroys some mechanism necessary for multiplication. However, some mutations don't cause death and occasionally even make the microorganism more virulent or more difficult to kill. Two such examples have already been mentioned: *V. cholerae* O139 and *E. coli* O157:H7.

Another well known example of microbial change is the influenza virus that changes constantly. About every year everyone becomes susceptible to the influenza virus regardless of past bouts with the virus. The immune system of those who have had influenza usually doesn't recognize the new virus and offers little or no protection. Likewise, last year's vaccine usually doesn't work against this year's new strain of virus, so annual "flu shots" are necessary to achieve the maximum protection.

Another major cause of disease emergence is the development of drug resistance (resistance to antibiotics) among several bacteria. Some of the changes that occur in bacteria involve the development of resistance to one or more antibiotics. For example, if resistance to penicillin has developed in a bacterium causing an infection and penicillin (which has always taken care of the infection in the past) is administered to the infected patient, the bacterium will not only continue to make the person sick but also will continue to multiply to higher numbers, enhancing its spread to others. As this continues with subsequent patients, the resistant bacterium reaches more and more people, causing the same disease that can no longer be treated with the original antibiotic. With time a large percent of those susceptible to this bacterium become infected with the antibiotic resistant strain. This usually causes delays in effective therapy, giving the bacterium a sometimes dangerous foothold in the early stages of disease.

Several pathogenic antibiotic-resistant bacteria have emerged, including drug-resistant *Streptococcus pneumoniae* (DRSP), vancomycin-resistant entercococci (VRE), methacillin-resistant *Staphylococcus aureus* (MRSA), and multiple drug-resistant *Mycobacterium tuberculosis* (MDRTB), all of which are important in dentistry and are further described in Chapter 6.

BREAKDOWN IN PUBLIC HEALTH MEASURES

Countless public health measures to protect against the spread of infectious diseases have been instituted in the U.S. but they must be maintained to remain effective. One measure is the production of safe drinking water (referred to as *potable water*). The breakdown of a water treatment process in the city of Milwaukee in 1993 resulted in about 400,000 cases of an intestinal infection caused by the protozoan *Cryptosporidium parvum*. This protozoan exists in the intestines of animals and thus ends up in ground water that empties into the streams that serve as the source of the nation's drinking water. If water treatment plants do not effectively remove this protozoan (and many other microorganisms) from the drinking water, problems can occur. Other municipal waterborne outbreaks of cryptosporidiosis have occurred in Texas, Georgia, and Oregon.

Many major cities periodically issue "boil water" notices indicating that tap water should be boiled before it is consumed or used in cooking. These usually result from a temporary problem at the water treatment plant or with the lines that distribute the water from the plant to homes and workplaces. Commonly, a notice will be generated if a water main (a large water distribution pipeline) breaks as a result of below freezing temperatures, earthquakes, settling of the ground, or age of the water distribution system. These events can allow potentially contaminated ground water into the drinking water that flows downstream from the break.

With the recent formation of the New Independent States from the former Soviet Union, some public health vaccination programs were relaxed. This resulted in the development of 45,000 new cases of diphtheria in 1994, with a prediction of 200,000 cases in the following year unless action was taken. Strengthening of the vaccination programs resulted in "only" 60,000 cases in 1995. Diphtheria in the U.S. is rare because of our effective vaccination program involving DPT inoculations (D stands for diphtheria; P stands for *Pertussis*—the bacterium that causes whooping cough; T stands for tetanus). There have been about five cases a year since 1980, and since 1988 all the cases in the U.S. have been imported. However, if the U.S. were to relax its vaccination program as occurred in the former Soviet Union, we would experience similar problems because the bacterium *(Corynebacterium diphtheriae)* is still present, living in the throats of asymptomatic carriers.

UNEXPLAINED EMERGENCE

Ebola hemorrhagic fever was first recognized in 1976 in two outbreaks (one in Northern Zaire and one in Southern Sudan) that killed hundreds in Africa. This rapidly progressing virus disease causes a high fever with bleeding from multiple sites and the ultimate shutdown of the major organs. The Zaire strain of the Ebola virus was fatal in 90% of the cases and the Sudan strain had a lower case fatality rate of 50%. The third outbreak of Ebola hemorrhagic fever was in Sudan in 1979 and involved 34 people. The most recent outbreak involved about 315 cases in and around Kikwit, Zaire, and resulted in 244 deaths, which is a case fatality rate of 77%. Kikwit has a population of about 400,000 and is about 1,000 kilometers south of the site of the original 1976 outbreak in the small village of Yambuku, Zaire. The Ebola viruses involved in both the Kikwit and the Yambuku outbreaks (even though the outbreaks occurred 19 years apart) have been shown to be almost identical. A different Ebola virus was isolated in 1994 from a single nonfatal human case in Cote d'Ivoire, which is in Western Africa. No other cases involving this Ebola strain have been reported.

Great fear exists that this disease will break out in a small village and those infected will carry the virus to a site of a larger population, causing a major epidemic and even a pandemic. In the 1995 outbreak, it was feared that the disease would spread from Kikwit to the capital of Zaire, Kinsasha, about 240 miles to the east. Maybe the reason this did not occur is because the disease progresses so rapidly that the victims die in a matter of days, which limits their contact with others. In both the 1976 and 1995 outbreaks, person-to-person spread occurred through close personal contact with infected blood and other body fluids. Those infected included family members and health-care providers, although the exact modes of spread still need to be better defined. An obvious problem in these outbreaks is the lack of modern medical facilities and barrier products that could have better protected health-care workers from exposure to their infected patients.

The natural reservoir (source) where the Ebola virus "hides out" in Zaire between outbreaks is unknown but attempts to identify the source are being made by culturing local animals, insects, and the environment. The index patient in the 1995 outbreak is thought to have been a charcoal maker that worked in the forest near Kikwit, so this area is being carefully analyzed. The cause of Ebola emergence is still unknown.

SELECTED READINGS

Centers for Disease Control and Prevention: Hantavirus pulmonary syndrome—United States, 1993, *MMWR* 43(No 3):45-48, 1994.

Centers for Disease Control and Prevention: Update: *Vibrio cholerae* O1—Western hemisphere, 1991-1994, and *V. cholerae* O139—Asia, 1994, *MMWR* 44(No 11):215-219, 1995.

Centers for Disease Control and Prevention: Diphtheria epidemic—New Independent States of the former Soviet Union, 1990-1994, *MMWR* 44:177-181, 1995.

Centers for Disease Control and Prevention: Hantavirus pulmonary syndrome—United States, 1995 and 1996, *MMWR* 45(No 14):291-295, 1996.

Coyle PK (editor): *Lyme Disease,* St. Louis, Mosby, 1993.

Morse SS: Factors in the emergence of infectious diseases, *Emerg Infect Dis* 1(No 1):7-15, 1995.

Wilson ME: Travel and the emergence of infectious diseases, *Emerg Infect Dis* 1(No 2):39-46, 1995.

Chapter 5

ORAL MICROBIOLOGY AND PLAQUE-ASSOCIATED DISEASES

The mouth contains the normal oral microbiota that have colonized and are continually maintained on the teeth and soft tissues and in saliva. These microorganisms usually cause no harm except when they are allowed to accumulate in the form of dental plaque or are displaced from the mouth to deeper tissues such as the tooth pulp or to other body sites such as the bloodstream.

NORMAL ORAL MICROBIOTA

The human mouth is usually first exposed to microorganisms at birth during passage through the birth canal. Most of the mother's vaginal bacteria that enter the child's mouth are transient (short-lived) and do not establish themselves as regular members of the oral microbiota. With time, the child is exposed to microorganisms from the environment and it appears that the main sources of microorganisms that colonize the child's mouth are the mouths of other people, particularly the mother and other close family members.

For microorganisms to become established members of the oral microbiota, they must attach to oral surfaces and be able to multiply in the oral environment. Eruption of the primary teeth results in a major change in this environment, now providing tooth surfaces, gingival crevices, and more opportunity for bleeding into the mouth. New bacteria, such as *Streptococcus mutans,* appear that can survive only on the teeth. Anaerobes increase in number because of the added anaerobic sites around the teeth. Thus, different sites in the mouth (tongue, buccal epithelium, supragingival tooth surfaces, subgingival tooth surfaces, and crevicular epithelial surfaces) support different combinations of microorganisms. As one grows older, more and more microorganisms colonize the mouth and, in general, the composition stabilizes by approximately the early teen years.

The normal oral microbiota consists mostly of bacteria, although approximately one third of the population also has the yeast *Candida albicans* in their mouths. The oral microbiota is very complex, with approximately 30 genera of bacteria represented (Box 5-1), although not every person has all of these genera present all of the time. Each genus may be represented by several species, resulting in a very complex group of gram-positive and gram-negative bacteria. A gram of dental plaque (about one quarter of a teaspoonful) contains approximately 200 billion bacteria, and saliva contains approximately 10 million to 100 million bacteria per milliliter.

Box 5-1   Bacterial Genera in the Mouth

GRAM-NEGATIVE	GRAM-POSITIVE
Bacteroides	Streptococcus
Porphyromonas	Actinomyces
Prevotella	Lactobacillus
Mitsuokella	Arachnia
Fusobacterium	Propionibacterium
Actinobacillus	Bifidobacterium
Capnocytophaga	Micrococcus
Eikenella	Peptostreptococcus
Wolinella	Eubacterium
Campylobacter	Rothia
Treponema	Corynebacterium
Neisseria	
Leptotrichia	
Selenomonas	
Centipeda	
Haemophilus	
Veillonella	
Cardiobacterium	
Moraxella	

MICROBIOLOGY OF CARIES

Dental caries is an infectious disease. It is caused by a *demineralization* of tooth structure by acids produced during metabolism of dietary sugars by bacteria associated with the tooth surfaces (Figure 5-1). As with any infectious disease, there are four factors that are necessary for caries to occur: susceptible host, microorganisms, substrate, and time.

Susceptible Host

Not all people are susceptible to all infectious diseases. Resistance may be attributable to many factors (other than specific immunity) that are not well understood. In the case of caries-free people, resistance has not been clearly explained but may involve characteristics of saliva, anatomic differences in the teeth, or the nature of the oral microbiota. Nevertheless, for caries to occur, the person must be susceptible to the disease.

Microorganisms

Bacteria capable of causing caries must be present in the mouth and must be closely associated with the teeth. This association may be in the form of *dental plaque,* a microbial mass that accumulates on the teeth in the absence of oral hygiene, or may result from an

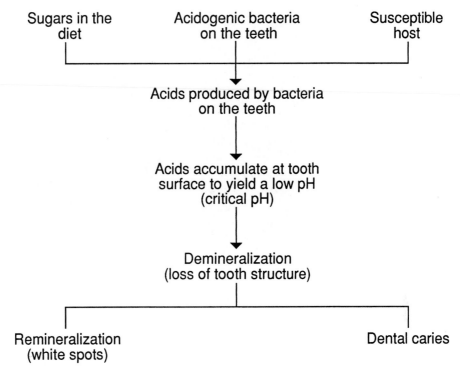

FIGURE 5-1   Formation of dental caries. In a person susceptible to dental caries, the acidogenic bacteria on the teeth ferment sugars in the diet to acids (mainly lactic acid). The acids accumulate on the tooth surface, lowering the pH to a critical level of about 5.2. This starts dissolving the minerals in the tooth, causing loss of tooth structure (demineralization). A natural body defense mechanism called remineralization attempts to restore the lost calcium and phosphate in the tooth, which will appear as a white spot on the tooth. If remineralization occurs more slowly than demineralization, dental caries occurs.

impaction of bacteria and food in the *nonself-cleansing areas* of the dentition (pits and fissures, interproximal sites, gingival crevices).

Dental Plaque

Plaque is composed of bacterial cells embedded in an intercellular matrix (Figure 5-2). The matrix contains macromolecules and small molecules that:

- are produced by the multiplying bacteria
- may enter the mouth in the diet
- originate from mammalian cells, saliva, or blood

Plaque formation begins to reform within seconds after the teeth are cleaned. Glycoproteins from saliva are first absorbed onto the tooth surface to a thin proteinaceous layer, called the *pellicle,* that coats all tooth surfaces exposed to saliva. Next, the bacteria attach to the pellicle, and these serve as an initial "layer" to which other bacterial cells attach. These other cells may come from saliva or they may be the daughter cells formed from previously attached cells that are multiplying. Plaque accumulates most rapidly in the nonself-cleansing areas of the dentition where the tip of the tongue, the musculature of the

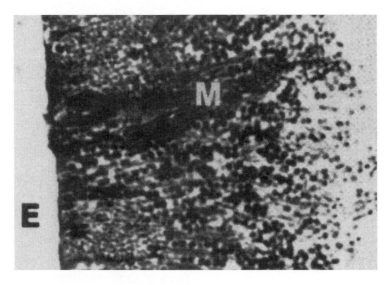

FIGURE 5-2   Relatively thin predominantly coccal flora (plaque) on the enamel surface associated with nondisease gingival tissue. *E,* Enamel; *M,* columnar microcolony. *(From* Listgarten MA: *Periodontal* 47:3, 1976.)

cheeks, and the occlusion of the teeth cannot remove the accumulating bacteria. As the plaque accumulates in the absence of oral hygiene, potentially harmful products from the multiplying bacteria accumulate and may cause damage to the teeth (caries) or to the nearby periodontal tissues (*gingivitis* or *periodontitis*).

There are many mechanisms by which the bacteria attach to the tooth surfaces or to each other during plaque formation. Some mechanisms involve interactions of the bacteria with glycoproteins or calcium from saliva or pellicle, some involve fimbriae or special receptors on the surfaces of the bacteria, and others involve extracellular macromolecules produced by the bacteria that can then bind to cell surfaces. One approach to prevention of plaque-associated diseases (caries, periodontal diseases) other than brushing and flossing is to develop special mouth rinses that interfere with bacterial attachment to the teeth to prevent plaque from accumulating.

Caries-conducive Bacteria

Although dental plaque contains many different species of bacteria, some are more important than others in directly contributing to the initiation or progression of dental caries (Table 5-1).

A group of closely related streptococci called the *mutans streptococci* consist of the most caries-conducive bacteria in the mouth. Members of this group that are most commonly present in the human mouth are *Streptococcus mutans* and *Streptococcus sobrinus.* Other species in this group occur in the mouth less frequently. The mutans streptococci have all three pathogenic properties important for caries formation:

- Producing acids from carbohydrates (being *acidogenic*)
- Surviving at low pH (being *aciduric*)
- Accumulating on teeth

Table 5-1   Important Caries—Conducive Bacteria in Humans

BACTERIUM	PATHOGENIC PROPERTIES
Mutans streptococci	Acidogenic; aciduric; accumulates on teeth
Streptococcus mutans	
Streptococcus sobrinus	
Streptococcus rattus	
Streptococcus cricetus	
Lactobacillus species	Acidogenic; aciduric
Actinomyces naeslundii	Accumulates on teeth; slightly acidogenic

The mutans streptococci are thought to be the most important oral bacteria in initiating caries, particularly on smooth tooth surfaces where plaque that can resist the cleansing action of the tongue and cheeks "rubbing" against the teeth is needed for caries to develop. Mutans streptococci are very important plaque-formers and can rapidly accumulate in plaque in the presence of *sucrose* (table sugar). The mutans streptococci have special enzymes (glucosyltransferases) that split sucrose, linking together the glucose units of the sucrose molecules to form polysaccharides called glucans (Figure 5-3). The remaining fructose part of sucrose is taken into the cell and processed through catabolic fermentation reactions to produce energy with mainly lactic acid as a waste product (see Chapter 2). The glucans bind to the cells and act as bridges that bind to other cells. This permits new daughter cells to attach to the cell mass and accumulate in the developing dental plaque. The mutans streptococci not only produce acids (acidogenic) from sugar metabolism but also are capable of surviving and metabolizing in the presence of these acids at a low pH (aciduric), whereas most bacteria die at a low pH.

Lactobacillus species such as *L. acidophilus* and *L. casei* are thought to be more important in the progression of a carious lesion after other bacteria (mainly mutans streptococci) have initiated the tooth destruction. Although lactobacilli are highly acidogenic and aciduric, they do not have very effective attachment mechanisms to allow them to accumulate in plaque that develops over noncarious teeth. Thus the other bacteria present in plaque (e.g., mutans streptococci) are more important in the initial attack on the tooth. Low numbers of lactobacilli, however, are accidentally "trapped" in plaque as it develops and may be present in saliva. If acids are produced by the plaque bacteria, causing demineralization of the tooth, the aciduric bacteria such as lactobacilli and mutans streptococci are given an advantage to multiply more rapidly. The nonaciduric bacteria begin to die, leaving more nutrients available for the acidurics. The best place for lactobacilli to thrive is within the highly acidic carious lesion itself. As it thrives, it and the mutans streptococci produce even more acids, if sugars are present, causing the lesion to progress.

Actinomyces naeslundii is a good plaque former and can accumulate to high numbers in plaque. It is not as caries conducive as the mutans streptococci, likely because it is only slightly acidogenic and not aciduric. However, *A. naeslundii* is important in root caries formation but the mechanisms of its involvement have not been clearly defined.

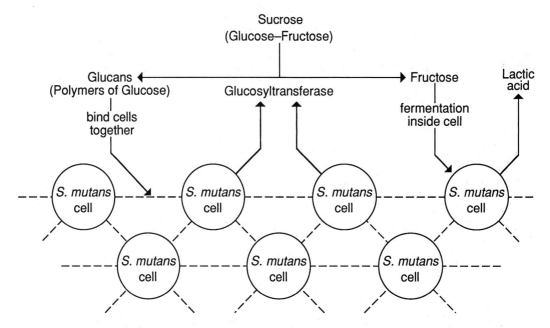

FIGURE 5-3   Plaque formation—*Streptococcus mutans. S. mutans* produces enzymes called glucosyltransferases that degrade sucrose into free fructose and polymers of glucose called glucans. The glucans bind to the surfaces of the *S. mutans* cells, linking them together into a mass in the plaque. The fructose is taken into the cells and metabolized through fermentation with production of energy for multiplication and lactic acid as a waste product. *Dashed lines* indicate glucans.

Substrate

The third factor needed for caries development is a dietary substrate that is metabolized by oral bacteria through catabolic fermentation to produce acids. Sucrose is the most caries-conducive component of our diet but other sugars such as fructose, glucose, lactose, and starch also can be fermented by bacteria and contribute to the disease.

Time

As with any infectious disease, time is needed for the disease to become recognized. This time can be called the incubation time, as described in Chapter 3. Dental checkups are frequently scheduled at 6-month intervals because this approximates the usual incubation time for clinically detectable caries.

MICROBIOLOGY OF PERIODONTAL DISEASES

Like dental caries, periodontal diseases are also infectious diseases caused by members of the normal oral microbiota that have been allowed to accumulate in gingival sulcus plaque (Figure 5-4). As the bacteria multiply, they produce histolytic enzymes, toxic metabolites, exotoxins, endotoxins, and immunosuppressive and antiphagocytic factors (all are de-

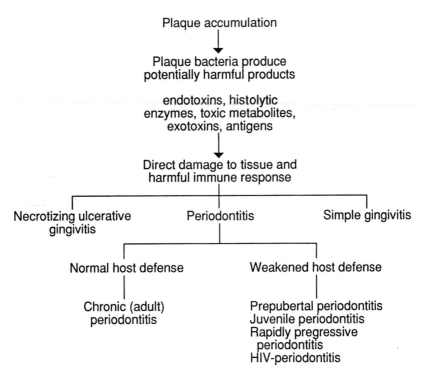

FIGURE 5-4   Development of plaque-associated periodontal diseases. As plaque accumulates in the gingival crevice, the bacteria multiply and produce harmful products that can cause direct damage to the periodontal tissues and that continually stimulate the immune system, resulting in tissue damage. The types of bacteria in the plaque and/or the nature of the body defense mechanisms combating the infection determine which form of periodontal disease may result.

scribed in Chapter 3). The accumulation of these bacteria and their potentially harmful products and antigens then produce periodontal diseases by the following mechanisms:

- Direct damage to the tissue
- Inflammation
- Interference with some host defense mechanisms
- Stimulation of the immune response in the periodontal tissues, which can cause damage

Types of Periodontal Diseases

If the disease process affects only the gingival tissue, resulting in an inflammatory response, including swelling, redness, and maybe spontaneous bleeding, the disease is called *simple* or *acute gingivitis*. This disease is reversible. When the plaque (and its tissue damaging products) is removed, the gingival tissue returns to normal. Another gingivitis, called *necrotizing ulcerative gingivitis* (NUG) or trench mouth, is associated with plaque accumulation and predisposing factors such as stress. This gingivitis also is reversible if the predisposing factors are eliminated and plaque accumulation is controlled.

If the disease process affects the bone in which the teeth are set, the disease is called *periodontitis*. This involves the development of periodontal pockets around the teeth where the gingival tissue has separated from the teeth. These pockets are filled with plaque bacteria and limit access to cleaning. Some of the plaque products directly or indirectly destroy the periodontal tissues and the alveolar bone, which can result in a loosening or loss of the teeth involved. Periodontitis is not reversible. Removal and subsequent control of the plaque, however, can stop further progress of the disease in many instances.

The type of periodontal disease that develops from the accumulation of plaque is influenced by the specific types of bacteria present in the plaque and by how the body responds to the infection. For example, the continuous presence of plaque in people with normal body defense mechanisms likely leads to *chronic periodontitis,* a slowly progressing destruction of the bone in which the teeth are set that occurs over a period of years. This is the most common form of periodontitis that usually occurs in people older than age 35.

In those with some defect in body defenses (usually decreased phagocytosis), the bone destruction that occurs in periodontitis may occur rapidly, within months or weeks, as in *rapidly progressive periodontitis* (most commonly seen in those younger than age 35), *juvenile periodontitis* (most common during the early teen years), or *prepubertal periodontitis* (occurring in those with primary teeth). Immunosuppression resulting from human immunodeficiency virus (HIV) infection also may predispose to a rapidly progressing periodontitis.

Microorganisms in Periodontal Diseases

Subgingival plaque associated with all forms of periodontal disease contains many bacteria that possess a wide variety of pathogenic properties. Thus many species can contribute to the disease processes but some appear to be more important than others and are often called *periodontopathogens* (Box 5-2). Although caries-conducive bacteria are all gram-positive, most of the periodontopathogens are gram-negative; the exceptions are *Peptostreptococcus, Streptococcus,* and *Actinomyces.* The latter two genera are mostly associated with gingivitis rather than with periodontitis. Although some research has discovered strong associations of specific species with specific types of periodontitis (e.g., *Actinobacillus actinomycetemcomitans* with juvenile periodontitis and *Porphyromonas gingivalis* with chronic periodontitis), this is not always true in every case of the diseases.

Box 5-2   Important Periodontopathogens

Porphyromonas gingivalis	*Eikenella corrodens*
Actinobacillus actinomycetemcomitans	*Capnocytophaga ochracea*
Prevotella intermedia	*Bacteroides forsythus*
Wolinella recta	*Peptostreptococcus micros*
Treponema denticola	*Streptococcus* species
Fusobacterium species	*Actinomyces* species

PREVENTION OF PLAQUE-ASSOCIATED DISEASES

Regular brushing and flossing have long been used for preventing plaque-associated diseases. Also, fluoride and pit and fissure sealants are effective against caries. Caries and periodontal diseases still occur, however, and other preventive approaches are being used or studied. A current approach involving microbiology is the use of antimicrobial mouth rinses. Other approaches still under investigation include more effective means of delivering antimicrobial agents to sites of infection, developing new antimicrobial agents, replacement of oral pathogens with nonpathogenic strains, and use of vaccines or other chemical agents that may prevent bacterial attachment or disrupt preformed plaque.

ACUTE DENTAL INFECTIONS

As carious lesions progress and approach the tooth pulp, microbial byproducts may enter the pulp and cause inflammation called *pulpitis.* As the disease continues, the bacteria enter the pulp chamber, enhancing the inflammation and destroying the pulp tissue. Further progression may extend the infection through the tooth apex, causing a *periapical infection.* Depending on the host response and probably the types of bacteria involved, the surrounding facial tissues may become infected, producing a *cellulitis.* Endodontic treatment, in general, involves removing necrotic (dead) pulp tissue, killing and removing the remaining bacteria in the root canals, and filling the canals with inert material to prevent further access of bacteria to the periapical tissues. Treatment with antibiotics also may be necessary to slow down bacterial growth involved with periapical infections and cellulitis. Thus the normal oral bacteria present in carious lesions that extend to the pulp tissues become the causative agents of these acute dental infections.

OTHER INFECTIONS

Members of the normal oral flora may be involved in other harmful infections if given the opportunity to invade tissues as in pulpitis. For example, *Actinomyces israelii,* a gram-positive anaerobic, rodshaped bacterium, or other *Actinomyces* species found in plaque, may cause a harmful infection in the jaw and neck area called cervicofacial *actinomycosis.* This is a rare disease resulting from entrance of these bacteria into oral tissues as a result of tooth extractions or some other trauma. Actinomycosis of the lung is another rare disease that results from aspiration (breathing in) of *Actinomyces* species into the lung from the mouth.

The slightest trauma in the mouth that results in bleeding (e.g., tooth brushing, biting the cheek, dental procedures) may permit members of the normal oral microbiota to enter the bloodstream, causing a *transient bacteremia.* Normally, the phagocytes in the blood rapidly destroy these bacteria before they have a chance to cause problems. If a person has had previous damage to their heart valves, however, such as in rheumatic heart disease, certain oral bacteria in the blood may induce further damage to these valves or cause *subacute bacterial endocarditis* (inflammation of the inside of the heart). This is why some dental patients with previous heart damage must be given antibiotics prophylactically (for prevention) when they receive dental care. When bacteria do enter the bloodstream and cause damage to tissues, it is referred to as septicemia rather than bacteremia.

Other harmful infections caused by oral microorganisms are those resulting from a bite or a puncture or cut with a contaminated dental instrument. Several microorganisms are implanted through the skin in these instances, which can lead to a harmful infection that sometimes needs antibiotic treatment. Thus many members of the normal oral microbiota have pathogenic potential, if they are allowed to gain entrance to deeper tissues or if they gain entrance to the bodies of others.

SELECTED READINGS

Baehni PC, Guggenheim B: Potential of diagnostic microbiology for treatment and prognosis of dental caries and periodontal diseases, *Crit Rev Oral Biol Med* 7:259-277, 1996.

Bowen WH, Tabak LA: *Cariology for the nineties,* Rochester, 1993, University of Rochester.

Miller CH: Periodontal microbiology. In Willett NP, White RR, and Rosen S, editors: *Essential dental microbiology,* Norwalk, Conn, 1991, Appleton & Lange.

Miller CH: The oral microbial flora. In Schuster G, editor: *Oral microbiology and infectious diseases,* Philadelphia, 1990, BC Decker.

II
PART

INFECTION CONTROL

Chapter 6

BLOODBORNE PATHOGENS

As described in Chapter 3, the patient's mouth is the most important source of potentially pathogenic microorganisms in the dental office. Pathogenic agents may occur in the mouth as a result of four basic conditions: bloodborne diseases, oral diseases, systemic diseases with oral lesions, and respiratory diseases. The bloodborne diseases will be presented here (Table 6-1) and the oral and respiratory diseases will be pesented in Chapter 7.

BLOODBORNE PATHOGENS

Bloodborne pathogens may infect different blood cells or other tissue of the body but during infection the pathogens exist or are released into the blood or other body fluids, which may include semen, vaginal secretion, intestinal secretions, tears, mothers' milk, synovial (joint) fluid, pericardial (around the heart) fluid, amniotic fluids (surround the developing fetus), and saliva in dentistry. Because blood or other body fluids may contain the pathogens, the disease may be spread from one person to another by contact with the fluids. Thus the diseases are called bloodborne diseases. Bloodborne pathogens may enter the mouth during dental procedures that induce bleeding. Thus contact with saliva during such procedures may result in exposure to these pathogens if present. Because it is very difficult to determine if blood is actually present in saliva, saliva from all dental patients should be considered potentially infectious.

Viral Hepatitis

There are at least six hepatitis viruses that cause clinically similar diseases: hepatitis A, B, C, D, E, and G (Table 6-2). Hepatitis A and E are mainly transmitted through contaminated food and water (fecal-oral route of spread); hepatitis B, C, D, and G are bloodborne diseases usually transmitted by direct contact with infected body fluids. Hepatitis also may be caused by excessive alcohol consumption, exposure to some hazardous chemicals, and as a complication of other viral infections such as cytomegalovirus.

Hepatitis B

Hepatitis B, an inflammation of the liver, is a major health problem in the United States and is endemic (occurs regularly) in other parts of the world. Between 200,000 and 300,000 people are infected with the hepatitis B virus (HBV) each year. Approximately 10,000 will require hospitalization, approximately 250 will die of fulminant hepatitis (an overwhelming and rapidly destructive form of the disease), and approximately 15,000 will become chronic carriers of the virus. About 4,000 people die each year of hepatitis B-related cirrhosis of the liver, and an additional 800 die of related liver cancer. Current esti-

Table 6-1 Bloodborne Diseases

DISEASE	PATHOGEN
Hepatitis B	Hepatitis B virus (HBV)
Hepatitis C	Hepatitis C virus (HCV)
Hepatitis D	Hepatitis D virus (HDV)
Hepatitis G	Hepatitis G virus (HGV)
HIV disease*	Human immunodeficiency virus (HIV)

*Includes HIV infection and AIDS.

mates by the Centers for Disease Control and Prevention suggest that there are approximately 1.0 to 1.25 million HBV carriers in the United States that have some potential to spread the virus to others.

Hepatitis B virus.   The HBV is an enveloped DNA virus that infects and multiplies in human liver cells. During the course of an infection, the virus and cells containing the virus are released in high numbers into the bloodstream and other body fluids, explaining its description as a bloodborne disease agent. A milliliter of blood from an infected person may contain as many as 100 million virus particles, meaning that only small amounts of blood or other body fluids are necessary to transmit the disease to others. The virus has three components that are important antigens; some are on its surface (HBsAg) and two are inside the virus (HBcAg and HBeAg) (Table 6-3). The hepatitis B vaccines consist of the HBsAg that is synthesized in the laboratory by genetic engineering techniques. Hepatitis B virus has been shown to be killed or inactivated by commonly used methods of sterilization and disinfection, including the steam autoclave, and 10-minute exposure to 1:100 diluted bleach, 1:16 diluted phenolic glutaraldehyde, 75 parts per million iodophor, and 70% isopropyl alcohol. Thus HBV is relatively easy to kill when outside the body, provided the killing agent comes into direct contact with the virus. Hepatitis B virus is more easily killed than *Mycobacterium tuberculosis* and bacterial spores.

Disease states.   Approximately 90% of those infected with HBV undergo complete recovery without developing a carrier state (Figure 6-1). Approximately 5% to 10% become carriers of the virus, with approximately one half eliminating the virus from their bodies within 2.5 years. The other one half (2.5%-5% of all those originally infected) become chronic carriers. The carrier state is defined as being HBsAg-positive on at least two occasions when tested at least 2 months apart or being HBsAg positive and IgM anti-HBc negative at a single test. Anyone who is positive for HBsAg has a potential to spread the disease to others. Those who are also HBeAg positive have very high concentrations of the virus in their blood and, therefore, are considered as being highly infectious. Persons who have chronic hepatitis have approximately a 200 to 300 times greater chance of later developing liver cancer.

Transmission.   Hepatitis B virus is spread percutaneously (through the skin) or permucosally (through mucous membranes) by contact with infected body fluids, for exam-

Table 6-2 Types and Characteristics of Viral Hepatitis

	A	B	C	D	E
Other name	Infectious	Serum	Parenterally transmitted non-A, non-B	Delta	Enterically transmitted non-A, non-B
Route of spread	Fecal-oral (food, water)	Parenteral, Sexual contact, Perinatal	Sexual contact, Perinatal	Parenteral, Sexual contact	Fecal-oral (food, water)
Incubation period	2-6 weeks	4-26 weeks	2-21 weeks	4-24 weeks	2-9 weeks
Carrier state	No	Yes (5%–10%)	Yes (10%–50%)	Yes	No
Mortality	About 0.15%	About 1.5%	About 1.5%	2%–20%	About 1.5%
Vaccine	Yes	Yes	No	No*	No

From Miller CH: *Calif Dent Inst J Cont Ed* 40:18–28, 1992.
*Since a previous or simultaneous infection with the hepatitis B virus is required for infection with hepatitis D virus, vaccination against hepatitis B may help protect against hepatitis D.

Table 6-3 Hepatitis Terminology

	ABBREVIATION	TERM	DEFINITION/COMMENTS
Hepatitis A	HAV	Hepatitis A virus	Etiologic agent of "infectious" hepatitis; a picornavirus; single serotype
	Anti-HAV	Antibody to HAV	Detectable at onset of symptoms; lifetime persistence
	IgM anti-HAV	IgM class antibody to HAV	Indicates recent infection with hepatitis A; detectable for 4–6 months after infection
Hepatitis B	HBV	Hepatitis B virus	Etiologic agent of "serum" hepatitis; also known as Dane particle
	HBsAg	Hepatitis B surface antigen	Surface antigen(s) of HBV detectable in large quantities in serum; several subtypes identified
	HBeAg	Hepatitis Be antigen	Soluble antigen; correlates with HBV replication, high titer HBV in serum, and infectivity of serum
	HBcAg	Hepatitis B core antigen	No commercial test available
	Anti-HBs	Antibody to HBsAg	Indicates past infection with and immunity to HBV, passive antibody from HBIG, or immune response from HB vaccine
	Anti-HBe	Antibody to HBeAg	Presence in serum of HBsAg carrier indicates lower titer of HBV
	Anti-HBc	Antibody to HBcAg	Indicates prior infection with HBV at some undefined time
	IgM anti-HBc	IgM class antibody to HBcAg	Indicates recent infection with HBV; detectable for 4–6 months after infection
Hepatitis C	HCV	Hepatitis C virus	Diagnosis by exclusion. At least two candidate viruses, one of which has been proposed as hepatitis C virus; shares epidemiologic features with hepatitis B
	Anti-HCV	Antibody to HCV	Indicates past or present infection with HCV
Hepatitis D	HDV	Hepatitis D virus	Etiologic agent of delta hepatitis; can cause infection only in presence of HBV
	HDAg	Delta antigen	Detectable in early acute delta infection
	Anti-HDV	Antibody to delta antigen	Indicates present or past infection with delta virus
Hepatitis E	HEV	Hepatitis E virus	Diagnosis by exclusion. Causes large epidemics in Asia, Africa, and Mexico; fecal–oral or waterborne
Immune globulins	IG	Immune globulin (previously ISG, immune serum globulin, or gamma globulin)	Contains antibodies to HAV, low-titer antibodies to HBV
	HBIG	Hepatitis B immune globulin	Contains high-titer antibodies to HBV

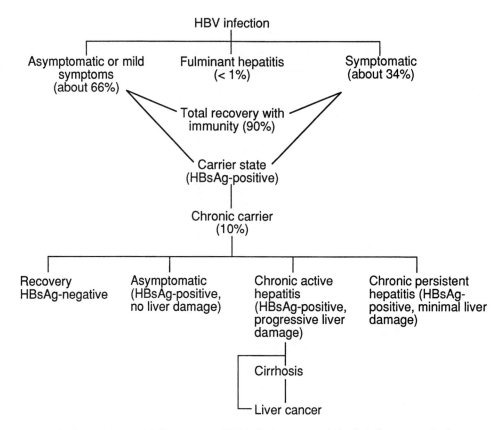

FIGURE 6-1   Hepatitis B outcomes. HBV infection may result in clinical symptoms in about one third of the cases and no symptoms or unrecognizable symptoms in about two thirds of the cases. A rapidly progressing fulminant disease leading to death occurs in less than 1% of the cases. About 90% of all infected recover. The remaining 10% develop chronic infection and become carriers, evidenced by being positive for HBsAg. Those with chronic infection may carry the virus for up to six months and then have complete recovery. Others will remain as chronic carriers, being asymptomatic, having chronic active hepatitis, or having chronic persistent hepatitis.

ple, at birth, during sexual activities, or with contaminated needles or other sharp objects. Also, the virus may be spread in environments involving frequent close contact with an infected person, as in households or institutions for developmentally disabled children. This latter route of spread likely involves unnoticed contact of infected body fluids with skin lesions or mucosal surfaces. Thus high-risk behaviors for acquiring hepatitis B include:

- Sharing contaminated needles during intravenous drug abuse
- Homosexual, bisexual, or heterosexual behaviors with multiple partners
- Injuries with sharp objects contaminated with blood or other body fluids
- Exposure of nonintact skin or mucous membranes to blood or other body fluids

Spread of HBV through transfused blood or blood products is now rare because of routine testing of blood for HBsAg and donor screening. Hepatitis B is not commonly transmitted by the fecal-oral route. In approximately 40% of the hepatitis B cases, however, the exact mode of transmission is not identifiable.

Symptoms.   If symptoms develop after infection, they begin to appear approximately 2.5 to 6 months after exposure. Roughly one third of those infected (see Figure 6-1) exhibit the more easily recognizable symptoms of yellowing of the skin (jaundice) and whites of the eyes, light-colored stools, dark urine, joint pain, fever, a rash, and itching. Approximately another one third develop less descript mild symptoms that may include malaise ("not feeling good"), loss of appetite, nausea, and abdominal pain. The other one third develop no symptoms at all. Thus two-thirds of all those infected develop no symptoms or have mild nondescript symptoms that are often unrecognized as being related to hepatitis. Yet symptomatic and asymptomatic cases can spread the virus to others. This unrecognizable infection with HBV and with other viruses (such as human immunodeficiency virus [HIV], described later) serves as the basis for universal precautions—applying infection control procedures during care for all patients not just for those who are known to be infected.

Development of a hepatitis B chronic carrier state may occur more commonly in those who are asymptomatic and is more likely to occur in the young. As many as 90% of newborns infected by their mothers become chronic carriers and from 25% to 50% of children infected before age 5 become carriers. Women who are pregnant should seek the advice of their personal physician about being tested for hepatitis B, so that, if infected, proper procedures can be instituted to protect the newborn. Approximately 5% to 10% of infected adults become carriers. Chronic carriers are at high risk of developing chronic hepatitis that may lead to cirrhosis of the liver or primary liver cancer. Thus one could be unknowingly infected with HBV, not develop any recognizable symptoms, become a chronic carrier, unknowingly spread the virus to others, and die years later of HBV liver damage. Hepatitis B is an insidious disease.

Risk for the dental team.   In the early to mid 1980s, approximately 10,000 to 12,000 cases of hepatitis B a year (approximately 4% of all cases) occurred in people who had an occupational risk for exposure to body fluids. In 1994, this number dropped to about 1,000 cases, showing approximately a 90% decrease in hepatitis B among health care workers. The greatest dental occupational risks for exposure are:

- Injuries from contaminated sharps (needlesticks, instrument punctures, cuts, bur lacerations)
- Blood and saliva contamination of cuts and cracks on the skin or ungloved hands or hands with torn gloves
- Spraying of blood and saliva onto open lesions on the skin or onto mucous membranes

Several blood testing surveys of dental workers conducted between 1975 and 1982 attempted to determine how many of the different types of dental workers had been infected with HBV. Although some of the studies involved only small groups of workers, the results suggested that approximately 13% of dental assistants, 17% of dental hygienists, 14% of dental laboratory technicians, and 9% to 25% of dentists had been infected. It is estimated that approximately 5% of the general population has been infected. Thus unvaccinated members of the dental team are at least two to five times more likely to become infected with HBV than the general population. Use of infection control barriers of masks, gloves, and protective eyeglasses that prevent exposure to blood and saliva help prevent hepatitis in health-care workers but some are still being infected through injuries with contaminated sharp instruments and needles.

Risk for dental patients.   The chances of a patient acquiring any disease in a dental office is extremely low. In the past, HBV has been spread from dentists to patients, as documented in ten separate instances. In each instance, the dentist was highly infectious (HBeAg-positive) and apparently did not routinely wear gloves. These instances occurred between 1974 and 1985, with none, as yet, being reported since. This coincides with the time (approximately 1984) when infection control in dentistry was reemphasized as a result of the advent of acquired immunodeficiency syndrome (AIDS).

Hepatitis B vaccine.   It is extremely fortunate that safe and effective vaccines for hepatitis B are available. Because there is no successful medical treatment to cure this disease, prevention is of paramount importance. Details on the vaccines and the vaccination series are presented in Chapter 8. The vaccines are strongly recommended for all members of the dental team. The Occupational Safety and Health Administration (OSHA) of the U.S. Department of Labor actually requires dentist-employers to offer the hepatitis B vaccine series free of charge to office staff who may have any potential for exposure to blood or saliva. OSHA requires this of employers in all health-care and other professions related to body fluid exposures. Also, in late 1991, the Centers for Disease Control and Prevention recommended hepatitis B vaccination for all newborns, and in 1995 the CDC recommended vaccination for 12 year olds who were not previously vaccinated.

Hepatitis C

Hepatitis C was previously called parenterally transmitted non-A, non-B hepatitis (see Table 6-2). The hepatitis C virus (HCV) is thought to cause approximately 30% of acute viral hepatitis cases in the United States. Hepatitis C is a bloodborne disease. It is estimated that about 170,000 people in the U.S. become infected with HCV every year but only about 25% of those infected have any recognizable symptoms (Figure 6-2). Approximately 50% of hepatitis C cases are associated with intravenous drug abuse, 13% are associated with sexual activity, 3% with blood transfusions, and 1% with occupational exposure in health-care workers. The remaining cases have unidentified routes of transmission. Hepatitis C has been transmitted to health-care workers through needlestick injuries.

An alarming fact about hepatitis C is that at least 50% of those infected (about 85,000 persons per year) apparently become chronic carriers, which may involve 1% to 3% of the population (see Figure 6-2). This disease is thought to cause from 8,000 to 10,000 deaths per year. Until recently, hepatitis C was diagnosed by indirect means showing that the patient did not have type A or type B hepatitis. The causative virus was first isolated in 1989, and a blood test for antibodies to HCV was designed in 1991. This test aids in diagnosing the disease, identifying those who are or have been infected, and in screening potential blood donors. As yet there is no vaccine for hepatitis C but development of the badly needed test for HCV is leading to more firm information on modes of spread of this virus. Neither the hepatitis A nor the hepatitis B vaccines provide any protection against hepatitis C.

Hepatitis D

Infection with hepatitis D virus (HDV), also known as the Delta agent, can apparently be regarded as a complication of hepatitis B (see Table 6-2). This virus may cause infection only in the presence of an active HBV infection. Hepatitis D virus is a defective virus that needs a part of the HBV to complete its life cycle. Infection with HDV may occur as a coinfection with HBV (both HDV and HBV infect simultaneously) or as a superinfection of HDV in an HBV carrier. Both instances usually result in clinical acute hepatitis and coinfection usually resolves, whereas superinfection frequently causes chronic HDV

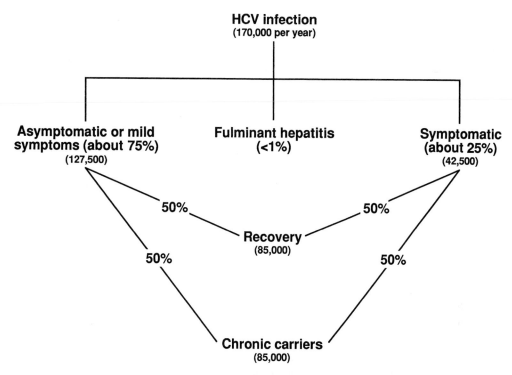

FIGURE 6-2 Hepatitis C outcomes. Hepatitis C may result in clinical symptoms in about one quarter of those infected and no symptoms in about three quarters of the cases. Of the estimated 170,000 new cases of hepatitis C infection that develop each year, 50% to 85% will apparently become chronic carriers of the virus.

infection and chronic active hepatitis. Hepatitis D virus is transmitted by routes similar to those of HBV, and outbreaks of hepatitis D have been reported in the United States. Thus those who are susceptible to HBV infection, occupationally or otherwise, are also susceptible to HDV infection. Successful vaccination against hepatitis B also should prevent hepatitis D.

Hepatitis G

Hepatitis G is the most recently described viral hepatitis, being first recognized in 1995. Very little information is available about the virus or the disease but transmission is thought to at least involve bloodborne spread.

Hepatitis A and E

Hepatitis A does not pose a particular risk to dental workers or patients because this form of hepatitis is primarily spread by the fecal-oral route involving consumption of contaminated food or water (see Table 6-2). There is a vaccine available for hepatitis A; it is recommended for people who may travel to countries with poor sanitation systems. Isolated instances of hepatitis A spread by contact with body fluids other than feces have been reported.

Hepatitis E also is spread by contaminated food or water, and only a handful of cases have been reported in the U.S. In contrast, hepatitis E is a problem in the Middle Eastern countries.

HIV Disease

The human immunodeficiency virus (HIV) causes HIV disease, which involves HIV infection that progresses to a final phase called acquired immunodeficiency syndrome (AIDS). AIDS was reported as a new clinical disease in the summer of 1981, and the Centers for Disease Control and Prevention now estimate that approximately 1.25 million people in the United States have been infected with HIV. Worldwide, HIV is thought to have infected about 31 million people.

HIV disease involves destruction of the body's immune system, making the individual susceptible to life-threatening opportunistic infections or cancers. Progression from the initial phase of the disease (HIV infection) to the terminal phase of the disease (AIDS) may take from approximately 2 to 12 or more years, with an average of approximately 10 years.

HIV

Human immunodeficiency virus is a member of a group of RNA viruses called retroviruses. Human immunodeficiency virus type 1 is the most common worldwide cause of HIV disease. Human immunodeficiency virus type 2 causes another less aggressive immunodeficiency syndrome in Western Africa. Infection with HIV-2 in the United States is uncommon, with most cases occurring in immigrants from Africa and in injection drug abusers.

Human immunodeficiency virus type 1 primarily infects T_4 lymphocytes but also can infect macrophages and a few other cell types. These special lymphocytes are the cells that regulate the immune response. Human immunodeficiency virus type 1 selectively attaches to and enters T_4 lymphocytes (also called CD_4 lymphocytes), where the virus RNA is quickly converted into viral DNA, which is incorporated as viral genes into the lymphocyte chromosomes. Thus the lymphocyte and its succeeding generations of cells are permanently infected with the HIV-1 genes. These genes may remain latent (delayed) for prolonged periods but they induce the production of new virus particles within the lymphocytes. This virus production occurs throughout HIV disease but at widely different rates in different patients. Virus production destroys the lymphocytes and yields more viruses that can infect and destroy more lymphocytes. This eventually depletes the body of T_4 cells. Thus HIV-1 produces a latent infection in which the infected person is usually asymptomatic until the level of T_4 lymphocytes becomes critically low. Human immunodeficiency virus type 1 may undergo mutations that produce several different genetic forms as the virus replicates inside lymphocytes and other cells. This genetic variation may explain the difference in the course of HIV disease in different individuals, with some strains of HIV-1 being more virulent than others. This genetic variation also is one reason why a vaccine for prevention has not yet been developed. A vaccine made against one HIV type 1 strain may not protect against other strains. Although there is no known approach to kill HIV type 1 after it is in the body, it can be easily killed when outside the body. It is readily killed by all forms of heat and gas sterilization and by the commonly used liquid sterilants and surface disinfectants, provided the killing agent comes into direct contact with the virus. Human immunodeficiency virus type 1 is much more easily killed on instruments and surfaces than *Mycobacterium tuberculosis* and bacterial spores.

Disease States and Symptoms

HIV infection. At approximately 4 weeks after initial infection with HIV type 1, a person may experience sore throat, fever, swollen glands, diarrhea, joint pain, and fatigue. This is called a retroviral syndrome, or acute HIV syndrome, signifying acute HIV-infection but is not unlike that which occurs with many viral infections. These symptoms may be slight or may be unnoticed. Antibodies to HIV type 1 usually develop within 6 to 12 weeks after initial infection, and by 6 months 95% of those infected have developed antibodies (seroconverted). Unfortunately, these antibodies do not protect against the disease; they do provide a means to diagnose HIV disease. A person with antibodies to HIV is referred to as being "HIV-positive," indicating that the person is infected with the virus.

After acute HIV infection has occurred, most people infected have no further clinical symptoms until months or years later, when the killing of T_4 lymphocytes or other cells becomes prominent. Nevertheless, people with asymptomatic HIV infection still can transmit the virus to others. Some HIV-positive persons experience persistent swollen glands under the arms and in the groin but are otherwise asymptomatic. The condition is referred to as generalized lymphadenopathy.

AIDS. Replication of HIV type 1 in T_4 lymphocytes kills the lymphocytes, and as more and more cells are killed the immune system becomes progressively weaker. This immunodeficiency results in increased susceptibility to opportunistic disease agents that normally do not cause infections or cause less severe infections in those with healthy immune systems. When an HIV-positive patient experiences one or more of these indicator opportunistic infections or a cancer, the patient is diagnosed as having AIDS. The symptoms experienced depend on the type of infection or cancer that occurs, examples of which are listed in Box 6-1. Eventually, one of these diseases causes death. The infectious diseases may be caused by bacterial, viral, fungal, or protozoan agents; the leading cause of death in an AIDS patient is *Pneumocystis carinii* pneumonia.

Oral Manifestations of AIDS

In many instances, early manifestations of AIDS occur as oral lesions. Oral manifestations include fungal diseases, such as candidiasis (thrush), histoplasmosis, geotrichosis, or cryptococcosis; viral diseases such as warts, hairy leukoplakia, or human herpesvirus type 1 (herpes simplex) infection; bacterial diseases such as rapidly progressing periodontitis or gingivitis; cancerous diseases such as Kaposi's sarcoma (recently associated with human herpesvirus type 8) and non-Hodgkin's lymphoma.

Transmission

Human immunodeficiency virus type 1 is transmitted from an infected person through:

- Intimate sexual contact (vaginal, anal, oral) involving contact or exchange of semen or vaginal secretions
- Exposure to blood, blood-contaminated body fluids, or blood products
- Perinatal contact (from infected mother to child)

Other exposures resulting in HIV-infection are variations of these three basic modes of

---

Box 6-1   Examples of Diseases Associated With HIV Disease

Bacterial
Infections with
Mycobacterium avium-intracellulare
Mycobacterium tuberculosis
Salmonella sp.
Shigella flexneri
Clostridium difficile
Streptococcus pneumoniae
Norcardia asteroides
Legionella pneumophila

Viral
Herpes simplex infections
Cytomegalovirus infections
Hairy leukoplakia

Protozoan
Pneumocystis carinii pneumonia
Toxoplasmosis
Giardiasis
Cryptosporidiosis

Fungal
Candidiasis
Histoplasmosis
Cryptococcosis
Coccidiodomycosis

Cancers
Kaposi's sarcoma
Non-Hodgkin's lymphoma

Others
HIV encephalopathy
Aseptic meningitis
Persistant generalized lymphadenopathy
HIV wasting syndrome

---

transmission. Human immunodeficiency virus infection is not spread by casual contact. Risk factors for acquiring AIDS are listed in Table 6-4.

Sexual contact.   Nationwide, unprotected sex has resulted in the greatest number of AIDS cases. The risk of exposure to HIV type 1 is present when unprotected genital or anal intercourse is performed with individuals whose HIV status is not known, be it homosexual, bisexual, or heterosexual contact. Having multiple sex partners of unknown HIV status even further increases this risk. Clearly, HIV disease is a sexually transmitted disease, as are genital herpes, gonorrhea, syphilis, nongonococcal urethritis, genital warts, and several other conditions. The presence of a sexually transmitted disease, particularly herpes, syphilis, or chancroid, increases 100 to 200 times the chance of acquiring HIV infection if exposed.

Although AIDS was first recognized in the male homosexual population in the U.S., spread through heterosexual activity occurs. In fact, between 1990 and 1991, the largest increase in the number of reported AIDS cases (21.0%) occurred among heterosexuals, with the second highest increase (15%) among women. Approximately 12% of all AIDS cases in the U.S. have occurred in women. Injection drug abuse results in the highest number of AIDS cases in some parts of the country, such as New York City, whereas it is ranked second to sexual contact in other geographical areas such as Indiana and several other states.

Table 6-4 Relationship of Risk Factors to the Number of AIDS Cases in the U.S.

EXPOSURE CATEGORY	TOTAL AIDS CASES (%)	
	1993*	1996[†]
Cases in Adults or Adolescents		
Homosexual	56	50
Injection drug user (IDU)	23	26
Homosexual and IDU	6	6
Heterosexual	7	9
Transfusion	2	1
Hemophilia	1	1
Not yet identified	5	7
Cases Involving Persons Age 12 or Under		
Mother with HIV disease	87	90
Transfusion	7	5
Hemophilia	4	3
Not yet identified	2	2

*Based on 289,320 AIDS cases reported through March, 1993 (CDC: HIV/AIDS Surveillance Report 5[No 1]:1-19, 1993).
[†]Based on 581,429 AIDS cases reported through December, 1996 (CDC: HIV/AIDS Surveillance Report Vol. 9 [No. 1]:1-37, 1998).

Exposure to blood. Intravenous drug abuse is a high-risk behavior when injection needles are shared, allowing the transfer of blood remaining in the used needles from one person to another. Injection of infected blood directly into the bloodstream is a very efficient route of transmission. Percutaneous (through the skin) injuries with contaminated needles or other sharp objects and contamination of skin or mucous membranes containing small cuts or abrasions or dermatitis are variations of this "shared needles" mode of transmission.

Administration of infected blood products (e.g., to those with bleeding disorders such as hemophilia) or transfusions with infected blood have caused approximately 3% of the total reported cases of AIDS. In 1985, however, tests were developed that detect HIV infected blood, and since then these modes of transmission have essentially been eliminated.

Human immunodeficiency virus type 1 has been isolated from numerous body fluids, including blood, semen, vaginal and cervical secretions, cerebrospinal fluid, synovial fluid, amniotic fluid, pericardial fluid, saliva, tears, breast milk, and urine. Although HIV type 1 has been isolated from saliva, so far no cases of transmission have been documented by this route in casual or household contact. Also, transmission was shown not to occur in a 2.5-year follow-up study of 198 health-care workers, 30 of whom were bitten or scratched by an HIV-infected patient. The extremely low risk for transmission through saliva may be attributable to the low concentration of the virus in the saliva of infected persons. A proteinaceous factor in human saliva also has been shown to interfere with the

HIV type 1 infection process. Nevertheless, "saliva in dentistry" is still considered potentially infectious because of the intimate contact with the patient's mouth during dental care and because most dental procedures result in varying degrees of bleeding into the mouth. Also, some natural bleeding may occur in the mouths of dental patients who have gingivitis or other oral soft tissue lesions. Thus, "saliva in dentistry" commonly contains blood.

Mother to child.   Approximately one half of infants who have HIV-positive mothers are infected before birth by passage of the virus across the placenta, at the time of birth by contact with mother's blood during delivery, or, less commonly, through breast milk. Approximately 1.7% of all reported AIDS cases in the United States have occurred in children younger than age 13 (pediatric AIDS cases), and 85% of these occurred by spread from infected mothers, with the remainder involving hemophilia or transfusion cases.

Risk for the Dental Team

The risk of HIV disease transmission from dental patients to members of the dental team is extremely low. Nevertheless, there is some small potential for this to occur. Through June 1997, the Centers for Disease Control and Prevention received reports of 52 healthcare workers in the U.S. with documented, occupationally acquired HIV infections and an additional 111 with possible occupationally acquired HIV-infection (Table 6-5). In 1992, these numbers were 32 and 69. A "documented" case involves seroconversion (HIV-negative at the time of exposure, later becoming HIV-positive) following a percutaneous or mucocutaneous (mucous membrane and skin) occupational exposure to blood, body fluids, or tissues. A "possible" case involves persons with no determined behavioral or transfusion risks who report past percutaneous or mucocutaneous occupational exposure to blood, other body fluids, or tissues but did not have a documented seroconversion. Although there are no documented cases of occupational spread to dental workers, there are seven cases in which this may have occurred (see Table 6-5).

Of the 52 "documented" cases described in Table 6-5, 86% had percutaneous exposure (e.g., sharps injuries), 10% had mucocutaneous exposure, and 2% had both; 90% were exposed to HIV-infected blood, 3% to a concentrated HIV-1 culture in the laboratory, and 3% were exposed to an unknown body fluid. Most of the 114 "possible" cases involved exposure to body fluids of unknown infectivity.

Risk for Dental Patients

The risk for a dental patient of acquiring HIV disease in the office from a member of the dental team must be extremely low. Although the bloodborne HBV has been spread in rare instances from dentist to patient (described early in this chapter), spread of HIV type 1 is suggested in only one instance. Apparently, a dentist with HIV infected six of his patients being treated in his Florida dental office during the years 1987 to 1990. The investigation of this case involved a comparison of the HIV type 1 from the dentist with the viruses isolated from the infected patients, and this demonstrated significant similarity in the viruses. Unfortunately, the investigation did not discover the mode of virus spread from the dentist to the six patients but the final conclusion by the investigators from the Centers for Disease Control and Prevention and the Florida Department of Health suggested that direct spread from the dentist to the patients was most likely rather than spread from contaminated instruments, equipment, or surfaces.

Table 6-5 Health-Care Workers With Documented and Possible Occupationally Acquired HIV Disease by Occupation—U.S., Through June 1997

OCCUPATION	1992*		1996†	
	DOCUMENTED	POSSIBLE	DOCUMENTED	POSSIBLE
Dental workers, including dentist	0	6	0	7
Embalmer/Morgue technician	0	3	0	2
Emergency medical technician/Paramedic	0	7	0	10
Health aide/Attendant	1	5	1	12
Housekeeper/Maintenance worker	1	5	1	7
Laboratory technician, clinical	11	12	16	16
Laboratory technician, nonclinical	1	1	3	1
Nurse	12	14	21	29
Physician, nonsurgical	4	7	6	10
Physician, surgical	0	2	0	6
Respiratory therapist	1	1	1	2
Surgical technician	1	1	2	2
Other technician or therapist	0	3	1	8
Other health-care occupations	0	2	0	2
TOTAL	32	69	52	114

*Centers for Disease Control and Prevention: *MMWR* 41 (No 43):823-825, 1992.
†Centers for Disease Control and Prevention: HIV/AIDS Surveillance Report Vol. 9 (No. 1):1-37, 1988.

Until recently, this Florida dentist case was the only known instance in all of dentistry and medicine of possible spread of HIV disease from a health-care worker to patients. It still remains the only known instance in dentistry, but in February of 1997, the French government reported that a woman patient contacted HIV disease from a physician in France in 1992. All of the details are not available but evidence released so far supporting this transmission (comparing the viruses from the patient and the physician) is compelling. The available information suggests that the physician (an orthopedic surgeon) may have contracted the disease from a patient in 1983 but was not tested for HIV status until 1994. The physician performed an orthopedic procedure of some 10 hours in length on the woman patient in 1993; it is assumed that this is when the transmission occurred. To date, 968 of this physician's surgery patients have been tested and only the one woman has been found to be HIV-positive. Further attempts have been made to identify and define the low risk of spread from health-care workers to patients by performing HIV testing on patients who have been cared for by other HIV-positive health-care workers. Of approximately 28,000 medical and dental patients tested so far, none have been shown to have acquired HIV diseases from any of the 63 infected dentists or physicians involved. Nevertheless, it is important to maintain proper infection control during care for all patients.

Prevention

Sexual contact.   Recommendations for preventing the spread of HIV type 1 through sexual contact include abstinence or limiting sexual activities to one partner who is not infected and who does not have any other sex partners. A lesser level of protection is offered by safer sex practices such as the use of condoms to eliminate or minimize contact of each partner with body fluids that may contain HIV type 1.

Blood contact.   Injection drug abusers must not use blood-contaminated needles. Continued screening for HIV-infectivity of blood for tranfusion and of blood products began in June of 1985 and must continue. All members of the dental team and other health-care workers must protect themselves from exposure to blood, saliva in dentistry, and other potentially infectious body fluids. Contaminated sharps must be handled and disposed of properly. Gloves, mask, and protective eyewear and clothing must be used during the care of all patients and in other instances to prevent direct or indirect contact with body fluids. Also, all health-care workers must prevent their blood or body fluids from coming into contact with the patients being treated and instruments and equipment used on more than one patient must be properly decontaminated before reuse. The infection control procedures involved in these approaches to disease prevention are described in Chapter 8 and in Chapters 10 through 15.

AZT Prophylaxis.   Zidovudine (ZDV), also known as azidothymidine or AZT, is a nucleoside analog used in AIDS therapy that inhibits HIV reverse transcriptase and may prolong survival of patients with HIV disease. There is also some evidence that post-exposure use of AZT may reduce the risk for HIV infection in health-care workers following percutaneous exposure to HIV-infected blood. Thus the management of occupational exposures to body fluids should include counseling regarding risks and benefits of AZT therapy for HIV disease prophylaxis. If such prophylaxis is to be taken, it should begin within hours after the exposure, so a rapid post-exposure response is important.

SELECTED READINGS

American Dental Association: *Facts about AIDS for the Dental Team,* ed. 3, Chicago, Illinois, 1991, American Dental Association.

American Health Consultants: CDC—French HIV surgical case will not affect U.S. policy on infected providers, *Hosp Infect Contrl* 24 (No 3):33-36, 1997.

Centers for Disease Control and Prevention: Case-control study of HIV seroconversion in health-care workers after percutaneous exposure to HIV-infected blood—France, United Kingdom, and United States, January 1988-August 1994, *MMWR* 50 (No 44):929-933, 1995.

Centers for Disease Control: Hepatitis B virus: A comprehensive strategy for eliminating transmission in the United States through universal childhood vaccinations, *MMWR* 49 (No RR-13):1-25, 1991.

Centers for Disease Control: Protection against viral hepatitis, *MMWR* 39 (No RR-2):1-26, 1990.

Centers for Disease Control: Update: acquired immunodeficiency syndrome: United States, 1991, *MMWR* 41 (No 26):463-468, 1992.

Cottone JA, Puttaiah R: Hepatitis B virus infection: current status in dentistry, *Dent Clin No Amer* 40 (No 2):293-307, 1996.

Glick M: The role of the dentist in the era of AIDS, *Dent Clin No Amer* 40 (No 2):343-357, 1996.

Mandell GL, Douglas RG, Bennett JE (editors): *Principles and Practice of Infectious Diseases,* ed. 3, New York, New York, 1994, Churchill Livingstone.

Miller CH:Viral hepatitis, *Calif Dent Inst Cont Ed J* 40:18-28, 1992.

Molinari JA: Hepatitis C virus infection, *Dent Clin No Amer* 40 (No 2):309-326, 1996.

Younai FS: Postexposure protocol, *Dent Clin No Amer* 40 (No 2):457-486, 1996.

Chapter 7

ORAL AND RESPIRATORY DISEASES

ORAL DISEASES

Chapter 5 discussed the plaque-associated diseases of caries and periodontal diseases. This chapter presents information on other oral diseases and respiratory diseases that may be spread in a dental office (Table 7-1). A key aspect of the potential for spread of respiratory diseases in the dental office is that dental patients (and many other people) are asymptomatic carriers of a variety of pathogens present in their oral or respiratory fluids (Table 7-2).

Human Herpes Virus Types 1 and 2

Human herpes viruses (HHV) cause several diseases (Table 7-3). Human herpes virus type 1 (herpes simplex virus 1 [HSV-1]) may cause infections of the mouth, skin, eyes, and genitals, and those who have depressed immune systems (immunocompromised) may have a widespread (systemic) infection.

About 90% of adults have been infected with HHV-1. Only 10% of infected persons (usually children) experience the typical symptoms of oral herpes (primary herpetic gingivostomatitis). In this disease, vesicle-type lesions occur in the mouth. Most (if not all) herpes viruses cause *recurrent diseases* (periodic re-occurrence of the disease). An example is herpes labialis, sometimes called fever blisters, with lesions periodically appearing on the lips. Vesicles during active HHV-1 infections at any site of the body contain the virus that may be spread to others by direct contact with these lesions. Also, the HHV-1 may be present in saliva in those with oral or lip lesions and in a small percent of those who are infected but have no active lesions (see Table 7-2). In such instances, direct contact with lesions may cause infection of the skin or sprays or aerosols of the saliva may result in spread of the virus to unprotected eyes of the dental team. Entrance of the virus through breaks in the skin on unprotected hands and fingers can lead to vesicle development at these sites called *herpetic whitlow*. A vivid example of how the HHV-1 may be spread from a lip lesion of one patient to the mouths of other dental patients via the ungloved hands of a dental hygienist is described in Chapter 10. HHV-1 causes about 10% of genital herpes cases.

Human herpes virus type 2 (herpes simplex virus 2 [HSV-2]) causes about 90% of genital herpes infections but occasionally causes oral infections. Although most infections are asymptomatic, HHV-2 can cause vesicle type lesions in the mouth or on the skin in the male and female genital and anal areas or internally in the female. As with other herpes virus infections, these vesicles may periodically recur. The vesicles contain the virus and are contagious on contact but the virus can also be spread in the absence of symptoms. Genital herpes is one of the most common sexually transmitted diseases.

Table 7-1 Important Infectious Diseases and Pathogens Associated with the Mouth

DISEASE	PATHOGEN
Oral Diseases	
Bacterial	
Gonoccal pharyngitis	*Neisseria gonorrhoeae*
Syphilis	*Treponema pallidum*
Viral	
Primary herpetic gingivostomatitis	Human herpes virus 1 or 2
Recurrent herpes (e.g., herpes labialis)	Human herpes virus 1 or 2
Hand-foot-and-mouth disease	Coxsackievirus
Herpangina	Coxsackievirus
Hairy leukoplakia	Human herpes virus type 4
Fungal	
Candidiasis (thrush)	*Candida albicans*
Denture stomatitis	*Candida albicans*
Systemic Diseases with Oral Lesions	
Bacterial	
Secondary syphilis	*Treponema pallidum*
Viral	
Chickenpox	Human herpes virus type 3 (varicella–zoster virus)
Infectious mononucleosis	Human herpes virus type 4 (Epstein-Barr virus)
Other Diseases Spread by Respiratory/Oral Fluids	
Bacterial	
Streptococcal pharyngitis ("strep throat") and scarlet fever	*Streptococcus pyogenes*
Tuberculosis	*Mycobacterium tuberculosis*
Diphtheria	*Corynebacterium diphtheriae*
Pneumonia	*Streptococcus pneumoniae, Staphylococcus aureus Mycoplasma pneumoniae, Chlamydia pneumoniae Moraxella catarrhalis, Hemophilus influenzae*
Meningitis, sinusitis, conjunctivitis	*Hemophilus influenzae* type b
Meningitis	*Neisseria meningitidis*
Bronchitis	*Hemophilus influenzae, Moraxella catarrhalis*
Viral	
Common cold	Rhinoviruses and several others
Influenza	Influenza viruses
Bronchitis	Influenza A, parainfluenza virus, coronavirus
Pneumonia	Influenza virus, adenovirus, respiratory syncytial virus

Continued

Table 7-1 Important Infectious Diseases and Pathogens Associated with the Mouth—cont'd

DISEASE	PATHOGEN
Other Diseases Spread by Respiratory/Oral Fluids—cont'd	
Viral—cont'd	
CMV disease	Cytomegalovirus
Infectious mononucleosis	Human herpes virus type 4 (Epstein-Barr virus)
Erythema infectiosum (5th disease)	Human parvovirus B19
Measles	Rubeola (measles) virus
Rubella	Rubella virus
Mumps	Mumps virus

Table 7-2 Estimated Asymptomatic Rates for Some Pathogens Present in Oral or Respiratory Fluids

MICROORGANISMS	DISEASE	CARRIER RATE
Streptococcus pneumoniae	Pneumonia, middle ear infection, meningitis, sinusitis	Preschoolers (33%) Adults (5%-70%)
Streptococcus pyogenes	"Strep throat," scarlet fever, skin infections	Children (0%-20%) Adults (0%-5%)
Staphylococcus aureus	Skin infections, secondary pneumonia	Adults (20%-40%)
Hemophilus influenzae type b	Meningitis, middle ear infection, sinusitis, conjunctivitis	Population (3%-5%)
Neisseria meningitidis	Meningitis	Adults (3%-30%)
Corynebacterium diphtheriae	Diphtheria	Population (0%-5%)
Human herpes virus type 4	Infectious mononucleosis	Adults (10%-20%)
Human herpes virus type 1	Oral, occular herpes	Adults (0.5%-15%)
Candida albicans	Thrush, denture stomatitis	Adults (33%)

Table 7-3 Human Herpes Viruses (HHV)

TYPE	OTHER NAME		DISEASE
HHV 1	Herpes simplex type 1	(HSV-1)	Oral herpes, occular herpes, some genital herpes
HHV 2	Herpes simplex type 2	(HSV-2)	Genital herpes, some oral herpes
HHV 3	Varicella-zoster	(VZV)	Chickenpox, shingles
HHV 4	Epstein-Barr	(EBV)	Infectious mononucleosis, hairy leukoplakia of tongue
HHV 5	Cytomegalovirus	(CMV)	CMV disease, retinitis
HHV 6	None		Roseola
HHV 7	None		Not yet known
HHV 8	None		Kaposi's sarcoma

Treatment of herpes virus infections with acyclovir usually reduces the severity and duration of the disease but does not prevent the recurrence of disease. Acyclovir is structurally similar to guanosine-triphosphate, which is a building block for DNA. When acyclovir is incorporated into the viral DNA being synthesized inside of body cells infected with the virus, that DNA becomes nonfunctional, and the virus does not survive.

Oral Candidiasis

Candida albicans is a yeast that occurs in the mouth asymptomatically in about one third of adults. It is an opportunistic pathogen usually causing a harmful infection only under special circumstances that give it an advantage to multiply to harmful levels. Such harmful infections are referred to as oral candidiasis and appear as whitish lesions (called thrush) or reddish areas (denture stomatitis). Circumstances that may result in oral disease might include:

- Conditions that disturb body defense mechanisms such as the systemic diseases of HIV infection and leukemia
- Long-term broad spectrum antibacterial therapy that gives the unaffected yeast a better chance to grow
- Trauma to the mouth from poorly fitting dentures causing the *C. albicans* to produce denture stomatitis
- Poor resistance in the mouth of newborns orally contaminated with the yeast during passage through mother's infected birth canal

Yeast infections with *C. albicans* may occur at other sites of the body, including the skin and the vagina, and is the cause of "yeast infections" in females.

Spread of *C. albicans* from a patient's mouth to the dental team is theoretically possible through direct contact with lesions or sprays or aerosols of infected saliva. However, unless the contaminated member of the dental team has lowered body defenses, the contamination will likely not lead to a harmful infection.

Oral candidiasis can be treated with one of several antifungal agents, which include nystatin, ketoconizole, and clotrimazole.

Oral Syphilis and Gonorrhea

Other important oral disease agents that may have some potential for spread to the dental team are *Treponema pallidum* and *Neisseria gonorrhoeae*.

Treponema pallidum is a spirochete bacterium and is the causative agent of syphilis. About 5% to 10% of the cases of syphilis first occur in the mouth in the form of a lesion called a primary chancre, an open ulcer frequently on the tongue or lip. These lesions contain the live spirochetes, which may be spread by direct contact. The possibility of the spirochete entering small cuts or breaks in the skin of unprotected hands of the dental team exists and has been documented in one instance causing syphilis of the finger.

Neisseria gonorrhoeae causes another sexually-transmitted disease: gonorrhea, which is an infection through the mucous membranes inside the penis or vagina. This gram-negative bacterium may be spread to the mouth during certain sex practices with an infected person, and the bacterium might cause an inflammation of the throat area. Although spread of *N. gonorrhoeae* from a patient with oral gonorrhea to a member of the dental team has never been documented, there may be some potential for this to occur during generation of dental aerosols. *N. gonorrhoeae* can cause eye infections.

Herpangina and Hand-Foot-and-Mouth Disease

Herpangina appears as vesicles on the soft palate or elsewhere in the posterior part of the mouth that break down to ulcers that last for about a week. Seldom do the vesicles appear on the gingiva, buccal mucosa, or tongue, which differentiates this disease from intraoral herpes infections. Fever, sore throat, and headache frequently accompany the vesicular stage. The lesions are caused by specific types of coxsackievirus (usually group A types 1 to 6, 8, 10, and 22). Coxsackievirus (usually type A16) may also cause a vesicular type of disease with vesicles occurring in the mouth, on the hands, and on the feet (hand-foot-and-mouth disease). In this instance, the oral vesicles occur primarily on the cheek mucosa and tongue but sometimes on the hard palate and anywhere else in the mouth. Usually children and young adults are affected; there is no specific treatment that attacks the virus.

SYSTEMIC DISEASES WITH ORAL LESIONS

Secondary Syphilis

In untreated syphilis, a secondary phase of the disease may appear 2 to 10 weeks after the initial lesion occurs and has subsided. This secondary phase results from spread of the *T. pallidum* bacterium from the initial lesion through the blood and may involve the appearance of mucous patches on mucous membranes in the mouth. The lesions contain the live spirochetes and may be spread to others by direct contact. Syphilis usually responds to penicillin therapy.

Chickenpox

Human herpes virus type 3 (varicella–zoster virus [VZV]) causes chickenpox as the primary disease (usually in the young) and shingles as the recurrent disease (usually in those over age 50). Although chickenpox commonly produces skin lesions, this disease is classified as a respiratory disease. HHV-3 enters the body by droplet infection, invades the respiratory tract, and is spread through the bloodstream to the skin and other organs. After about 2 weeks, vesicles frequently occur in the mouth in addition to those typically present on the skin. The virus is spread through saliva and nasal secretions in addition to contact with skin lesions.

The disease is highly contagious through droplet infection and is usually mild in children but it can be more severe in teenagers and adults. Occasionally an adult who escaped the primary infection as a child develops chickenpox, which is usually more severe and has a higher mortality rate due to an increased incidence of encephalitis. A vaccine for chickenpox was cleared by the U.S. Food and Drug Administration in 1996 and is further described in Chapter 9.

Infectious Mononucleosis

Human herpes virus type 4 (Epstein-Barr virus [EBV]) usually causes no or mild symptoms after infecting a child but may cause infectious mononucleosis (also known as the kissing disease) in adolescents and young adults. As might be suspected, this virus is spread from person to person through contact with saliva but also occasionally through blood transfusions. Symptoms of infectious mononucleosis commonly include fever, malaise, anorexia, fatigue, sore throat, oral ulcers, and enlarged cervical lymph nodes (those under the jaw). Other oral manisfestations may include palatal petechiae (small red areas), widespread erythema (reddening) of the oral mucosa, and swelling of the uvula. This virus also is associated with hairy leukoplakia (whitish lesions on the tongue) and with malignancies such as Burkitt's lymphoma, B-cell lymphoma in the immunocompromised, and nasopharnygeal carcinoma.

RESPIRATORY DISEASES

Streptococcal Pharyngitis

Streptococcus pyogenes (sometimes called β-hemolytic, group A streptococcus) causes streptococcal pharyngitis ("strep throat") and scarlet fever. Scarlet fever is "strep throat" with a skin rash. *Streptococcus pyogenes* is spread by droplet infection from mouth to mouth, and a few people who become infected experience poststreptococcal complications resulting in rheumatic fever or kidney damage. Each subsequent infection with *S. pyogenes* or with some other streptococci can result in progressively more damage to the heart (rheumatic heart disease) or the kidney. This is why patients with a history of post-streptococcal diseases are protected from possible reactivation by receiving antibiotics before dental or medical care.

Certain protease-producing strains of *Streptococcus pyogenes* (sometimes referred to as "flesh-eating" bacteria) can cause a condition called necrotizing fasciitis, which produces rapidly spreading damage to muscle tissue. Fortunately, only about 1,000 cases of this disease occur each year.

Children and adults carry *S. pyogenes* in their nose and throat area without having any symptoms and can spread the organism to others in respiratory droplets (see Table 7-2). Most harmful streptococcus infections respond well to penicillin therapy.

Tuberculosis

Occurrence

Tuberculosis (TB) is a lung infection caused by the bacterium *Mycobacterium tuberculosis*. Although TB is not a particular problem among dental professionals, it is a major health problem worldwide, including within the U.S. About 10 million new cases of TB and 3 million associated deaths occur annually worldwide. In the United States, TB is increasing among racial/ethnic groups (non–Hispanic Blacks, Hispanics, Asian-Pacific Islanders, American Indian/Alaskan Natives) but the overall number of cases has reached a plateau for the last 3 years. In 1990, almost 70% of all reported cases of TB in the U.S. occurred among these minorities. Between 1953 and 1984, the number of reported cases of TB in the U.S. steadily declined. This number began to increase through 1995 when it began to level off. In 1996 the Centers for Disease Control and Prevention (CDC) indicated that about 22,000 active TB cases were reported in the U.S.

Adverse social conditions and economic factors, the AIDS epidemic, and immigration of people with tuberculosis are contributing factors to the occurrence of TB in the U.S. Tuberculosis is a major problem among the homeless, people infected with HIV, and drug abusers. Tuberculosis in those with HIV disease is commonly a reactivation of an earlier asymptomatic infection, as described below.

Tuberculosis in the Dental Office

The risk for the dental team of acquiring TB is low because prolonged exposure to an infectious environment is usually required for infection to occur and brief contact appears to be of little risk. Spread from one person to another relates to closeness of contact and the duration of exposure to infectious droplets. Thus the key factor in spread is the concentration of infectious particles in the inhaled air. Respiratory aerosols remain airborne for several hours but the concentration of the infectious particles decreases with time from dilution with "clean" air and eventual settling. Nevertheless, TB is acquired by breathing in respiratory droplets from an infectious person with active pulmonary TB, and this must be given concern by the dental team.

The dental office should have a protocol for identifying patients who possibly have active pulmonary TB. These patients should be immediately referred for medical evaluation and have their dental care deferred until the TB is inactive or has been treated and is no longer infectious. Dental personnel should not treat patients with active TB unless they institute special isolation precautions that are usually only available in hospital clinics. The approach to the management of possible active TB patients is that described by the CDC. The CDC has published guidelines for the prevention of TB in health care facilities, and the Occupational Safety and Health Administration is in the process of developing a standard based on these CDC guidelines (Chapter 10).

Risk factors for TB and the symptoms of active TB are shown in Box 7-1. This box also describes questions on a medical history that may help identify dental patients that possibly have active TB.

Disease Process

If enough inhaled *M. tuberculosis* bacteria reach the lung alveoli and begin to multiply, one is said to be infected. In most people, the inflammatory and immune responses will control the infection with the only evidence of infection being a positive tuberculin skin test (see below). Cells of *M. tuberculosis* initially resist destruction after being engulfed by macrophages during the inflammatory response. However, after immunity develops (CMIR: cell-mediated immune response, see Chapter 3), the macrophages are activated to be able to kill the engulfed bacteria and the infection does not progress to active disease. However, most infected people (even if the infection is initially controlled by the CMIR) cannot completely rid the body of the TB bacteria unless they take antituberculosis drugs. This is why those with positive TB skin tests, even if they have never had any TB symptoms, are usually placed on a course of anti-TB drug therapy. Patients not placed on anti-TB drug therapy retain the bacteria in their bodies and may later progress to active disease (*latent TB infection* or *reactivation TB*).

About 10% of persons infected with *M. tuberculosis* will progress from infection to active disease with symptoms. About half of these progress to active disease soon after the primary infection and about half progress later in their lives. Symptomatic pulmonary TB begins with the development of an exudative condition in the lung, like pneumonia. Continued disease results in a granulomatous reaction (consolidation of tissue around the lung infection site), referred to as tubercle formation. As the disease progresses these tubercles enlarge, may become necrotic (casseation necrosis), and break down, producing cavities (open spaces) in the lung tissue. In persons who are infected but are asymptomatic and in those with symptomatic TB, healing may occur with or without the formation of calci-

---

Box 7-1   Risk Factors, Symptoms, and Medical History Questions Related to Tuberculosis

Risk Factors
Close/prolonged contact with known active TB case
Residency in prisons, mental institutions, nursing homes, certain health-care facilities
HIV disease
Alcoholism
Intravenous drug abuse
Homelessness
Old age

Symptoms
Malaise
Productive cough for more than 3 weeks
Blood in sputum
Headache
Fever, night sweats
Weight loss

Medical History Questions
Previous diagnosis of TB?
Previous treatment for TB?
Positive TB skin-test?
Productive cough for more than 3 weeks?
Blood in your sputum?
Headache, fever, chills, night sweats?
Recent weight loss, anorexia, fatigue?
HIV-disease?
Other systemic diseases?
Immunosuppressive therapy?
Alcoholism?
Intravenous drug use?
Relatives or close friends with active TB?
Visited anyone in hospital with active TB?

---

fied lung lesions or nodules, or development of fibrous tissue with calcium deposits.

Since *M. tuberculosis* can survive inside of macrophages early in the infection, this bacterium can be disseminated throughout the body (wherever the macrophages go). If active disease occurs, complications may develop that can involve infections in essentially any organ of the body.

Multiple Drug-resistant Mycobacterium Tuberculosis

Another disturbing fact about TB is that strains of *M. tuberculosis* that are resistant to the normal drugs used to treat this disease have recently emerged. These strains are causing outbreaks of multiple drug-resistant tuberculosis (MDRTB). The CDC reported that about 15% of all tuberculosis cases tested involved strains resistant to at least one antituberculosis drug (e.g., isoniazid [INH], rifampin, ethambutol) and 4% were resistant to both of the two most effective antituberculosis drugs. Most of the patients involved in outbreaks of MDRTB have been AIDS patients, others include hospital patients and institutionalized inmates. Transmission of MDRTB to hospital workers and prison guards is documented. The key approach to managing these infections is to diagnose the infection and analyze the causative strain of *M. tuberculosis* as soon as possible so that the proper anti-TB drugs can be administered at the earliest possible moment.

Tuberculin Skin Test

The Mantoux test, or PPD test, is used to screen for TB infection. *PPD is a purified protein derivative* prepared from cultures of *M. tuberculosis* that is used in the skin testing. The testing involves injecting a small amount of the PPD just under the skin (intradermally) on the under side of the forearm. The injection site is observed 48 to 72 hours later for any reaction to the PPD, although a positive reaction in some may be delayed for a week. A positive reaction is the occurrence of induration (a hardening, small nodule) at the injection site, and the degree of the positive reaction is determined by measuring the diameter of the indurated site. The CDC guidelines for interpreting the tuberculin skin-test results are given in Box 7-2.

Vaccination

A vaccine for prevention of TB has not been cleared for use in the U.S. However, the bacillus Calumett-Guérin (BCG) vaccine is widely used throughout the rest of the world. This vaccine consists of a live attenuated (weakened) bovine strain that probably causes a non-progressing infection that is a substitute for infection with virulent TB strains. Not everyone who receives the vaccine is protected but those who are vaccinated become PPD-tuberculin skin-test positive. In such people, the skin-test becomes useless as an aid in the diagnosis of the genuine *M. tuberculosis* infection.

Streptococcal Pneumonia

Many bacterial and viral agents can cause pneumonia but *Streptococcus pneumoniae* is of particular importance. This bacterium causes about 500,000 cases of lobar pneumonia a year in the United States and is particularly dangerous to the elderly or to others with weakened immune systems. *S. pneumoniae* normally exists in the nose and throat area of humans and is carried asymptomatically in preschoolers and adults (see Table 7-2). It is spread by droplet inhalation of respiratory/oral droplets. This bacterium also is the leading cause of middle ear infections in children and can cause bacterial meningitis, an inflammation of the membranes around the brain. A vaccine is available for the most common types of *S. pneumoniae* and is recommended for the elderly or others who may be predisposed to lung infections.

Human Herpes Virus Type 5

Human herpes virus type 5 (cytomegalovirus [CMV]) usually causes no symptoms on primary infection but occasionally causes disease in newborns and immunocompromised

---

Box 7-2 CDC Guidelines for Interpreting PPD-tuberculin Skin-test Reactions

1. An induration of ≥5 mm is classified as positive in:
   - Persons who have HIV infection or risk factors for HIV infection but unknown HIV status
   - Persons who have had recent close contact with persons who have active TB
   - Persons who have fibrotic chest radiographs (consistent with healed TB)
2. An induration of ≥10 mm is classified as positive in all persons who do not meet any of the criteria above but who have other risk factors for TB, including:
   - High-risk groups
   - Injecting drug users known to be HIV seronegative
   - Persons who have other medical conditions that reportedly increase the risk for progressing from latent TB infection to active TB (e.g., silicosis, gastrectomy, or jejuno-ileal bypass; being ≥10% below ideal body weight; chronic renal failure with renal dialysis; diabetes mellitus; high-dose corticosteroid or other immunosuppressive therapy; some hematologic disorders, including malignancies such as leukemias and lymphomas; and other malignancies)
   - Children <4 years of age
   - High-prevalence groups
   - Persons born in countries in Asia, Africa, the Caribbean, and Latin America that have high prevalence of TB
   - Persons from medically underserved, low-income populations
   - Residents of long-term care facilities (e.g., correctional institutions and nursing homes)
   - Persons from high-risk populations in their communities, as determined by local public health authorities
3. An induration of ≥15 mm is classified as positive in persons who do not meet any of the above criteria
4. Recent converters are defined on the basis of size of induration and age of the person being tested:
   - ≥10 mm increase within a 2-year period is classified as a recent conversion for persons <35 years of age
   - ≥15 mm increase within a 2-year period is classified as a recent conversion for persons ≥35 years of age
5. PPD skin-test results in health-care workers (HCWs)
   - In general, the recommendations in sections 1, 2, and 3 of this table should be followed when interpreting skin-test results in HCWs.
   - A recent seroconversion in an HCW should be defined generally as a ≥10 mm increase in size of induration within a 2-year period. For HCWs who work in facilities where exposure to TB is very unlikely, an increase of ≥15 mm within a 2-year period may be more appropriate for defining a recent conversion because of the lower positive-predictive value of the test in such groups

From CDC: Guidelines for preventing the transmission of *Mycobacterium tuberculosis* in health care facilities, 1994, *MMWR* 43(No RR-13):62, 1994.

persons. It can be spread by contact with saliva, vaginal secretions, semen, breast milk, blood, and transplanted tissue. HHV-5 can cause a congenital disease called cytomegalic inclusion disease that has a high fatality rate and causes mental retardation, neurological problems, deafness, and possible damage to many internal organs. Infection in otherwise healthy adults is usually asymptomatic but may cause symptoms like those of infectious mononucleosis. Infection of the immunosuppressed person or those with AIDS can be devastating and may involve transplant patients receiving immunosuppressive drugs. Conditions that may develop in such persons include pneumonia, gastroenteritis, and hepatitis. CMV retinitis occurs in about 10% to 15% of AIDS patients and CMV colitis or CMV esophagitis in about 10% of AIDS patients.

Human Herpes Viruses Types 6, 7, and 8

Human herpes virus type 6 is commonly isolated from saliva and was recently identified as the cause of roseola (exanthema subitum). Roseola occurs as a high fever and a skin rash in infants. This virus also may cause infectious mononucleosis symptoms in some adults. Human herpes virus type 7 is also isolated from saliva in as many as 70% to 80% of adults and children but has not yet been clearly associated with any particular disease state. Human herpes virus type 8 has been associated recently with Kaposi's scaroma, a condition seen in many AIDS patients.

Other Respiratory Diseases

Table 7-1 lists other respiratory diseases that are spread by inhalation of infected respiratory/oral droplets. These include diseases caused by about 170 different types of viruses and involve influenza, the common cold, pneumonia, croup, bronchitis, erythema infectiosum, measles, mumps, and rubella. Additional bacteria are involved in causing bacterial pneumonias, meningitis, and diphtheria.

WATERBORNE DISEASE AGENTS

There are many disease agents that may be spread through contaminated water, including those that cause cholera, *Shigella* and amebic dysentery, salmonellosis, *E. coli* colitis, cryptosporidiosis, and Hepatitis A and E. Since these disease agents are not known to be spread in dental offices, they will not be further discussed. However, numerous studies show that the water inside dental units and hoses for water-spray handpieces and the air/water syringes are heavily contaminated with bacteria. The level of these bacteria in dental unit water is much greater than that of tap water. When waterborne bacteria enter the dental unit, they attach to the inside walls of the waterlines. These bacteria then form a *biofilm* on the inside of waterlines that releases bacteria as the water flows out of the lines (for further discussion see Chapter 15). Although there are 30 to 40 different bacteria that may be present in dental unit water, there are two of particular interest because of their potential for causing opportunistic infections. One *(Legionella pneumophila)* causes legionnaire's disease and Pontiac fever and the other *(Pseudomonas aeruginosa)* is an opportunistic pathogen that can cause several harmful infections.

Legionnaire's Disease

Legionella pneumophila is a gram-negative rod-shaped bacterium that causes about 70% of the cases of *legionnaire's disease*. This disease is a pneumonia and was named after first being recognized among attendees of an American Legion convention in Philadelphia in 1976. The *L. pneumophila* and over 30 other species of *Legionella* commonly exist in natural and domestic waters but it is presumed that most of the cases of legionnaire's disease results from inhalation of water from water-handling systems rather than from lakes or streams. Such handling systems include air conditioning cooling towers, humidifiers, ultrasonic nebulizers, vegetable misters, respiratory therapy equipment, shower heads, industrial sprayers, and water distribution systems in some buildings.

One acquires lung infections with *L. pneumophila* by inhaling contaminated water or by aspirating the bacterium after it has colonized the oropharnygeal area. The infection progresses to pneumonia mostly in those who have some weakened body defenses. Erythromycin is used for treatment, and spread of the disease from person-to-person has not been documented.

Pontiac fever (named after the site in Michigan of the first recognized outbreak) is also caused by *L. pneumophila* but this disease is not a pneumonia. Instead, it is an acute self-limiting condition involving flu-like symptoms of fever, chills, muscle aches, headache, mild cough, and sore throat.

Although there is no scientific documentation for spread of legionnaire's disease in the dental office, about 10% of dental offices apparently have *Legionella* in their dental unit water that is being used for patient care. Thus it is possible that some patients may at least be exposed to this bacterium from some dental units. Also, comparison of past antibody response to *Legionella* in dental personnel with the same antibody response in nondental personnel in two separate studies reveals that the dental personnel had a higher exposure incidence to *Legionella*. Thus some dental personnel at least may be exposed to *Legionella* by contact with aerosols from dental unit water coming out of high speed handpieces, ultrasonic scalers, and air/water syringes.

Pseudomonas Infection

A report from England shows that two cancer-weakened dental patients acquired oral infections with *Pseudomonas aeruginosa* that originated from dental unit water. The same study also showed that an additional 78 patients treated at the same dental unit were orally colonized for 4 to 10 weeks by the *P. aeruginosa* present in the dental unit water. However, none of these patients developed harmful infections with the *Pseudomonas,* presumably, because they were not cancer-weakened or otherwise compromised. *Pseudomonas aeruginosa* is a very important opportunistic pathogen (see Chapter 3). It occurs widely in nature and is present in low numbers in the municipal water used in a dental unit.

In addition to waterborne bacteria, dental unit water may contain low numbers of oral bacteria. Retraction of oral bacteria back into the handpiece and air/water syringes and their connecting water lines may occur when these instruments are turned off after use in the mouth. Some dental units (depending on how they are constructed) contain anti-retraction valves to prevent this from occurring but these valves fail periodically.

The CDC and the American Dental Association indicate that:

- Dental unit water should not be used to irrigate surgical sites exposing bone
- Water lines should be flushed at the beginning of the day to temporarily reduce the number of waterborne bacteria that may have accumulated in the water overnight
- Water lines should be flushed between patients to reduce the numbers of oral microorganisms that may have been retracted into the lines after each patient

Information on how to improve the microbial quality of dental unit water is given in Chapter 15.

SELECTED READINGS

Centers for Disease Control and Prevention: Guidelines for prevention of the transmission of *Mycobacterium tuberculosis* in health-care facilities, 1994, *MMWR* 43(No RR-13), 1994.

Glick M (editor): *Dental Clinics of North America—Infectious Diseases in Dentistry,* vol 40 (No 2), Philadelphia, Pennsylvania, April, 1996, Saunders.

Glick M, Goldman HS: Viral infections in the dental setting, *J Amer Dent Assoc* 124:79-86, 1993.

Merchant VA: An update on herpesviruses, *J Calif Dent Assoc* 24(No 1): 38-46, 1996.

Miller CH: Microbes in dental unit water, *J Calif Dent Assoc* 24(No 1): 47-52, 1996.

Miller CH, Cottone, JC: The basic principles of infectious diseases as related to dental practice. *Dent Clin No Amer* 37(No 1):1-20, 1993.

Chapter 8

INFECTION CONTROL RATIONALE AND REGULATIONS

RATIONALE

The logic for routinely practicing infection control is that the procedures involved interfere with the steps in development of diseases that may be spread in the office. The diseases that may be spread are described in Chapters 6 and 7; the steps in development of such diseases (source, escape, spread, entry, infection, and disease) are described in Chapter 3.

Pathways for Cross-Contamination

A total office infection control program is designed to prevent or at least reduce the spread of disease agents from:

- Patient to dental team
- Dental team to patient
- Patient to patient
- Dental office to community, including the dental team's families
- From community to patient

These subdivisions of infection control are based on the five pathways for cross-contamination, and their relationship to modes of disease spread and infection control procedures are described in Table 8-1.

Patient to Dental Team

There are numerous opportunities for spread of patient microorganisms to members of the dental team, and this pathway is more difficult to control than the other three pathways. *Direct contact* (touching) with patient's saliva or blood may lead to entrance of microorganisms through a nonintact skin resulting from cuts, abrasions, or dermatitis. There are also invisible breaks in the skin, especially around the fingernails. Sprays, spatter, or aerosols from the patient's mouth may lead to *droplet infection* through nonintact skin, mucosal surfaces of the eyes, nose, and mouth, or inhalation. *Indirect contact* involves transfer of microorganisms from the source (e.g., the patient's mouth) to an item or surface and subsequent contact with the contaminated item or surface. Examples include cuts or punctures with contaminated sharp objects (e.g., instruments, needles, burs, files, scalpel blades, wire) and entrance through nonintact skin as a result of touching contaminated instruments, surfaces, or other items. Another opportunity for disease spread occurs by direct contact with infectious skin lesions or other nonintact skin of the patient with entrance of microor-

Table 8-1 Mechanisms of Disease Spread and Prevention

PATHWAY OF CROSS-CONTAMINATION	SOURCE OF MICROORGANISM	MODE OF DISEASE SPREAD	MECHANISM OR SITE OF ENTRY INTO BODY	INFECTION CONTROL PROCEDURE
Patient to dental team	Patient's mouth	Direct contact	Through breaks in skin of dental team	Gloves/handwashing Immunizations
		Droplet infection	Inhalation by dental team	Mask Rubber dam Mouthrinsing
			Through breaks in skin of dental team	Gloves/handwashing Protective clothing Faceshield Rubber dam Mouth rinsing
			Through mucosal surfaces of dental team	Mask Eyewear Faceshield Rubber dam Mouth rinsing Immunizations
		Indirect contact	Cuts, punctures, or needle-sticks in dental team	Needle safety and waste management Heavy gloves for clean-up Ultrasonic cleaning rather than handscrubbing Instrument cassettes to reduce direct handling during cleaning Antimicrobial holding solution Antimicrobial cleaning solution

			Through breaks in skin of dental team	Heavy gloves for clean-up Protective clothing Immunizations
	Patient's skin lesions	Direct contact	Through breaks in skin of dental team	Gloves/handwashing Immunizations
Dental team to patient	Dental team's hands (lesions or bleeding)	Direct contact	Through mucosal surfaces of patient	Gloves/handwashing Care in handling sharp objects Immunizations
		Indirect contact	Bleeding on items used in patient's mouth	Gloves/handwashing Instrument sterilization Surface disinfection Immunizations
	Dental team's mouths (oral or respiratory fluids)	Droplet infection	Inhalation by patient	Mask Faceshield
			Through oral mucosal surfaces of patient	Mask Faceshield
Patient to patient	Patient's mouth	Indirect contact (instruments, surfaces, hands)	Through oral mucosal surfaces of patient	Instrument and handpiece sterilization Sterilization monitoring Surface covers Surface disinfection Handwashing and proper gloving Changing mask Decontaminating protective eyewear Changing protective clothing when needed Use of sterile or clean supplies

Continued

Table 8-1 Mechanisms of Disease Spread and Prevention—cont'd

PATHWAY OF CROSS-CONTAMINATION	SOURCE OF MICROORGANISM	MODE OF DISEASE SPREAD	MECHANISM OR SITE OF ENTRY INTO BODY	INFECTION CONTROL PROCEDURE
				Flushing dental unit waterlines
				Monitoring water line antiretraction valves
				Use of disposable items
Office to community	Patient's mouth	Indirect contact	Cuts, punctures, breaks in skin of dental lab, waste disposal or laundry personnel	Waste management
				Disinfection of impressions and appliances
				Proper management of contaminated laundry
				Handwashing
				Immunization
Dental team families	Dental team body fluids	Direct/indirect contact	Intimate contact	
Community to patient	Municipal water	Direct contact	Patient's mouth	Use new and separate water source
				Periodically disinfect inside of dental unit waterlines
				Use water containing an approved antimicrobial agent
				Filter the water

U.S. Department of Labor, OSHA: *Controlling occupational exposure to bloodborne pathogens,* OSHA 3127 (revised), Washington, DC, 1996, OSHA.

ganisms through nonintact skin on the dental member's hands. This latter route of disease spread in the office is not common.

Infection control procedures to prevent patient to dental team spread are listed in Table 8-1 and described in detail in subsequent chapters.

Dental Team to Patient

Spread of disease agents from the dental team to patients is a rare event but could happen if proper procedures are not followed. If the hands of dental team members contain lesions or other nonintact skin, or if the hands are injured while in the patient's mouth, blood-borne pathogens or other microorganisms could be transferred by direct contact with the patient's mouth, and they may gain entrance through mucous membranes or open tissue. The patient may have indirect contact with bloodborne pathogens or other agents if a member of the dental team bleeds on instruments or other items that are then used in the patient's mouth. Apparent spread of bloodborne diseases from dentists to patients is described in Chapter 6. Droplet infection of the patient from the dental team could occur but this can occur in everyday life and is certainly not unique to the dental office.

Infection control procedures that interfere with this pathway of cross-contamination are listed in Table 8-1 and described later.

Patient to Patient

Disease agents might be transferred from patient to patient by indirect contact through improperly prepared instruments, handpieces and attachments, operatory surfaces, and hands. Although at the time of this writing, disease transmission from contaminated instruments or surfaces to dental patients has not been documented, the potential for such transfer does occur, and it has been documented to occur in the medical field. Conversely, transfer of the herpes simplex virus from a patient to the hands of a hygienist and then to the mouths of several patients has been documented, as described further in Chapter 10 under the discussion on gloves.

Patient to patient spread of HIV.   There is a report of the apparent spread of HIV from patient to patient in a medical/surgical practice in New South Wales, Australia. Five of nine patients seen in that medical office on the same day in November, 1989, became HIV-positive but the surgeon was HIV-negative. All five of these patients had minor surgeries that day involving the removal of moles or small cysts. Four of the five patients who became HIV-positive did not have any apparent risk factors for acquiring HIV disease (e.g., intravenous drug abuse, multiple sex partners of unknown HIV status, blood transfusions, sexually transmitted diseases). These four patients also experienced sore throat, swollen glands under the chin, slight joint pains, and/or slight fever in December of 1989. These are the symptoms of an HIV infection, referred to as acute retroviral syndrome, that usually occur about a month after the initial infection. The fifth patient admitted to having sex with male partners of unknown HIV status—likely his source of HIV. This patient died of *Pneumocystis carinii* pneumonia (a leading cause of death in AIDS patients) in 1990. This strongly suggests that he was already infected in November, 1989, when he was in the New South Wales medical office and that this patient served as the source of HIV in this incident.

The surgeon in this practice indicated that he ran the office by himself and that he didn't use multiple dose injection vials (an important mode of disease spread), didn't reuse scalpel blades but did reuse the handles, and that he changed gloves for every patient. He stated that he processed his contaminated instruments by soaking them in 1% glutaraldehyde, washing them in water, and placing them in boiling water for 5 to 10 minutes. There are several problems with these procedures (the correct procedures for processing contaminated instruments are described in Chapter 11). Since glutaraldehyde disinfectant/sterilant is commercially available only at concentrations between 2.0% and 3.4%, the surgeon apparently diluted his glutaraldehyde before using it, which saves money but also dilutes microbial effectiveness. Apparently, the instruments were not scrubbed or ultrasonically cleaned in a detergent, which suggests that blood could have remained on them after "washing in water." Although boiling can likely kill most microorganisms on instruments, if the instruments are clean, it is not a recognized method of sterilization. It is obvious that the instruments were not wrapped before processing, so they may have become recontaminated as a result of improper handling after the boiling step but before they were reused on another patient.

The surgeon also stated that the instrument processing area was about 9 feet away from where the surgeries were performed. Without a physical separation between "clean" areas and "dirty" areas, chances increase for cross-contamination. Thus there appears to have been several breeches in infection control procedures in this medical practice that may have resulted in the spread of HIV from one patient to four others that day. Unfortunately the appointment schedule for that day was not available to confirm that the HIV-positive man was an early patient of the day. The infection control procedures used to prevent patient-to-patient spread of disease agents are listed in Table 8-1 and described in more detail later.

Dental Office to Community

The dental office to community pathway may occur if microorganisms from the patient contaminate items that are sent out or are transported away from the office. For example, contaminated impressions or appliances or equipment needing service may in turn indirectly contaminate personnel or surfaces in dental laboratories and repair centers. Dental laboratory technicians have been occupationally infected with hepatitis B virus (HBV).

This pathway also may occur if members of the dental team transport microorganisms out of the office on contaminated clothing. In addition, if a member of the dental team acquires an infectious disease at work, the disease could be spread to personal contacts outside the office.

Regulated waste that contains infectious agents and is transported from the office may contaminate waste haulers if it is not in proper containers. Immunity from hepatitis B vaccination protects the dental team from acquiring the disease and passing it along to family members. Other infection control procedures that interfere with the office to community pathway are listed in Table 8-1 and described in later chapters.

Community to Patient

The community to patient pathway involves the entrance of microorganisms into the dental office in the water that supplies the dental unit. These waterborne microorganisms colonize the inside of the dental unit waterlines and form a film of microorganisms (biofilm) on the inside of these lines. As water flows through the lines during use of the air-water syringe, high-speed handpiece, or ultrasonic scaler on some units, it "picks up" microorganisms shed by the biofilm. While municipal water may have a dozen or so bacteria per milliliter of water as it enters the dental unit, the water exiting a dental unit through the air-water syringe or through the spray from a high-speed handpiece may contain over 100,000 per milliliter.

There is no evidence that this contaminated water is making people sick but it is not good infection control practice to use heavily contaminated water during dental care. It certainly must not be used during surgery. Potential pathogens (e.g., *Pseudomonas aeruginosa* and *Legionella pneumophila*) may be present in the incoming water and in the dental unit waterline biofilm. There is one report from England describing how in 1988 two cancer-compromised patients acquired oral infections with *P. aeruginosa* that was later found to be present in water from a dental unit previously involved in the care of those patients. More details about contaminated dental unit water are presented in Chapter 13, and suggested infection control procedures to improve the microbial quality of dental unit water is given in Table 8-1.

Goal of Infection Control

After microorganisms enter the body, there are three basic factors that determine if an infectious disease will develop: virulence (pathogenic properties of the invading microorganism), dose (the number of microorganisms that invade the body), and resistance (body defense mechanism of the host). These factors are called determinants of an infectious disease and their interaction determines the outcome of an infection, as follows:

$$\text{Health or disease} = \frac{\text{Virulence X Dose}}{\text{Body resistance}}$$

Health is favored by low virulence, low dose, and high resistance; disease is favored by high virulence, high dose, and low resistance. Prevention of infectious diseases involves influencing the determinants to favor health.

Unfortunately, virulence of microorganisms in their natural environments cannot be easily changed. Thus our body defenses must deal with whatever microorganism presents itself, be it one with high virulence or low virulence. We can enhance our resistance to infectious diseases through specific immunization (e.g., hepatitis B, tetanus) but immunizations are not available against all of the diseases we would like to prevent. Thus the only disease determinant we can effectively manage is the dose, and management of the dose is called infection control.

Therefore the goal of infection control is to eliminate or reduce the dose of microorganisms that may be shared between individuals or between individuals and contaminated surfaces. The more the dose is reduced, the better the chances for preventing disease spread. Procedures that minimize spraying or spattering of oral fluids (e.g., rubber dam, high-volume evacuation, preprocedure mouth rinse) reduce the dose of microorganisms that escape from the source. Hand washing and surface precleaning and disinfection reduce the number of microorganisms that may be transferred to surfaces by touching. Barriers such as masks, gloves, and protective eyewear and clothing reduce the number of microorganisms that contaminate the body or other surfaces.

Instrument precleaning and sterilization eliminate or reduce the number of microorganisms that may be spread from one patient to another. Proper management of infectious waste by using appropriate containers for disposal eliminates or reduces the number of microorganisms that may contaminate people or inanimate objects. Disease prevention is based on reducing the dose and increasing the body's resistance.

RECOMMENDATIONS AND REGULATIONS

Recommendations are made by individuals or groups who have no authority for enforcement. *Regulations* are made by groups who do have the authority to enforce compliance, usually under the penalty of fines, imprisonment, or revocation of professional licenses.

Recommendations may be made by anyone but regulations are made by governmental groups or licensing boards in towns, cities, counties, and states.

Infection Control Recommendations
Centers for Disease Control and Prevention

The current infection control recommendations for dentistry from the *Centers for Disease Control and Prevention* (CDC) are presented in Appendix B. Although the CDC began making general infection control recommendations many years ago, their first set of complete recommendations directed specifically toward dentistry was in 1986, with an update in 1993. Most infection control procedures practiced in dentistry today are based on the 1993 recommendations. The CDC is a part of the Public Health Service, which is a division of the United States Department of Health and Human Services. The CDC has an Oral Health Services section that studies oral diseases, fluoride applications, and infection control in dentistry. The CDC does not have the authority to make laws but many of the local, state, and federal agencies use CDC recommendations to formulate the laws. See Appendix A for further information on the CDC and how to access their voice information service on infection control in dentistry.

The CDC also has published guidelines on preventing the transmission of tuberculosis in health care settings, which include dental offices. Excerpts from these guidelines are presented in Appendix C.

American Dental Association

The *American Dental Association* (ADA) makes infection control recommendations through its Councils on Scientific Affairs and Dental Practice. The most recent recommendations from the ADA were published in the August, 1996, issue of the *Journal of the American Dental Association* (see Appendix G). The ADA main office is located in Chicago (see Appendix A).

Office Safety and Asepsis Procedures Research Foundation

The *Office Safety and Asepsis Procedures (OSAP) Research Foundation* (see Appendix A) is a not-for-profit professional organization composed of dentists, hygienists, assistants, university professors, researchers, manufacturers, distributors, consultants, and others interested in infection control. This broad-based group is the premier infection control education organization in dentistry. It publishes its official infection control recom-mendations annually to keep pace with new information and distributes information of continuing importance monthly in the form of newsletters, reports, position papers, announcements, and press releases. This organization also sponsors regional and national educational programs related to infection control for its members. All members of the dental team should join this organization to keep up-to-date in the area of infection control (see Appendix D).

Association for Advancement of Medical Instrumentation

The *Association for Advancement of Medical Instrumentation* (AAMI; see Appendix A) is another voluntary organization that is composed of manufacturers, distributors, researchers, regulators, and users of medical equipment. One component of this organization is devoted to developing sterilization standards, including recommended practices on how to properly use sterilizers and technical documents on the equipment itself. For example, two documents completed in 1992 and revised in 1997 and 1998 are of particular interest to the dental team in that they describe the proper use and monitoring of small office steam and dry heat sterilizers.

Infection Control Regulations

State and Local

Some state and local regulations exist in relation to medical waste management, instrument sterilization, and sterilizer spore testing in dentistry. Examples of states with such special dental infection control regulations include Ohio, Indiana, Washington, Oregon, California, Missouri, Connecticut, and Florida. In some instances, these regulations are made by the county health departments and in others by state legislatures, state boards of dental examiners, state dental disciplinary boards, or state departments of health.

Twenty-two states also have their own Division of Occupational Safety and Health Administration (OSHA) in their state Departments of Labor (see Appendix A). These states must administer regional OSHA standards, including those for occupational exposure to bloodborne pathogens and for management of hazardous materials, that are at least as stringent as the federal OSHA standards (see section on OSHA).

Because infection control regulations vary from state to state, particularly in the areas of instrument sterilization, waste management, and sterilizer spore testing, it is important to keep in contact with the various state agencies for the latest information that may affect infection control in the dental office. Two other sources of information may be the state dental association and the infection control officer in a school of dentistry located in the state.

Food and Drug Administration

The *Food and Drug Administration* (FDA; see Appendix A) is a part of the United States Department of Health and Human Services. In relation to infection control, the FDA regulates the manufacturing and labeling of medical devices (such as sterilizers, biologic and chemical indicators, ultrasonic cleaners and cleaning solutions, liquid sterilants [e.g., glutaraldehydes] gloves, masks, surgical gowns, protective eyewear, handpieces, dental instruments, dental chairs, and dental unit lights) and of antimicrobial hand-washing agents and mouth rinses.

The purpose of the FDA is to assure the safety and effectiveness of drugs and medical devices by requiring "good manufacturing practices" and reviewing the devices against associated labeling to assure that claims can be supported. The FDA may require general controls, certain performance standards, or various items such as, for example, notification from a manufacturer that a device is about to be marketed to requiring certain performance standards or approval of the device before marketing. All medical devices to be sold in the U.S. must first be cleared by the FDA. To do this the manufacturers must submit to the FDA a 510(k) application (premarket notification) that describes the device and the manufacturing facilities, and presents the results of studies conducted to support any claims of effectiveness and safety made for the device. The FDA does not control the actual use of a medical device but indicates that misuse (using an item contrary to instructions on the device) transfers any liability for problems that develop from the manufacturer to the user.

Environmental Protection Agency

The United States *Environmental Protection Agency* (EPA; see Appendix A) is associated with infection control by attempting to ensure the safety and effectiveness of disinfectants. The EPA also is involved in regulating medical waste after it leaves the dental office. Information on the safety and effectiveness of disinfectants must be submitted by manufacturers to the EPA for review to make sure that safety and the antimicrobial claims stated for the products are supported with scientific evidence. If the claims meet the criteria, the disinfectant product receives an EPA Registration number that must appear on the product label. EPA involvement with waste management is discussed in Chapter 16.

Occupational Safety and Health Administration

The Occupational Safety and Health Administration (OSHA; see Appendix A) is a division of the United States Department of Labor, and its charge is to protect the workers of America from physical, chemical, or infectious hazards in the workplace. The OSHA standard for protection against hazardous chemicals is described in Chapter 19. OSHA began to develop its standard for protection against occupational exposure to bloodborne pathogens in 1986 and published the final rules in 1991. The standard is known as the *Bloodborne Pathogens Standard,* and it became effective Nationwide in 1992. OSHA requires that a copy of the regulatory text of this standard be present in every dental office and clinic. This regulatory text is provided in Appendix H.

This standard indicates that it is the employer's responsibility to protect employees from exposure to blood and other potentially infectious materials (OPIM) in the workplace and that proper care must be given if such exposure does occur. It applies to employers in any type of facility where employees have a potential for exposure to body fluids, including dental and medical offices; dental, clinical, and research laboratories; hospitals; funeral homes; emergency medical services; nursing homes; and others.

Compliance with this standard is monitored through investigations of facilities by OSHA compliance officers after a complaint by an employee of the facility to OSHA. Also, compliance officers may investigate a facility with eleven or more employees in the absence of an employee complaint. Noncompliance with any rule in the standard can result in a fine.

The standard is effective throughout the United States and in 22 states is administered by the state OSHA programs. In the other states, it is administered through regional branches of the federal OSHA (see Appendix A for details).

OSHA BLOODBORNE PATHOGENS STANDARD

The Bloodborne Pathogens Standard (see Appendix H) is the most important infection control law in dentistry. General steps for employer compliance with this standard are described in Box 8-1 and the seven major sections of the standard are discussed below.

Exposure Control Plan

Each dental office, clinic, or school must prepare a written *Exposure Control Plan* that contains the elements listed in Box 8-2. This plan must be reviewed and updated at least annually and a copy must be accessible to all employees.

Box 8-1 The OSHA Bloodborne Pathogen Standard: General Steps for Compliance

1. Review the standard
2. Prepare a written Exposure Control Plan
3. Train the employees
4. Provide employees everything needed to comply with the standard
   a. Offer hepatitis B vaccination series
   b. Provide, maintain, dispose of or clean and ensure use of personal protective equipment and/or engineering controls
   c. Establish appropriate work practices and decontamination procedures
   d. Establish post-exposure medical evaluation and follow-up
   e. Provide appropriate biohazard communication
5. Maintain appropriate records

Box 8-2 The Written Exposure Control Plan

Prepare a written plan that documents the components listed below
1. Exposure Determination
   Determine which employees may have occupational exposure and are therefore covered under the standard
2. Schedule of Implementation
   Describe how and when the provisions of the standard will be implemented, including:
   a. Communication of hazards to employees
   b. Hepatitis B vaccination
   c. Post-exposure evaluation and follow-up
   d. Recordkeeping
   e. Methods of compliance such as engineering and work practice controls, personal protective equipment, housekeeping
3. Evaluation of Exposure Incidents
   Describe how the circumstances surrounding an exposure incident will be evaluated

Exposure Determination

An occupational exposure is defined as any reasonably anticipated skin, eye, mucous membrane, or parenteral (e.g., needlestick, cut, abrasion, instrument puncture) contact with blood or other potentially infectious material (OPIM) such as saliva that may result from the performance of an employee's duties. For the exposure determinations, survey all tasks performed by all employees and make a list (I) of all job classifications in the office in which all of the employees in that classification have occupational exposure (e.g., "dentist," "dental hygienist," "clinical dental assistant"). Then make a second list (II) of job classifications in which some of the employees in that classification may have occupational exposure (e.g., "receptionist," "bookkeeper," "office manager"). Make these determinations as if gloves, masks, eyeglasses, and protective clothing are not being used.

Now make a list of all tasks and procedures or groups of closely related tasks and procedures in which occupational exposure occurs (without regard to personal protective equipment or clothing) and that are performed by employees in job classifications noted in list II described above.

Employees in these job classifications on lists I and II are covered under the standard.

Schedule of Implementation

Prepare a schedule of when and how each provision of the standard will be implemented. The provisions to be included are listed in Box 8-2 and described further in this chapter. One approach in a small office is to simply make notes on a copy of the standard of when (a specific date) and how each provision will be implemented. Larger facilities may wish to prepare a more extensive document covering all health and safety provisions that includes the Exposure Control Plan.

Evaluation of Exposure Incidents

If an employee is exposed to blood, saliva, or OPIM, the circumstances surrounding the incident must be evaluated. The route of exposure needs to be documented (e.g., splash in the eyes, needle stick in left thumb), and the source patient, types of protective barriers worn at the time of exposure, and what the employee was doing at the time of exposure should be documented. This can best be accomplished by using an Exposure Incident Report form (see example in Appendix E). Evaluation of this information will assist in the postexposure medical evaluation (described later) of the employee and will determine if the employee may need further training in attempts to prevent future exposures.

Communication of Biohazards

Informing employees of biohazards is to occur in two general ways: by giving specific information and training and by using labels and signs that identify hazards. The goal of this communication is to eliminate or minimize exposure to bloodborne and other pathogens.

Information and Training

The OSHA standard indicates that employers shall ensure that all employees with occupational exposure participate in a training program on the hazards associated with body fluids and the protective measures to be taken to minimize the risk of occupational exposure. Box 8-3 gives the minimum content of the required training program. The train-

---

Box 8-3   Minimum Content of OSHA-required Training

- An accessible copy of the regulatory text of the bloodborne pathogen standard and an explanation of its contents
- A general explanation of the epidemiology and symptoms of bloodborne diseases
- An explanation of the modes of transmission of bloodborne pathogens
- An explanation of the employer's exposure control plan and the means by which the employee can obtain a copy of the written plan
- An explanation of the appropriate methods for recognizing tasks and other activities that may involve exposure to blood and OPIM
- An explanation of the use and limitations of methods that will prevent or reduce exposure, including appropriate engineering controls, work practices, and personal protective equipment
- Information on the types, proper use, location, removal, handling, decontamination and disposal of personal protective equipment
- An explanation of the basis for selection of personal protective equipment; information on the hepatitis B vaccine, including information on its efficacy, safety, method of administration, the benefits of being vaccinated, and that the vaccine and vaccination will be offered free of charge
- Information on the appropriate actions to take and persons to contact in an emergency involving blood or other potentially infectious materials
- An explanation of the procedure to follow if an exposure incident occurs, including the method of reporting the incident and the medical follow-up that will be made available
- Information on the postexposure evaluation and follow-up that the employer is required to provide for the employee after an exposure incident
- An explanation of the signs and labels and/or color-coding required by the standard
- An opportunity for interactive questions and answers with the person conducting the training session

---

ing is to be provided at no cost to the employee at the time of initial appointment (before the employee is placed in a position in which occupational exposure may occur) and at least annually thereafter, as well as whenever job tasks change that may reflect the employees' potential for exposure. The training must be given to full-time, part-time, and temporary employees who have a potential for exposure.

A person must conduct the training or at least be available during the training to answer questions. Training solely by means of a film or video tape or written material without the opportunity for a discussion period is not acceptable. Likewise, a generic computer program, even an interactive one, is not considered appropriate unless it is supplemented with the site-specific information required (e.g., the location of the Exposure Control Plan, the procedures to be followed if an exposure incident occurs) and a person is accessible for interaction.

The OSHA standard requires that the person conducting the training be knowledgeable about bloodborne pathogens and about infection control procedures related to the dental workplace. The dentist-employer, hygienists, assistants, dental school professors, or others may conduct the training, provided they are familiar with bloodborne pathogen

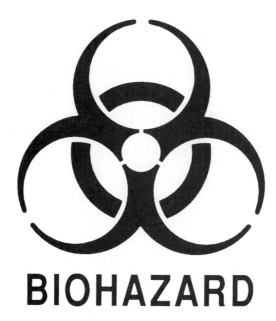

FIGURE 8-1   Biohazard symbol.

control and the subject matter required to be presented. The trainer must be able to answer questions related to the information presented.

The manner of the training must be at a level that is appropriate for the employees being trained (e.g., employee's education, language, literacy level). If an employee is proficient only in a foreign language, the trainer or an interpreter must convey the information in that language.

The required record keeping (described below) on the training session includes a description of the qualifications of the person providing the training. OSHA compliance officers will verify the competency of the trainer based on the completion of specialized courses, degree programs, or work experiences, if the officer determines during an investigation that deficiencies in training exist.

Use of Signs and Labels

Warning labels containing the biohazard symbol and the word "Biohazard" are fluorescent orange or orange-red with the lettering and symbol in a contrasting color (Figure 8-1). Such labels must be affixed to containers of regulated waste, refrigerators and freezers containing blood or OPIM, and other containers used to store, transport, or ship blood or OPIM. Red bags or red containers may be substituted for labels (if employees are trained as to the meaning of the red bags or containers). Individual containers of blood or other potentially infectious materials that are placed in a labeled container during storage, transport, shipment, or disposal are exempt from the labeling requirement. Contaminated equipment that is to be shipped for service must be labeled, however, and the label must include a description of the part of the equipment that is contaminated.

Contaminated laundry also must be properly labeled, as described later in this chapter.

Box 8-4   Hepatitis B Vaccination

EMPLOYER	EMPLOYEE	HEALTH CARE PROFESSIONAL (HCP)*
1. Gives a copy of the OSHA standard to the HCP	1. Receives the vaccine-related training	1. Receives a copy of the OSHA standard from employer
2. Provides vaccine-related training to employee	2. Receives the offer for free vaccination from the employer	2. Evaluates employee for vaccination, prior immunity, or contraindication
3. Offers vaccination series to employee	3a. Accepts the offer and sees the HCP, or	3a. Vaccinates employee, or
	3b. Declines the offer and signs the declination statement†	3b. Explains contraindication or prior immunity to employee
4a. Receives and maintains the signed statement if employee declines the offer, or	4. Is evaluated for vaccination by the HCP and receives vaccine or explanation for not being administered vaccine	4. Gives written opinion to employer on evaluation and if vaccine was administered
4b. Receives written opinion from HCP on evaluation and administration of vaccine and gives copy to employee		
5. Maintains written opinion or declination statement in confidential employee medical records file		

*Physician or other licensed health-care professional such as a nurse practitioner. Evaluation and vaccination is provided according to recommendations from the U.S. Public Health Service.
†May later request and obtain the vaccination series free of charge.

Hepatitis B Vaccination

Employees covered by the standard must be offered the hepatitis B vaccination series free of charge after they have received the training required by the OSHA standard and within 10 days of their employment. Booster dose or doses also must be made available free of charge if recommended by the U.S. Public Health Service. However, as yet booster doses have not been recommended. If the employee received the complete vaccine series previously, or if antibody testing discloses immunity, or if the vaccine is contraindicated for medical reasons, vaccination need not be offered. The employer must not make participation in a prescreening program a prerequisite for receiving hepatitis B vaccination. The vaccine is to be administered by or under the supervision of a licensed physician or other licensed health-care professional (e.g., a nurse practitioner), and this professional must be provided with a copy of the OSHA bloodborne pathogens standard (Box 8-4).

If the employee initially declines vaccination but at a later date, while still covered under the standard, decides to accept the offer, the employer must make the vaccine available at no charge at that time. Employers must ensure that employees who decline vaccination sign a specifically worded statement of declination that is printed in the OSHA standard. This statement is reproduced in Chapter 9.

To document compliance, the employer must obtain a written opinion from the physician responsible for the vaccination as to whether the hepatitis B vaccination is indicated for an employee and if the employee received the vaccination series. This written opinion of employee vaccination status must be retained by the employer with a copy given to the employee and must be made available to a physician who later may be involved in providing a postexposure medical evaluation of the employee. This will help the evaluating physician determine the need for prophylaxis or treatment related to such an exposure. Maintenance of these records also provides documentation for the employer that a medical assessment of the employee's ability and indication to receive hepatitis B vaccination was completed.

Postexposure Medical Evaluation and Follow-up

Documentation of Exposure

After a report of an exposure incident, the employer must make immediately available to the exposed employee a confidential medical evaluation and follow-up at no cost to the employee, at a reasonable time and place and performed or supervised by a licensed physician or other licensed health-care professional (HCP) (Box 8-5). The employer must document the exposure and surrounding circumstances. This is best accomplished by using an Exposure Incident Report form as previously mentioned (see Appendix E). This documentation as well as a job description of the employee as related to the incident, any information documenting the exposed employee's hepatitis B vaccination status (e.g., past written opinions from the HCP), any HCP-written opinions from past exposure incidents, and a copy of the OSHA standard are given to the evaluating HCP.

Testing of the Source Individual

The source individual is any patient whose body fluid is involved in the exposure incident. After an employee exposure, the employer must promptly request that the source individual's blood be tested (with consent) to determine HBV and human immunodeficiency virus (HIV) infectivity, unless this person is already known to be infected with HBV or HIV. If the source individual does not give consent for testing or if it is not feasible to obtain consent, the employer shall establish that this consent cannot be obtained. If consent is given, the source individual may be sent to the HCP or an appropriate accredited laboratory or testing site for the testing. The results of the source individual's tests are confidential and are to be directed only to the HCP evaluating the exposed employee. The employer must ensure that the exposed employee is confidentially informed of these results by the attending HCP but the employer does not have the right to know the source individual's test results.

Testing the Exposed Employee

The employer must make available collection and testing of blood from the exposed employee for HBV and HIV status with the employee's consent. This can be arranged through

---

Box 8-5 Post-exposure Medical Evaluation and Follow-up

EMPLOYER	EMPLOYEE	HEALTH CARE PROFESSIONAL (HCP)*
1. Sends exposed employee to HCP for testing (with consent)	1. Reports to the HCP for evaluation	1. Receives the following from the employer:
2. Sends source individual to HCP or arranges for other testing (with consent). If HBV and HIV status is already known or consent is not given, informs the HCP	2. Gives or withholds consent for testing	Copy of standard
		Incident report
	3. Receives own and source individual's test results from HCP	Employee's job description
		Past written opinions on employee's vaccination status and any past exposure incidents
3. Gives the following to the HCP:	4. Is told by HCP of any conditions resulting from exposure that require further evaluation or treatment	2. Arranges for testing of source individual (with consent) OR receives test results from employer-arranged testing OR receives other information about source individual's HBV and HIV status or that consent for testing was not given
• copy of OSHA standard		
• incident report		
• employee's job description as related to the exposure incident		
• past written opinions on employee's hepatitis B vaccination status and any past exposure incidents		3. Evaluates exposed employee for testing with consent and arranges for testing when indicated†
4. Assures that test resul of source individual are given to the HCP and that HCP informs employee of these results stressing confidentiality		4. Informs exposed employee of:
		Source individual's test results stressing confidentiality
5. Receives written opinion from HCP		Results of the evaluation
6. Maintains written opinion in confidential employee medical records file		Any condition that requires further evaluation or treatment
		5. Gives written opinion to employer that employee was informed of results and of any further evaluation or treatment needed

*Physician or other licensed health-care professional such as a nurse practitioner. Evaluation and vaccination is provided according to recommendations from the U.S. Public Health Service.
†If blood is drawn but consent for testing is not given, arrangements are to be made to store blood sample for 90 days should employee change his/her mind.

the HCP. If the employee consents to blood collection but does not give consent for testing for HIV, the blood sample is to be preserved for 90 days, in case the employee later consents to testing. The HCP is to provide medical evaluation and follow-up according to the U.S. Public Health Service recommendations and to provide the employer with a written opinion within 15 days after the evaluation. This written opinion shall include only the following information: (1) that the employee has been informed of the results of the evaluation and (2) that the employee has been told about any medical conditions resulting from exposure that require further evaluation or treatment. All other findings or diagnoses shall remain confidential and shall not be included in the written opinion.

This written opinion is to be kept in a confidential employee medical records file with the hepatitis B vaccination written opinion for that employee.

Record Keeping
Training Records

Records documenting that employees covered under the standard received the required training must contain: (1) dates of the training sessions, (2) contents or summary of the training, (3) names and qualifications of the persons conducting the training, and (4) names and job titles of all persons attending the training sessions. The records are to be kept for three years from the date on which the training occurred.

Employee Medical Records

Medical records for each employee covered under the standard are to include: (1) name and social security number of the employee; (2) the hepatitis B vaccination status, including the dates of vaccination and the written opinion from the HCP regarding the vaccination or the signed statement that the employee declined the offer to be vaccinated; and (3) reports documenting occupational exposure incidents, as well as the written opinion from the HCP who made the evaluation.

These medical records are confidential and are not to be disclosed except to the employee, anyone having written consent of the employee, representatives of the Secretary of Labor (on request), or as required or permitted by state or federal law. The records must be maintained for 30 years past the last date of employment.

Employers with eleven or more employees also must maintain OSHA Form 200, which is a log of occupational injuries, including needlestick, cuts, and instrument injuries.

Universal Precautions

Universal precautions is the concept that all human blood and certain human body fluids are treated as if known to be infectious for HIV and HBV and other bloodborne pathogens. Justification for this concept is based on the inability to easily identify most of those infected with HIV, HBV, or HCV, as described in Chapter 6. Universal precautions are to be observed under the rules of the standard.

Engineering and Work Practice Controls

Engineering and work practice controls are to be used to minimize or eliminate employee exposure. If exposure remains after institution of these controls, personal protective equipment also is to be used.

Engineering controls generally act on the hazard itself so that the employee may not have to take self-protective action. An example is use of a sharps container. Work practice controls alter the manner in which a task is performed, reducing the likelihood of exposure, such as safe handling techniques for needles. All engineering controls should be examined and maintained or replaced and work practices reviewed on a regular basis to ensure their effectiveness.

Handwashing

Readily accessible handwashing facilities are to be provided to employees. In the rare instances when this is not feasible, antiseptic towelettes or an antiseptic hand cleaner and cloth or paper towels are to be provided, with soap and water handwashing to follow as soon as feasible. Employers are to ensure that employees wash their hands as soon as possible after removal of gloves or other personal protective equipment. Hands and other skin are to be washed with soap and water, and mucous membranes are to be flushed with water as soon as feasible after contact of these body sites with blood/saliva.

Handling Disposable Contaminated Sharps

Contaminated needles and other sharps are not to be bent, recapped, or removed unless the employer can demonstrate that no alternative is feasible or that such action is required by a specific medical procedure. It is quite clear that disposable needles must be removed from the nondisposable dental anesthetic syringes. Recapping is to be accomplished using a one-handed technique or a mechanical device. Also, shearing or breaking of contaminated needles is prohibited.

Handling Reusable Contaminated Sharps

Contaminated reusable sharps (e.g., special needles, sharp instruments) are to be placed in appropriate containers as soon as possible after use. The containers shall be puncture-resistant and color coded or labeled with a biohazard symbol and be leakproof on the sides and bottom. The sharps shall not be stored or processed (prior to decontamination) in a manner that requires employees to reach blindly into containers where these sharps have been placed.

Restricted Activities in the Work Area

Eating, drinking, smoking, applying cosmetics or lip balm, and handling contact lenses are prohibited in work areas where there is a chance for occupational exposure. Food and drink cannot be stored in refrigerators or freezers or kept on shelves or on countertops or in cabinets where blood or saliva is present.

Minimizing Spatter

All procedures involving blood or saliva are to be performed in such a manner that will minimize splashing, spraying, spattering, and generation of droplets of these substances. Although OSHA does not mention specific procedures that limit spatter and generation of droplets in dentistry, consideration might include use of the rubber dam, high volume evacuation, and pre-procedure mouthrinsing.

Specimen Containers

Specimens of blood or saliva or other potentially infectious material are to be placed in a container that prevents leakage during collection, handling, processing, storage, or shipping.

The container is to be closed and color-coded or labeled with a biohazard symbol for storage, transport, or shipping. A second container with the same characteristics is to be used if the outside of the primary container is contaminated. If the specimen could puncture the primary container, a second container with the same characteristics plus being puncture-resistant is to be used.

Servicing Contaminated Equipment

Equipment that may become contaminated with blood or saliva or OPIM is to be examined before servicing or shipping and decontaminated as necessary unless the employer can demonstrate the decontamination of such equipment or portions of such equipment is not feasible. If portions remain contaminated, these portions are to be identified and labeled with a biohazard symbol. This identification and labeling information is to be conveyed to all affected employees, the servicing representative and/or the manufacturer, as appropriate, before handling, servicing, or shipping so that proper precautions will be taken.

Personal Protective Equipment

When there is a potential for occupational exposure, the employer shall provide, at no cost to the employee, appropriate personal protective equipment such as gloves, protective clothing, masks, face shields or eye protection, and mouthpiece, resuscitation bags, pocket masks, or other ventilating devices. Such equipment will be considered appropriate if it does not permit blood or saliva to pass through or to reach the employee's work clothes, street clothes, undergarments, skin, eyes, mouth, or other mucous membranes under normal conditions of use.

The employer is to: (1) ensure that the employee uses the personal protective equipment; (2) ensure that the regular personal protective equipment in the appropriate sizes is readily accessible in the office (including hypoallergenic gloves, glove liners, powderless gloves, or other alternatives for those who are allergic to the regular gloves); (3) clean, launder, and when appropriate dispose of personal protective equipment; and (4) repair or replace personal protective equipment as needed to maintain its effectiveness.

All personal protective equipment is to be removed before leaving the work area. If a garment is penetrated by blood or saliva, it is to be removed immediately or as soon as feasible. When personal protective equipment is removed, it is to be placed in an appropriately designated area or container for storage, washing, decontamination, or disposal.

Gloves

Gloves are to be worn when the employee may have hand contact with blood or saliva, mucous membranes, nonintact skin, or when handling or touching contaminated items or surfaces. Handwashing is required after glove removal. Surgical or examination gloves are to be replaced as soon as practical when contaminated or as soon as feasible if they are torn, punctured, or otherwise compromised. Disposable gloves are not to be washed or decontaminated for reuse. Utility gloves may be decontaminated for reuse if the integrity of the glove is not compromised. However, they must be discarded if cracked, peeling, torn, punctured or they become deteriorated in any way.

Masks, Eye Protection, and Face Shields

Masks in combination with eye protection devices such as goggles or glasses with solid side shields, or chin-length face shields, are to be worn whenever splashes, spray, spatter, or droplets of blood or saliva may be generated and eye, nose, mouth contamination may occur. If face shields are used, they need to be curved to give protection to the sides of the eyes. If regular prescription glasses are used as protective eyewear, they should have clip-on side shields.

Protective Clothing

Appropriate protective clothing such as gowns, aprons, lab coats, clinic jackets, or similar outer garments are to be worn in occupational exposure situations. The employer must evaluate the task to determine the appropriate nature of the protective clothing to be used. Examples of different levels of exposure given by OSHA are "soiled" (low level, requiring laboratory coats), "splashed, splattered or sprayed" (medium level, requiring fluid-resistant garments), "soaked" (high level, requiring fluid-proof garments).

Protective clothing must not permit blood or saliva to pass through or reach the employees' work clothes, street clothes, undergarments, or skin. If an item of clothing is intended to protect the employees' person or work clothes or street clothes against contact with blood or saliva, then it would be considered as personal protective clothing. If a uniform is used to protect the employee from exposure, the uniform is considered personal protective clothing. If a lab coat or protective gown is placed over the uniform, the uniform is not protective clothing; the lab coat or gown is. Thus it is the outer covering that is the protective clothing that must be provided by the employer.

Also, the employer is required to maintain, clean, launder, and/or dispose of all personal protective equipment, including protective clothing, at no cost to the employee. Furthermore, employees cannot launder the protective clothing at home. Thus employers must provide disposable protective clothing or reusable protective clothing that is laundered in the office or is cleaned by a laundry service. OSHA reasons that with these options, the employer has control over the protective clothing to ensure proper disposal or cleaning.

Housekeeping

Employers are to assure that the worksite is maintained in a clean and sanitary condition. All equipment and environmental and working surfaces are to be cleaned and decontaminated after contact with blood or OPIM. OSHA states that this must be done "after completion of procedures, immediately or as soon as feasible when surfaces are overtly contaminated or after any spill of blood or OPIM, and at the end of the work shift if the surface may have become contaminated since the last cleaning."

The employer must prepare and implement a **written schedule** for cleaning and method of decontamination of respective worksites within the facility, for example: All uncovered contaminated surfaces in the dental operatory will be sprayed with an iodophor (state the brand), wiped clean, resprayed with the iodophor, let stand for 10 minutes and wiped dry. This will be performed immediately after care is completed for each patient.

Other statements must be written for other worksites such as the sterilizing room, x-ray room, darkroom, in-office lab, restroom, or any other site where surfaces may be contaminated with blood or OPIM. OSHA does not specify which disinfectant must be used, only that it must be EPA-registered. Choose an EPA-registered product that is tuberculocidal (as further discussed in Chapter 12).

Protective coverings (such as plastic-wrap, aluminum foil, or imperviously backed absorbent paper) used to protect surfaces or equipment from contamination are to be removed and replaced as soon as possible after contamination or at the end of the workshift. Although not specified by OSHA, protective surface covers should be replaced between patients as discussed in Chapter 12.

All reusable containers that may become contaminated with blood or OPIM are to be inspected and decontaminated on a regularly scheduled basis and as soon as feasible if visibly contaminated.

Broken glassware that may be contaminated (e.g., an anesthetic capsule or glass beakers used in the ultrasonic cleaner) is not to be picked up directly with the hands. Mechanical means such as tongs, forceps, or a brush and dust pan should be used.

Regulated Waste

The management of regulated waste is fully described in Chapter 16. Several local, state, or federal laws may apply to various aspects of waste management in your specific locality. OSHA is primarily concerned with the handling and disposal of contaminated sharps; blood or OPIM that is in a liquid, semi-liquid, or caked state; and pathological or microbiological wastes contaminated with blood or OPIM.

Contaminated Sharps

Contaminated sharps (anything that could puncture the skin that contains blood or OPIM) are to be placed in containers that are closable, puncture-resistant, leakproof on the sides and bottom, and color-coded red or marked with a biohazard symbol. These are called sharps containers or sharps boxes. The containers are to be easily accessible and located as close as possible to where sharps are used or may be found (e.g., at chairside and in the sterilizing room). The containers are to be maintained in an upright position (so the contents do not spill out), and are to be replaced routinely and not allowed to overflow. The containers are to be closed during handling, storage, transport, or shipment. If the outside of the container is contaminated or if it could leak, it is to be placed in a second leakproof, puncture-resistant, color-coded or labeled container during handling, storage, transport, or shipping.

Other Regulated Waste

Other regulated waste that is nonsharp (e.g., any item that could release liquid, semiliquid, or caked blood or OPIM when compressed such as a blood- or saliva-saturated gauze square) is to be placed in containers that are leakproof, closable, and color-coded or labeled with a biohazard symbol. An example is a biohazard bag. The containers are to be closed prior to handling, storage, transport, or shipping and if the outside is contaminated it is to be placed in a second closable, leakproof, color-coded or labeled container that is closed before handling, storage, transport, or shipping.

Contaminated Laundry

Contaminated laundry (e.g., reusable protective clothing, towels, patient drapes) is to be handled as little as possible with a minimum of agitation. It is not to be bagged, containerized, sorted, or rinsed in the location of use. Contaminated laundry is to be placed and transported in bags or containers that are color-coded or labeled with a biohazard symbol. When a facility uses universal precautions in handling all laundry to be cleaned, alternative labeling is sufficient if it permits all employees to recognize the containers as requiring compliance with universal precautions. If the contaminated laundry is sent off-site for cleaning, it must be placed in bags or containers that are color-coded or labeled with a biohazard symbol, unless the laundry uses universal precautions in handling all soiled laundry.

Instrument Sterilization not Covered by OSHA

A very important area of infection control that is not covered under the OSHA blood-borne pathogens standard is instrument sterilization and associated sterilization monitoring in a clinical setting such as the dental office. These procedures are considered as patient-protection procedures rather than worker-protective procedures. Since OSHA is charged by the United States Congress to protect the workers of America, it cannot legally make or enforce rules that relate only to patient protection.

Appropriate procedures for processing reusable dental instruments and handpieces are described in recommendations from important organizations such as the CDC, ADA, OSAP Research Foundation, and AAMI. Also, several states, including Indiana, Ohio, Washington, Oregon, and Florida, have passed laws requiring sterilization of all reusable instruments and handpieces between patients and monitoring of sterilization processes. Specific details for instrument sterilization and sterilization monitoring are presented in Chapter 11.

SELECTED READINGS

American Dental Association, Councils on Scientific Affairs and Dental Practice: Infection control recommendations for the dental office and the dental laboratory, *J Amer Dent Assoc* 127:672-680, 1996.

Centers for Disease Control and Prevention: Recommended infection-control practices for dentistry, 1993, *MMWR* 42(no RR-8):1-12, 1993.

Miller, CH: Infection control strategies for the dental office. In Ciancio SG, editor: *ADA guide to dental therapeutics,* Chicago, 1998, American Dental Association, pp. 489-504.

Office Safety and Asepsis Procedures Research Foundation. Infection control in dentistry guidelines, Anapolis, Maryland, 1997.

U.S. Department of Health and Human Services, Centers for Disease Control and Food and Drug Administration: *Practical infection control in the dental office: a workbook for the dental team,* Washington, DC, 1989, Department of Health and Human Services.

U.S. Department of Labor, OSHA. 29 CFR Part 1910.1030: *Occupational exposure to bloodborne pathogens; final rule.* Federal Register 56 (No. 235):64004-64182, Friday, December 6, 1991 (actual regulatory text: p. 64175-64182).

U.S. Department of Labor, OSHA: *Controlling occupational exposure to bloodborne pathogens in dentistry,* OSHA 3129, Washington, DC, 1992, OSHA.

U.S. Department of Labor, OSHA: Controlling occupational exposure to bloodborne pathogens, OSHA 3127 (revised), Washington, DC, 1996, OSHA.

Chapter 9

IMMUNIZATION

In the United States, there are an estimated 8.8 million persons who work in the health care industry. About six million are employed in the nation's 6,000 hospitals. However, a significant portion of health care that in the past was provided only in hospitals now occurs in offices, freestanding clinics (e.g., surgery and emergency care clinics), nursing homes, and many dental specialty offices (e.g., oral surgery, periodontics, and endodontics). Health care workers in hospitals and at off-site locations are at risk for the occupational acquisition of infectious diseases. After infection, disease could be spread to patients, co-workers, household members, and possibly to the community at large.

Ensuring that dental personnel are immune to vaccine preventable diseases is an essential part of a successful infection control plan. Optimal use of vaccines can prevent transmission of disease and can help eliminate unnecessary work restrictions. Vaccination prevents illness and is far more cost effective than individual case management or outbreak control.

It is known that compliance with a vaccination scheme is greater when the program is mandatory, rather than voluntary. It is also known that when the employer pays for the vaccinations, compliance is markedly higher than if the employees must pay all or part of their immunization costs.

The decision as to which vaccines should be included in an immunization program is influenced by the types of health care provided, characteristics of the patient pool, and the age and experience of the health care workers. In some cases, screening can help determine susceptibility to certain vaccine preventable diseases. Hepatitis B (HBV) is an example.

Dental personnel are exposed daily to a variety of communicable diseases present in their work environments. Personal protective barriers such as gloves, masks, gowns, and protective eyewear help prevent the majority of cross-infections. Immunization when available, however, is the most effective method to reduce the chances of disease acquisition. Maintenance of immunity is an essential component of any effective infection control program. Current Occupational Safety and Health Administration (OSHA) standards require immunization records be maintained for all at risk employees.

Unfortunately, vaccines do not exist for all diseases (Box 9-1). Important "missing vaccines" for dentistry include immunization against hepatitis C, HIV-1, tuberculosis, and some forms of human herpesviruses.

To have the most effective and efficient office/clinic infection control program, a personnel health scheme must be an essential component. Vaccinations (including screenings and postexposure prophylaxis in some cases) must be teamed with occupational risk assessment and management, personnel health and safety education, and the proper handling of job-related illnesses and exposures. Proper record keeping and data management help generate valuable information, which report the vaccination histories of the personnel and could aid in the investigation and analysis of job-related illnesses and injuries.

Box 9-1 Diseases for Which Vaccines are Available for use in the United States*

Adenovirus	Pertussis
Anthrax	Plague
Cholera	Pneumococcal pneumonia
Diphtheria	Polio
Hemophilus influenzae type b	Rabies
Hepatitis A	Rubella
Hepatitis B	Tetanus
Influenza	Typhoid fever
Measles	Pertussis
Meningicoccal meningitis	Varicella (chickenpox)
Mumps	Yellow fever

---

*Refer to the current Immunization Practices Advisory Committee recommendations from the Centers for Disease Control and Prevention for more details and current vaccines available.

Topics in this chapter reviewed in depth are tetanus, influenza, and hepatitis B. Other vaccine-preventable diseases, however, will be discussed briefly.

TETANUS

Tetanus ("lockjaw") is a severe disease with a high case-fatality ratio. Tetanus in the U.S. is primarily a disease of older adults, who usually are unvaccinated or poorly vaccinated. It can be an infectious complication of any cut and/or puncture wound and is caused by the toxins (tetanospasmins) of *Clostridium tetani*. Proliferation of the implanted bacilli under the anaerobic conditions present in deep wounds results in the production of the tetanospasmins.

Tetanus is usually a clinical diagnosis based on acute onset of hypertonia and/or painful muscular contractions (usually of the muscles of the jaw and neck first) and generalized muscle spasms. Death is often an expected outcome of infection. However, other medical problems must first be ruled out by physical and serologic examination.

Worldwide, tetanus is an extremely important disease. In many developing countries, aseptic perinatal care and vaccination schemes are suboptimal. The result is an unacceptably high infant mortality rate. In contrast, tetanus has become rare in the United States. For example, in 1947 when reporting of tetanus started, there were 560 cases. Tetanus immunization became widely available in the mid-1940s. During the period 1991-1994, the Centers for Disease Control and Prevention (CDC) received notification of 201 cases. The impact of vaccination can be appreciated through a comparison of 1947's 560 cases to the 51 reported cases in 1994.

Only one case of neonatal tetanus has been reported in the United States during the last five years. Worldwide, an estimated 550,000 annual deaths can be attributed to neonatal tetanus. However, cases involving older adults who had never been vaccinated, improperly vaccinated, or had not received booster injections are also common worldwide.

Tetanus endospores are continually present in the environment and because they are quite resistant to disinfection procedures an overt effort must be made to control their spread. Meticulous handling of all wounds and the monitoring of immune status are essential. Chemoprophylaxis against tetanus is neither practical nor useful in the management of wounds.

Tetanus is a preventable disease. Tetanus toxoid is usually given as part of a triple childhood immunization that includes diphtheria and acellular pertussis vaccines (DTP). The initial DTP vaccine may be given as early as six weeks of age but always before the age of seven. A common regimen includes injections given at 2, 4, and 6 months. At least a four-week interval must be allowed between each injection. A fourth dose (first booster) is recommended at 15 to 18 months. It is designed to maintain protection during preschool years. A fifth dose (second booster) is given when the child is four to six years old (which will protect through most of the schoolyears).

Routine tetanus booster immunization, usually combined with diphtheria toxoid, is recommended for all persons over the age of seven. Traumatic injury (large/extensive wounds exposed to soil and bacterial spores) may necessitate the earlier application of a booster. Arthus–type hypersensitivity reactions to the tetanus toxoid are known, as well as adverse effects for those in their first trimester of pregnancy and for individuals who have a history of neurologic reaction or immediate hypersensitivity. If wounds are minor and uncontaminated, the CDC Advisory Committee on Immunization Practices recommends boosters need only be given every ten years. In individuals known to have been properly immunized, other types of wounds, even rather serious ones, often requires a booster if it is more than five years since the last injection. Many wounds, especially when received during the summer (when greater numbers of viable bacilli are present in the soil), can more readily transmit organisms. However, the injured often decide not to visit a physician's office or hospital for examination and possible treatment.

Protection against tetanus is based on the establishment and maintenance of adequate tetanus antitoxin levels. This is achieved only through proper primary and routine booster injections. The need for vaccination should be discussed regularly with one's primary health care provider.

INFLUENZA

Influenza is an acute respiratory disease caused by influenza type A or B viruses. Incubation ranges from one to four days. Maximum viral shedding occurs one day before the onset of symptoms and for the first three days of clinical illness.

Typical features of influenza include an abrupt onset of fever, coryza, a sore throat, and a nonproductive cough. Also commonly present are systemic symptoms such as headache, muscle aches, and fatigue. Unlike other common respiratory infections, influenza can cause extreme malaise for several days. More severe disease can result if viruses invade the lungs (primary viral pneumonia) or if a secondary bacterial pneumonia occurs. Complications (including hospitalization and even death) are most common among older adults and individuals with chronic health problems such as cardiopulmonary disease. Acute symptoms usually last for two to four days. However, malaise and cough may persist for up to two weeks.

During some influenza epidemics, over 20,000 adults (80% to 90% over 65 years old) in the U.S. will die. Several national health surveys indicate that less than 30% of persons 65 years or older are vaccinated annually.

Two measures available in the U.S. are capable of reducing the impact of influenza. These are immunoprophylaxis with inactivated (killed-virus) vaccine and chemoprophylaxis or chemotherapy. Although antiviral drugs are available, chemoprophylaxis cannot be considered a substitute for vaccination.

Influenza vaccine is a trivalent vaccine made from highly purified, egg-grown viruses rendered noninfectious by treatment with formaldehyde. The vaccine can not cause influenza. Each year's vaccine consists of three virus strains (usually two type As and one type B). The strains selected represent the influenza viruses most likely to circulate in the U.S. during the next winter. Usually one or two components are updated each year. This is to provide a better antigenic match with circulating viruses. The efficacy of the vaccine depends on the correct selection of viral types. Also important is patient age and immunocompetency.

When properly administered, most children and young adults produce high levels of protective antibodies. Some elderly recipients, especially those with chronic diseases (e.g., pulmonary or cardiovascular system diseases, diabetes mellitus, renal dysfunction or immune suppression, even when caused by medication) develop lower postvaccination antibody titers and may remain susceptible to infection. However, current information indicates that about 70% of healthy persons under the age of 65 are protected to the point that they will not become ill.

High-risk individuals, such as persons over 65, especially those in long-term care facilities or with a serious chronic disease, should be vaccinated each year. Other individuals who are clinically or subclinically infected and who live with, attend, or treat high-risk persons can transmit the virus. Therefore health care workers, including dental practitioners, who have contact (e.g., in a hospital, clinic, or residential care facility) with high-risk persons of all ages, including infants, should be vaccinated. Employees of long-term care (nursing home or chronic-care) facilities, home care providers, and household members who contact high-risk people should also be immunized. Most dental personnel, for their own well being and the health of their patients and families, should receive the vaccine annually.

Vaccination is a single deltoid injection of a trivalent vaccine ideally administered in early November. The vaccine should not be given to persons known to have anaphylactic hypersensitivity to eggs or some component of the vaccine without first consulting a physician. In some cases, desensitization may be attempted.

Annual vaccination of persons at high risk (and their close contacts) for influenza-associated complications is the most effective means of reducing the impact of influenza. Because influenza viruses undergo regular antigenic shifts, vaccination must be repeated annually. Last year's vaccine usually has little to no preventive ability against this year's prevailing influenza viruses. The need and regimen for vaccination should be discussed regularly with one's primary health care provider.

HEPATITIS B

The hepatitis B virus (HBV) is an infectious agent associated with acute and chronic inflammation of the liver. Worldwide, HBV is a major cause of necrotizing vasculitis, cirrhosis, and primary hepatocellular carcinoma. HBV can be found primarily in blood and blood products but can also be present in other body fluids, such as semen, tears, feces, urine, vaginal secretions, and saliva.

HBV is a bloodborne pathogen that is transmitted by percuntaeous or mucosal exposure (e.g., IV drug abuse and needlestick accidents by health care workers), by sexual contact, and from mother to fetus or infant. HBV is relatively environmentally stable, especially when surrounded by blood. This allows for the potential of indirect transmission such as contact with contaminated instruments.

Hepatitis B is one of the most frequently reported vaccine-preventable diseases in the United States. Each year between 15,000-20,000 cases of acute hepatitis B are reported. However, many persons with acute infections are asymptomatic, and many cases of symptomatic disease are not reported. Only 30% to 50% of cases have clinical symptoms indicating infection. It is estimated that approximately 150,000 persons in the U.S. are infected annually, with 11,000 hospitalizations and 300 to 450 deaths from acute fulminate hepatitis.

The CDC estimates that about 1,000 health care workers occupationally acquired hepatitis B in 1994. This represents a 90% decline since 1985. The decrease is attributable to the use of vaccine and adherence to other preventive measures (e.g., universal precautions).

Chronic HBV infection is defined as the presence of HBV viral markers in serum for at least six months. Risk of developing chronic infection is age dependent and is greatest for infants infected at birth (90% probability). Overall, 30% to 50% of children and 4% to 10% of adults with acute infections will develop chronic infections. Chronicity increases dramatically the chances for HBV transmission over extended intervals, of cirrhosis, of delta virus hepatitis infections, and for the development of primary hepatocellular carcinoma. It is estimated that 1 to 1.25 million people in the U.S. are chronically infected. Approximately 5,500 of these people die each year.

Hepatitis B is a major occupational hazard for dental personnel with attack rates among unvaccinated individuals 3 to 10 times the 4% rate present in the general population. Hepatitis B is an especially difficult problem because many dental workers have repeated intimate contact with patient body fluids and with items soiled with such fluids. HBV infection appears to be related more to the extent of exposure to blood than to the number or type of patients treated.

Personal protective barriers can not eliminate all body fluid exposures, especially needlestick accidents. Therefore the best protection against HBV infection is immunization. Two vaccines, *Recombivax HB* (Merck Sharp & Dohme) and *Engerix B* (SmithKline) are currently available. Both are recombinant fungal products and can be used interchangeably. The most common vaccine regimen consists of 1.0 mL doses given at 0, 1, and 6 months (Table 9-1). Vaccination of infants (often in the delivery hospital) is common. The goals are to vaccinate at a very young age (which usually positively influences seroconversion rates) and to attempt to prevent perinatal infection from an infected mother.

Injections given in the deltoid muscle have produced seroconversion rates over 95% to 97% in immunocompetent, seronegative younger adults. Lower conversion rates are noted in persons over 40 years of age, smokers, those who are overweight, and among individuals who received injections in the buttocks (as low as 70% seroconversion). Recent studies indicate that genetic factors may significantly influence seroconversion rates.

All at risk personnel need to be vaccinated. This includes clinicians, laboratory workers, and clean-up crews. A person such as an office receptionist may be considered as not being at risk. However, many dental offices practice multi-tasking because when there is an emergency or special patient need, "office workers" temporarily participate in chairside dentistry.

Table 9-1   Recommended Doses of Currently Licensed Hepatitis B Vaccines[*]

GROUP	RECOMBIVAX HB[†] DOSE IN μg (mL)	ENGERIX-B[†] DOSE IN μg (mL)
Infants of HBsAg-negative mothers and children <11 years of age[‡]	2.5 (0.5)	10 (0.5)
Infants of HBsAg-positive mothers; prevention of perinatal infection[‡]	5 (0.5)[§]	10 (0.5)
Children and adolescent 11-19 years of age	5 (0.5)[§]	10 (0.5)
Adults ≥20 years of age	10 (1.0)[§]	20 (1.0)
Dialysis patients and other immunocompromised persons	40 (1.0)	40 (2.0)

[*]Modified from Centers for Disease Control and Prevention (1997-October 15), *Chapter 4: Hepatitis B* (WWW document), URL *http://www.cdc.gov/nip/manual/hepb/hepb.htm*.
[†]Both vaccines are routinely administered in three-dose series. *Engerix-B* also has been licensed for a four-dose series administered at 0, 1, 2, and 12 months.
[‡]HBsAg, hepatitis B surface antigen.
[§]Usual adult formulation.

Unless there is some reason to suspect infection, serologic screening before vaccination is not recommended. Complete protection against HBV, however, does include postscreening for antibody levels. This procedure should be conducted one to two months after the final injection. If seroconversion occurs after vaccination, protective levels of antibodies have been shown to persist for at least eight years. If a vaccine recipient fails to seroconvert, a second series of three injections should be given. Continued failure to respond should be investigated. A chronic HBV infection may be present. One characteristic of a chronic infection is a person's inability to produce a defensive antibody response to HBV.

The need for a booster injection is still being debated. The CDC currently does not recommend boosters. This, however, is based on a proper immune response to vaccination verified through serologic postscreening. The antibody levels of thousands of individuals will have to be measured for a period of years before a booster recommendation could be made. However, if an individual was vaccinated over five years ago and was not serologically evaluated at that time, it probably would be best to have a single injection and then have his or her antibody titer determined.

Compliance with HBV vaccination among health care workers has not been universal. Concerns expressed include vaccine safety, cost, efficacy, pregnancy-related issues, lack of information on the vaccine, and consideration of oneself to be at low-risk. Hospital studies indicate vaccination levels improve markedly when the cost of the series is paid by the employer. National studies show that dentists (over 98% have been vaccinated or have been infected) are among health care worker groups with the highest rates of vaccination. Similar levels of compliance are noted for dental hygienists with lower vaccination rates for dental assistants.

Box 9–2   OSHA Bloodborne Pathogens Standard (29 CFR Section 1910.1030) Hepatitis B Vaccination Performance Standards

1. The employer shall make employees aware of their occupational risk for hepatitis B through formal training.
2. The employer shall inform all at risk employees (except those already properly vaccinated, those shown to be immune or for whom the vaccine is medically contraindicated) of the presence of a hepatitis B vaccine and shall make it available within ten working days of their initial assignment. The employer shall provide information on the vaccine, including the vaccine's efficacy, safety, method of administration, the benefits of being vaccinated, and the assurance that all medical records concerning the vaccination process will be kept confidential.
3. The employer may not require the employee to be serologically prescreened prior to receiving the vaccine.
4. Any employee may decline the vaccine, but if still covered by the Standard at a later date may request to be vaccinated. Employees who decline must sign Appendix "A".
5. All vaccinations must be performed under the supervision of a physician, be given in a manner according to current U.S. Public Health Service procedures, be made available at a reasonable time and place and be of no cost to the employee. The supervising physician shall provide the employee with written assurance that the vaccination was necessary and provided in the proper manner.
6. If in the future the U.S. Public Health Service recommends booster injections, the employer shall make such boosters available.
7. Laboratory costs associated with post-screening for seroconversion will be paid by the employer.
8. The employer must maintain all medical records (e.g., dates of vaccination and laboratory serology results) concerning an employee's hepatitis B vaccination processes for the duration of employment plus 30 years.

Despite the presence of a proven occupational risk and the availability of safe and effective vaccines, not all at risk health care workers have been vaccinated. There are several reasons why health care workers have not been universally vaccinated. Some still question the vaccines' safety and efficacy. Both vaccines have been shown to produce only minimal side effects. The most common complaints include transient injection site soreness and redness, headache, and fever. Individuals with severe allergies to yeast or iodine (the vaccines' preservative) must consult their physicians before being vaccinated. This also applies to individuals with pregnancy related concerns. Another major noncompliance factor is the cost of the vaccine series ($150–$200). It should be noted that OSHA's Bloodborne Pathogens Standard (29 CFR 1910.1030, *Occupational exposure to bloodborne pathogens, final rule,* December 6, 1991) specifically recognizes the important occupational hazard HBV presents for health care workers (see Chapter 6, Appendix D, and Box 9-2). The rule involves several employer and employee performance functions. All costs associated with HBV vaccination must be assumed by the employer. Employees have the right to refuse vaccination. However, a declination statement must be read and signed. The verbiage to be used must be as described in the Standard. A copy of the necessary statement is presented in Figure 9-1.

OSHA Bloodborne Pathogens Standard (29 CFR 1910.1030) Hepatitis B Vaccine Declination

I understand that due to my occupational exposure to blood and other potentially infectious materials I may be at risk of acquiring hepatitis B virus (HBV) infection. I have been given the opportunity to be vaccinated with hepatitis B vaccine, at no charge to myself. However, I decline hepatitis B vaccination at this time. I understand that by declining this vaccine, I continue to be at risk of acquiring hepatitis B, a serious disease. If in the future I continue to have occupational exposure to blood or other potentially infectious materials and I want to be vaccinated with hepatitis B vaccine, I can receive the vaccination series at no charge to me

_____   _____

Employee Signature   Date

_____   _____

Witness Signature   Date

FIGURE 9-1   Mandatory hepatitis B vaccine declination.

RISK OF MISSING AN IMPORTANT OPPORTUNITY

Immunization programs have been extremely successful in the prevention of diseases among children. However, most of us are not aware of the continuing need for vaccinations during adulthood. An important number of vaccine-preventable diseases occur today in the adult population. Anyone who passes through childhood without immunization or infection is at risk. Many diseases are considerably more severe when contracted as an adult. The occupations and/or social behaviors of adults also increase the chances of disease acquisition.

In addition to immunization against influenza, tetanus, and hepatitis B, dental personnel should discuss with their primary health care provider their immune status to other vaccine-preventable diseases. These include hepatitis A, pneumococcal pneumonia, measles, rubella, mumps, and poliomyelitis. Also, whenever possible, dental personnel should make themselves available for disease screenings. People are regularly screened for cholesterol and blood sugar levels, blood pressure, the presence of blood in feces, and heart rate. Screenings for infectious diseases also exist. Some are serologic, for example, antibody testing for hepatitis B and C, the AIDS virus, and herpesviruses. Others include external monitoring for pathogen exposure, the most important of these is an annual interdermal Mantoux tuberculin skin test.

SELECTED READINGS

ADA Council on Scientific Affairs and ADA Council on Dental Practice. Infection control recommendations for the dental office and the dental laboratory, *Journal of the American Dental Association* 127:672-80, 1996.

Advisory Committee on Immunization Practices. Use of vaccines and immune globulins in persons with altered immunocompetence, *MMWR* (RR-4):1-42, 1993.

Advisory Committee on Immunization Practices. Update: vaccine side effects, adverse reactions, contraindications, and precautions. Recommendations of the Advisory Committee on Immunization Practices (ACIP), *MMWR* 45 (RR-12):1-35, 1996.

Advisory Committee on Immunization Practices. Prevention and control of influenza: recommendations of the Advisory Committee on Immunization Practices (ACIP), *MMWR* 46 (RR-9):1-25, 1997.

Centers for Disease Control and Prevention (1997 - October 15), *Chapter 13: Tetanus* (WWW document), URL *http://www.cdc.gov/nip/manual/tetanus/tetanus.htm.*

Centers for Disease Control and Prevention (1997 - October 15), *Chapter 4: Hepatitis B* (WWW document), URL *http://www.cdc.gov/nip/manual/hepb/hepb.htm.*

Centers for Disease Control and Prevention (1997 - October 15), *Chapter 5: Influenza* (WWW document), URL *http://www.cdc.gov/nip/manual/influenz/influenz.htm.*

Centers for Disease Control and Prevention: Draft guidelines for infection control in health care personnel, 1997; notice, *MMWR* 62:47275-47327, 1997.

Cottone JA, Puttaiah R: Hepatitis virus infection - current status in dentistry, *Dent Clinics NA* 40(2):293-307, 1996.

Cottone JA, Puttaiah R: Viral hepatitis and hepatitis vaccines. In Cottone JA, Terezhalmy GT, Molinari JA: *Practical infection control in dentistry,* ed 2, Baltimore, 1996, Williams and Wilkins.

Miller CH, Palenik CJ: Infection Control in Dentistry. In Block S: *Sterilization, Disinfection, Preservation and Sanitation,* ed 4, 1991, Philadelphia, Lea & Febiger.

Occupational Health and Safety Administration: *Occupational exposure to bloodborne pathogens, final rule,* 29 CFR 1910.1030. Federal Register 56:64175-64182, 1991.

Chapter 10

PROTECTIVE BARRIERS

Chapter 3 describes the steps in development of an infectious disease, indicating that contamination of the body with microorganisms must occur before disease can develop. It is always better to prevent this exposure or contamination (when possible) than to rely totally on the body's resistance to fight off disease agents after contamination. Preventing exposure means to avoid contact with the microorganisms, and this is accomplished in two ways. One way is to prevent the microorganisms from escaping from their source (e.g., in the dental office the main source of microorganisms is the patient's mouth). Totally preventing microorganisms from escaping the patient's mouth during care is impossible because microorganisms exit the patient's mouth on instruments, fingers, and supplies used intraorally and they escape in aerosols and spatter droplets generated during the use of the air-water syringe, slow- and high-speed handpieces, and ultrasonic scalers. However, this escape from the patient's mouth can be reduced by using a rubber dam and preprocedure mouthrinsing, as described in Chapter 14.

The second way is the use of barriers to prevent exposure to microorganisms escaping from their sources. In dentistry this involves the use of protective barriers such as gloves, masks, protective eyewear, and protective clothing. The OSHA bloodborne pathogens standard (see Chapter 8) indicates that in facilities where exposure to bloodborne pathogens may occur (e.g., dental offices), the employer is responsible for providing, maintaining, cleaning/laundering, disposing of, and ensuring the use of protective barriers, sometimes referred to as *personal protective equipment (PPE)*.

GLOVES

Protective Value of Gloves

Gloves protect dental team members from direct contact with microorganisms in patients' mouths and on contaminated surfaces, and they also protect patients from microorganisms on the hands of the dental team.

Protection of the Dental Team

Although intact skin is an excellent barrier to disease agents, a small or even invisible cut appears like the Grand Canyon to these microorganisms. Thus small cuts and abrasions can serve as a route of entry of microorganisms into the body, causing a skin infection or other more widespread diseases. A study in 1982 showed that fourth-year dental students had an average of four areas of trauma on their hands; 12% of the traumas became painful on contact with alcohol, suggesting open skin (cut or abrasion). Also, some visually intact areas give a painful response with alcohol, particularly around the fingernails. Thus even a close visual inspection of the hands may not detect all possible portals of entry for microorganisms.

Cuts on unprotected hands is suggested by many to be an important reason for the high occurrence of hepatitis B in dental and medical personnel who do not routinely glove. Also, analyses of the disease herpetic whitlow (herpes simplex virus infection around the fingernails) before the routine gloving era of dentistry indicates that this condition occurred more frequently in dentists than in others. Another protective value of wearing gloves in the office is protection against contact with chemicals (such as cleaners, disinfectants, sterilants, x-ray developing solutions) and some dental materials that may irritate the skin. Also, heat-resistant gloves protect against burns when heat-processing instruments.

Protection of Patients

Microorganisms are present on just about every surface in the office that has not just been cleaned and disinfected. They are there because they settle out from the air or as a result of contact with other contaminated surfaces. Thus ungloved hands become contaminated with microorganisms upon touching just about any environmental surface and from direct contact with fluids or surfaces in a patient's mouth. If these contaminating microorganisms are not removed by handwashing (as described below) or covered up with gloves, they may be transmitted to a patient.

A study in 1982 has shown that a dental patient's blood can be retained under the fingernails of a dental team member for several days, even with handwashing. This could serve as a source of infection for subsequent patients. Thus routine gloving can prevent blood or saliva impaction in these areas (particularly around and under the fingernails) that are difficult to clean.

Microorganisms present in blood may exit the body through small cuts in the skin. This is probably enhanced if these cuts are moistened, as when a dental team member does not wear gloves when working in a patient's mouth. It is suggested that this route of disease spread from dental team member to patient may have been important in several of the 10 reported cases of hepatitis B spread from infected dentists to patients (see Chapter 6). These infected dentists did not routinely glove for patient care.

One of the most clearly documented cases of disease spread in a dental office occurred as a result of not routinely gloving for patient care. An ungloved hygienist with dermatitis on her hands and fingers cared for a patient with active herpes labialis (herpes simplex infection on the lips). About a week later, vesicles of herpetic whitlow developed on the hygienist's hands. Before any sign of her infection appeared, however, she unknowingly spread the virus to at least 20 other patients, who developed intraoral herpes lesions. When the vesicles appeared on the hygienist's hands, she began to routinely wear gloves, which prevented further spread of the virus to any more patients.

This case demonstrates three modes of disease spread in the office, as discussed in Chapter 8: first, from patient to dental team member; second, from dental team member to patient; and third, from patient to patient. In this instance, all three modes of disease spread could have been prevented by routine gloving with every patient. Another important point demonstrated by this case is that dermatitis greatly reduces the effectiveness of handwashing in removing contaminating disease agents. Less vigorous handwashing is performed because of the painful dermatitis, and the dermatitis itself provides additional places on the hands where microorganisms can "hide" from the mechanical action of handwashing.

Uses and Types of Gloves

Box 10-1 lists the several types of gloves available for various uses in the dental setting. Some have specific uses and others have multiple uses (Figure 10-1).

Patient Care Activities

Disposable gloves should be worn during all patient care activities where there is a potential for direct hand contact with saliva, blood, or other oral fluids, mucous membranes, nonintact skin, and when handling items or surfaces contaminated with body fluids or potentially infectious materials.

Box 10-1 Types of Gloves in Dentistry

Patient Care Gloves
Sterile latex surgical gloves
Sterile neoprene surgical gloves*
Sterile styrene surgical gloves*
Sterile synthetic copolymer gloves*
Sterile reduced protein latex surgeon's gloves
Latex examination gloves
Vinyl examination gloves*
Synthetic copolymer examination gloves*
Nitrile examination gloves*
Styrene-butadiene examination gloves*
Powderless gloves
Flavored gloves

Utility Gloves
Heavy latex gloves
Heavy nitrile gloves
Thin copolymer gloves
Thin plastic ("food handlers") gloves

Other Gloves
Heat-resistant gloves
Dermal (cotton) gloves

---

*Non-latex gloves, but review the labeling or check with the manufacturer to confirm.

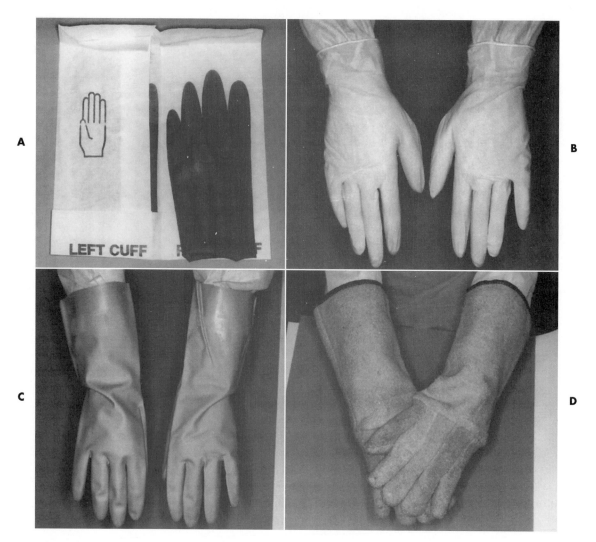

FIGURE 10-1   Gloves used in dentistry. **A,** Sterile surgeon's gloves; **B,** latex examination gloves; **C,** utility gloves; **D,** heat-resistance gloves.

Gloves used for patient care are not to be reused on a subsequent patient. Also, do not wash patient care gloves with any detergent or chemical; this may weaken stabilizers in the glove material or enhance penetration (cause wicking) of material through inherent defects. The powder (cornstarch) on fresh gloves may be rinsed off with plain water before patient care, if desired.

If you leave chairside during patient care, it is best to first remove your gloves and don a fresh pair on returning to chairside. This prevents contamination of any surfaces you may touch when away from chairside and prevents contaminating the patient with microorganisms already present on those same surfaces. Also, remember that any surface at chairside that is touched with contaminated gloves and also may be touched during the care of the next patient must have been previously covered to prevent cross-contamination or precleaned and disinfected before care of the next patient (see Chapter 12 on surface asepsis). An alternative to changing gloves in these situations is to use inexpensive copolymer or plastic gloves or a sheet of plastic wrap over the patient care gloves (overgloving) to prevent spread of the patient's microorganisms to surfaces that are touched. The overgloves are then removed before resuming care on the patient.

Another important aspect of glove use during patient care is that torn or punctured gloves must be removed as soon as possible, followed by immediate handwashing and fresh glove replacement.

Sterile latex or vinyl gloves are used during surgical procedures but nonsterile gloves are appropriate for most other dental procedures. Surgeon's gloves are provided in half-sizes ranging from approximately 5 to 9 and usually provide the best fit because the gloves are made for the right hand and left hand. Examination gloves are ambidextrous in that any glove can be used on the right or left hand. They usually are provided in extra-small, small, medium, and large sizes but some brands may be sized from 5 to 9. Latex gloves are thought by most to give a better fit than vinyl gloves but this may not always be true. It is important to use gloves that fit properly to ensure efficient handling of items and to prevent fatigue of the hands.

Use of powderless gloves, reduced protein latex gloves, and non-latex gloves and dermal gloves relates to the irritations and allergic reactions some people have to gloves. This area is discussed below under reactions to gloves.

Operatory Cleanup and Instrument Processing

It is best to provide more protection for your hands during operatory cleanup and handling instruments than that provided by the thin latex or vinyl patient care gloves or thin copolymer or plastic gloves.

Use utility gloves of nitrile or heavy latex when preparing and using chemicals, precleaning and disinfecting contaminated surfaces, and when handling contaminated items during instrument processing. Each person in the office needing these gloves should have his or her own pair or pairs. The heavy utility gloves are reusable and can be cleaned and disinfected or washed with an antimicrobial handwashing agent, rinsed, and dried. Some nitrile gloves are heat tolerant and can be steam sterilized.

Heat-resistant gloves for handling hot items should be used when unloading sterilizers or whenever there is a risk of burning the hands or forearms.

Other Activities

Gloves should be worn whenever there is a chance for contact with items potentially contaminated with pathogenic microorganisms. This includes handling appliances or equipment in the dental laboratory that have not been decontaminated. It also includes handling contaminated laundry, contaminated waste, tissue, or teeth, and containers of blood, saliva, or other infectious material if there is a risk of spilling or splashing.

Limitations of Gloves

The manufacturing process for patient care gloves may result in a low level of pinholes; however, the U.S. Food and Drug Administration has placed strict requirements on glove manufacturers to help ensure a high quality of these medical devices. Some manufacturers even test each glove for defects before they are sold.

Although gloves provide a high level of protection against direct contact with infectious agents through touching, they offer little protection against injuries with sharp objects such as instruments, needles, and scalpel blades. Thus contaminated sharps must still be handled safely even while wearing gloves. Sharps injuries also can and do occur through the heavy utility gloves during instrument processing.

Do not use gloves that are torn or have other noticeable defects. Do not reuse heavy utility gloves if they are peeling, cracking, discolored, torn, punctured, or show any other signs of deterioration.

Harmful Reactions to Gloves

Some health-care workers and patients have harmful reactions when they come into contact with latex gloves or with airborne glove materials. Since these reactions result from contact with latex proteins or other chemicals in the gloves, a brief description of glove manufacturing may help explain the origin of these chemicals.

Latex gloves are manufactured from latex extracted from the rubber tree *Hevea brasiliensis,* which grows in tropical areas throughout the world. The latex is in the form of a milky fluid to which anticoagulants and preservatives are first added. The latex fluid itself contains the rubber material (cis-1,4 polyisoprene), along with proteins, lipids, and carbohydrates. This latex material is then compounded by adding up to 200 different chemicals, depending on the desired characteristics of the final product. These chemicals are antidegradants, vulcanizing agents that make the latex elastic, accelerators, retarders, promoters, pigments, activators, and mold-releasing agents, and may also include fragrances, emulsifiers, stabilizers, biocides, and ultraviolet (UV) light absorbers. Hand-shaped porcelain formers coated with more chemicals and with cornstarch powder as a releasing agent are dipped into the compounded latex. The formers are then passed through ovens and a warm water leaching bath to remove some of the latex proteins and other chemicals. Further treatments include adding more cornstarch or a special chlorination treatment if powder-free gloves are desired. Items manufactured from natural latex are referred to as natural rubber latex (NRL) products.

Although allergies to the NRL in gloves are the major areas of concern, contact with other latex-containing products (Box 10-2) besides gloves also may induce a reaction. Currently it is estimated that about 1% to 6% of the general population and 8% to 12% of regularly exposed health-care workers are sensitive to latex.

There are three types of reactions that may occur with gloving. One is a skin reaction to irritants in the gloves called, *irritant contact dermatitis,* and the other two are the immunologic reactions of *allergic contact dermatitis* and *latex allergy.*

Irritant Contact Dermatitis

Most reactions from wearing gloves result from a nonimmunological irritation of the skin from non-latex chemicals in the gloves or applied to the hands. In these instances the skin on the hands becomes dry, reddened, itchy, and sometimes cracked in severe cases.

Conditions that may initiate or aggravate this dermatitis include handwashing with irritating cleaners or antiseptics, failure to completely rinse, failure to thoroughly dry hands after rinsing, excessive perspiration on the hands, and irritation from cornstarch powder.

To reverse and prevent recurrence of irritant contact dermatitis, attempt to identify the irritant by first making sure proper handwashing is performed (p. 125). Also consider changing glove and/or handwashing agent brands. When changing glove brands be sure

---

Box 10-2   Examples of Items That May Contain Latex*

Dental Products	**Other Products**
Gloves	Stethoscopes
Rubber dam	Tourniquets
Prophy cups	Electrode pads
Anesthetic carpules	Rubber aprons and sheets
Nitrous oxide masks	Intravenous ports
Orthodontic rings	Catheters and ventilator tubing
Bite blocks	Syringe stoppers
Mixing bowls	Automobile tires
Liquid droppers	Handlebar grips
Blood pressure cuffs	Carpeting and adhesives
Elastic bands	Racquet handles
Suction adapters	Dishwashing gloves
Some masks	Elastic bands
	Condoms and diaphragms
	Balloons and rubber toys
	Baby bottle nipples and pacifiers
	Hot water bottles and raincoats
	Erasers and rubber bands

---

*Some of these items are available in latex-free forms.

to determine if a different brand is really a different type of glove. Because the same glove may be sold under many different brands, compare samples before purchasing "new" gloves in large volumes.

Allergic Contact Dermatitis

There are four types of immunological hypersensitivities or allergies (I, II, III, IV). Two of these types (I and IV) are involved in reactions to gloves, and both types require a person to first become sensitized to an agent (called an allergen) that on subsequent contact will cause a harmful reaction. Allergic contact dermatitis (ACD) is type IV hypersensitivity, also called delayed hypersensitivity. It is the most frequently occurring immunologic reaction to gloves, accounting for about 80% of the cases. Type I hypersensitivity to glove latex is described below.

ACD is almost always limited to the areas of contact and is characterized by initial itching, redness, and vesicles within 24 to 48 hours, followed by dry skin, fissures, and sores. The reaction to poison ivy also is a type IV hypersensitivity. ACD caused by contact with gloves results from exposure to one of the many chemicals added during latex harvesting, processing, or glove manufacturing. The most common chemical sensitizers are the accelerators used in vulcanization: thiurams, carbamates, and mercaptobenzothiazoles. Vulcanization is the polymerizing process that makes the latex elastic. In two studies of patients with allergic reactions to gloves, 72% and 83% were patch test positive for thiurams and 25% and 22% were positive for carbamates. The patch test contains small amounts of different chemcials that when applied to the skin of an allergic person will produce a small reaction indicating the specific causative agent.

Eliminating contact with the sensitizing agent is the only way to prevent ACD. Glove manufacturers attempt to control the addition of chemicals to latex products but a confusing point is the labeling of gloves as "hypoallergenic" just because they may contain reduced levels of certain chemicals. Such gloves are not free of all potentially sensitizing chemicals and may still be able to induce harmful reactions. In the near future, the FDA will prohibit such labeling or at least require changes so it will be less confusing.

Latex Allergy

Mechanisms.   Latex allergy is the third type of reaction to gloves and the second type involving an immune response. Latex allergy is a type I hypersensitivity, also called an immediate hypersensitivity. In this instance, a person is allergic to the naturally occurring proteins present in latex. A person who develops a latex allergy first becomes sensitized by one or more exposures to latex protein allergens before reaction to a subsequent exposure can occur. In sensitization, IgE antibodies develop after exposure to the latex protein allergens. These antibodies bind to special cells in the body called mast cells, but a harmful reaction doesn't occur yet. When more latex protein allergen enters the body (with subsequent exposure), the mast cells are stimulated to produce substances that can cause skin reactions, and occasionally more serious systemic reactions that effect blood flow and breathing or cause anaphylaxis.

Symptoms.   The symptoms of a latex allergy reaction usually begin within 20 minutes or so after contact with NRL and may be skin reactions of urticaria (hives), redness, burning, and itching. More severe reactions may involve respiratory symptoms such as runny nose, sneezing, watery itchy eyes, scratchy throat, and asthma (difficult breathing, coughing spells, wheezing). Anaphylactic shock is rarely seen as the first sign of latex allergy but could occur with subsequent exposures. Of the 80 cases of anaphylactic shock to NRL reported in the medical literature up to 1995, 15 people died.

Airborne latex proteins.   Of particular concern in latex allergy is the potential for exposure to the NRL protein allergens present in the glove cornstarch powder. These proteins can migrate from the glove into the cornstarch, which causes more protein to be associated with the skin. This cornstarch becomes aerosolized when gloves are removed from boxes and when they are "snapped" during donning or removal. If a latex-sensitive person inhales airborne latex proteins, they may have a serious respiratory or systemic reaction. Another very important aspect of protein-laden cornstarch is that after it is airborne, it can "travel" extensively throughout the office, clinic, or building and expose many persons to these allergens. Studies of other allergy-causing substances have shown that the higher the overall exposure in a population, the greater the likelihood that more individuals will become sensitized. Unfortunately, the amount of latex exposure needed to produce sensitization or to produce a reaction is not known. However, reductions in exposure are known to decrease sensitization.

Preventing or Managing Latex Allergies

In the dental worker.   As with all other NRL allergies, avoiding contact/exposure with latex protein is necessary to prevent reactions in a sensitive person. In the dental setting this is hopefully accomplished by use of non-latex gloves and other items and establishment of a "latex-safe" environment (or at least a reduced presence of latex). If latex

---

Box 10-3   Recommendations From NIOSH* for Preventing Latex Allergies in the Workplace

What Workers Should Do

Use non-latex gloves when appropriate

If latex gloves are used, use powder-free gloves with reduced protein content

If latex gloves are used, do not use oil- or petroleum-based hand lotions unless they have been shown to reduce latex-related problems

After removing latex gloves, wash hands with a mild detergent and dry thoroughly

Frequently clean areas that may be contaminated with latex-powder (upholstery, carpets, ventilation ducts, and plenums)

Frequently change ventilation filters and vacuum bags used in latex-contaminated areas

Take advantage of latex allergy training provided by your employer and learn about procedures for preventing latex allergies and about latex allergy symptoms (skin rash; hives; flushing; itching; nasal, eye, or sinus symptoms; asthma; and shock)

If symptoms of latex allergy develop, avoid direct contact with latex-containing gloves and other items until after seeing a physician

If a latex allergy develops, consult a physician regarding the following precautions: avoid contact with latex-containing products; avoid areas where powder may be inhaled from latex gloves; tell employer about the latex allergy; wear a medical alert bracelet

Carefully follow physicians instructions for dealing with allergic reactions to latex

What Employers Should Do

Provide workers with non-latex gloves

If latex gloves are chosen, provide reduced protein, powder-free gloves

Assure that workers use good housekeeping practices to remove latex-containing dust from the workplace: identify areas contaminated with latex dust for frequent cleaning (upholstery, carpets, ventilation ducts, and plenums) and make sure that workers change ventilation filters and vacuum bags frequently in latex-containing areas

Provide workers with education programs and training materials about latex allergy

Periodically screen high-risk workers for latex allergy symptoms. Detecting symptoms early and removing symptomatic workers from latex exposure are essential for preventing long-term health effects

Evaluate current prevention strategies whenever a worker is diagnosed with latex allergy

---

*National Institute for Occupational Safety and Health. Department of Health and Human Service (NIOSH) Publication No. 97-135, June, 1997.

gloves are used, they should be the powder-free, reduced-protein type to eliminate airborne latex-protein allergens. The National Institute of Occupational Safety and Health, a division of CDC, has issued recommendations for preventing latex allergies (Box 10-3).

    In patients. The first approach to addressing latex allergies in dental patients is to include appropriate questions in the medical history (Box 10-4). Sensitivities to NRL-proteins are greater in certain individuals and this includes persons who have occupational ex-

> ### *Box 10-4* Questions About Latex Allergy to Include in the Patient Medical History
>
> 1. Are you allergic to latex or rubber products?
> 2. Have you ever had a reaction to balloons, gloves, dental dams, condoms, diaphragms, elastic bands, rubber toys?
> 3. Are you allergic to any foods (particularly bananas, chestnuts, avocados, kiwis), medications, or other things?
> 4. Did you have major surgical procedures as an infant?
> 5. Did you have more than two operations as a child?
> 6. Does your health bring you in to contact with latex-containing products (e.g., with catheterizations, dental work, enemas)?
> 7. Have you ever been tested for allergies?
> 8. Have you ever had asthma or hay fever?
> 9. Do you wear rubber gloves frequently at home or work?
> 10. Do you work around latex-containing products?
>
> Positive responses to questions 1 through 5 indicate the need for further skin testing unless a latex allergy was confirmed by testing. Positive responses to the other questions may indicate closer investigation, possibly skin testing.

posure to latex. Persons with spina bifida, urogenital anomalies, and spinal cord injuries are considered at high risk. A history of allergies in the patient or patient's family is also important to consider. The same is true if a person is allergic to foods, particularly bananas, chestnuts, avocados, or kiwis. Providing dental care for a latex allergic patient should be done in an environment with latex ALARP (as low as reasonably possible). The following will help achieve this.

- Provide treatment in a specially prepared room as first patient of the day
  —No latex worn by staff preparing treatment room
  —All items that will contact patient are to be handled with non-latex gloves
  —Do not let any one into the treatment room who has worn latex gloves that day
- Minimize previous contact of patient care items with latex containing materials
- Prevent latex from directly contacting the patient during treatment (use latex alternatives)
- Minimize patient exposure to airborne latex-protein in glove powder
- Have dental team wear non-latex–containing items that may contact the patient

HANDWASHING

Protective Value

Hands are one of the most important sources of microorganisms in disease spread. Handwashing is an important type of personal hygiene for everyone but it is a primary disease prevention procedure for health-care workers in dentistry and medicine.

There are two types of microbial flora on the hands: resident and transient skin flora. The *resident skin flora* consists of microorganisms that colonize the skin and become permanent residents. They are always there and can never be totally removed even with a surgical scrub (likely because the resident flora can exist even several layers under the surface in the stratum corneum) but their numbers can be reduced. Although members of the resident skin flora can cause infection when directly or indirectly spread to others, they are likely less important in disease spread than the second type of skin flora, the *transient skin flora*. The microorganisms of this flora contaminate the hands during the touching of or other exposure to contaminated surfaces. They do not usually colonize and survive on the hands for long periods; thus they are called members of the transient flora (they "come and go"). The transient flora serves as a source of disease spread because it can contain just about any pathogenic microorganism, depending on how the hands become contaminated. Fortunately, the transient flora can be removed or greatly reduced by routine handwashing, usually because the contaminating microorganisms remain primarily on the outer layers of the skin.

Although handwashing clearly reduces the spread of disease agents, it also reduces the number of microorganisms that may contaminate and subsequently cause a harmful infection of or through the hands. Thus handwashing protects patients and the dental team.

Handwashing Procedures and Agents

The mechanical action of handwashing is very important to suspend dirt and microorganisms from the skin surface so they can be rinsed away with water. Step-by-step procedures for routine handwashing and surgical scrubbing are given in Box 10-5.

Although plain soap without antimicrobial activity performs well in removing dirt and some transient microorganisms from the hands, it has little effect on the resident flora. *Health-care personnel handwashing products* contain low to medium levels of antimicrobial agents. Their frequent use in 10- to 30-second routine handwashing procedures minimizes the number of transient microorganisms on the hands and aids in reducing the number of resident bacteria by means of their bactericidal chemical activity. *Surgical scrub products* contain the highest levels of antimicrobial agents and are used in a more vigorous scrubbing procedure when maximum reduction in transient and resident flora are desired, such as before surgical procedures. Nevertheless, the surgical scrub procedure will not sterilize the hands.

Common antimicrobial agents in handwashing products include chlorhexidine digluconate (CHG), povidone iodine (PI), para-chlorometaxylenol (PCMX), and triclosan (TLS). Chlorhexidine digluconate is well known for its widespread antimicrobial activity and its residual activity (prolonged antimicrobial effect). CHG binds to the skin to give prolonged release of antimicrobial activity. TLS also may have a prolonged effect, whereas persistence of PCMX on skin may be less. PI does not exhibit prolonged activity. It is very important to wash hands every time before gloving and after removing gloves. When the skin is occluded (tightly covered up) with gloves, members of the resident flora, and to a lesser extent the transient flora, dramatically increase. This increase may be as great as 4,000-fold per hour. This increased growth of microorganisms in the warm, moist environment under gloves can cause skin irritation. Washing hands before gloving reduces the number of microorganisms to begin with, and washing after removing gloves reduces the number of those that have increased, as well as the transient microorganisms that may

---

Box 10-5   Handwashing **Step-by-Step Procedures**

At Beginning of Day

1. Remove jewelry and gently clean fingernails
2. Scrub hands, nails, and forearms with a liquid, antimicrobial, handwashing agent and soft sterile brush or sponge for one minute and rinse with cool to lukewarm water for 10 seconds
3. Vigorously lather hands and forearms with the germicidal agent for 20 seconds and rinse with cool to lukewarm water for 10 seconds
4. Dry hands, then forearms, with clean paper towels and use the towels to turn off hand-controlled sink faucets

Routine Handwashing During the Day

1. Vigorously lather hands and forearms with a liquid, antimicrobial, handwashing agent for 20 seconds and rinse with cool to lukewarm water for 10 seconds
2. Repeat lathering and rinsing
3. Dry hands, then forearms, with clean paper towels and use towels to turn off hand-controlled sink faucets

Before Surgery

1. Remove jewelry and gently clean fingernails
2. Scrub nails, hands, and forearms with an antimicrobial surgical scrub product and a soft sterile brush or sponge for 5 to 7 minutes using multiple scrub and rinse cycles
3. Rinse hands and forearms with cool to lukewarm water starting with the fingers and keeping your hands above the level of your elbows. Let the water drip from your elbows, not your hands
4. Dry with sterile towels
5. Put on sterile gloves by inserting hands into the gloves held around the wrists by an assistant wearing sterile gloves
6. Check the gloves for defects and do not touch contaminated items or surfaces before patient care

---

Adapted from Miller CH: Practical barrier techniques. In Cottone JC, Terezhalmy GT, Molinari JA, editors: *Practical Infection Control in Dentistry,* Philadelphia, Lea & Febiger, 1991.

have contacted the skin through defects in the gloves. Handwashing after gloves are removed also helps remove any powder containing latex protein.

The routine use of a handwashing product containing an antimicrobial agent with a prolonged effect maintains minimum levels of microorganisms on the skin. Aseptic techniques associated with handwashing include the use of faucets controlled by foot pedals, elbow handles, "electric eyes," or ultrasonics. Foot-operated or electric eye soap dispensers also prevent contamination of the hands from multi-use soap containers. "Squeeze-bottle" soap dispensers facilitate cross-contamination and are not recommended. Also, bar soaps in soap dishes tend to accumulate skin and environmental microorganisms and are not recommended for health care facilities.

MASKS

Protective Value

Masks were developed originally to reduce the chances of postoperative infections in patients that were caused by microorganisms in the respiratory tracts of the surgeons. Although some controversy exists as to the ability of masks to accomplish their original purpose, wearing a mask is still standard practice during surgery, or at any other time when it may be important to reduce the spread of potential respiratory disease agents. In recent years, a face mask has been viewed also as a means to protect the one who wears the mask from disease agents that might be present in sprays, splashes, or even some aerosol particles of body fluids or other potentially infectious materials. In dentistry, masks protect mucous membranes of the nose and mouth of the dental team from contact with sprays or splashes of oral fluids from the patient or from items contaminated with patient fluids. Also, some degree of protection to the dental team likely occurs from the prevention of inhaling aerosolized particles of oral fluids that may contain infectious disease agents. Masks worn by the dental team may give some protection to the patients.

Uses and Types of Face Masks

Face masks should be worn by the dental team any time there is a risk of spraying or splashing of fluids that may contain potentially infectious disease agents. This may occur during patient care activities involving high-speed or low-speed handpieces, ultrasonic scalers, air/water syringes, oral irrigators, and during grinding or splashing of items that may be contaminated with patient fluids. The mask should be changed with every patient because its outer surface becomes contaminated with droplets from sprays of oral fluids from the previous patient or from touching the mask with saliva-coated fingers. A mask also protects from splashes of contaminated ultrasonic or other cleaning solutions that may occur if the cleaning basket or instruments are accidentally dropped into the solution. Rinsing of instruments under tap water also may cause splashing.

Face masks are composed of synthetic material that serves to filter out at least 95% of small particles that directly contact the mask. In 1995, the National Institute of Occupational Safety (a part of the Public Health Service) indicated that it would certify three classes of filters, N-, R-, and P-series with three levels of filter efficiency: 95%, 99%, and 99.97% in each class. All filter tests are to employ particles that are of aerosol size: 0.3 mm aerodynamic mass median diameter. Some masks have a preformed dome shape and others are pliable. They may be secured with an elastic band, ear loops, or ties (Figure 10-2). Most are formfitting over the bridge of the nose to reduce fogging of eyewear from warm expelled air that escapes around the edge of the mask during breathing.

Limitations of Face Masks

Face masks do not provide a perfect seal around their edges, and exhaled and inhaled air that is not filtered can pass through these sites. Thus it is important to select a mask that fits the face well to minimize passage of unfiltered air. Also, when a mask is wetted from moist exhaled air, the resistance to airflow through the mask increases, causing more unfiltered air to pass by the edges of the mask. Thus wet masks should be replaced, maybe every 20 minutes, to maintain high filterability.

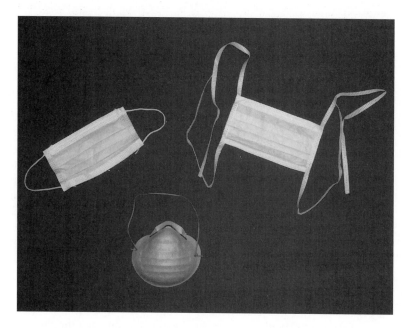

FIGURE 10-2   Facemasks. Other types not shown are available.

PROTECTIVE EYEWEAR

Protective Value

A variety of disease agents may cause harmful infection of the eyes or enter the associated mucous membranes and cause systemic infections. An example is the herpes simplex virus, which may be present in sprays or aerosols of oral fluids from a patient. Another example is the hepatitis B virus, which may use the eye as a portal of entry into the body and cause hepatitis B.

Besides protecting against infectious disease agents, eyewear also protects against physical damage to the eyes by propelled objects such as tooth fragments or small pieces of a restorative material exiting a patient's mouth during cavity preparation. Impact damage to the eyes can occur from any polishing, grinding, or buffing procedure, be it performed in a patient's mouth, at chairside, or in the dental laboratory. Eyewear also can protect against eye damage from ultraviolet irradiation and from splashes of chemicals used at chairside or for cleaning instruments and surfaces, disinfecting surfaces, developing radiographs, or for work in the dental laboratory.

Patients should be offered eye protection during treatment. Reports of eye damage to patients include impalement of a patient's eye by an excavator, corneal abrasion from an exploding anesthetic carpule and from a piece of acrylic denture tooth, and subconjunctival hemorrhage after a dentist hit a patient's eye with his thumb. Instruments and chemicals should not be passed over the head of the patient. If a patient wears prescription eyeglasses, they should be allowed to continue to wear them during care; other patients should be provided with eye protection. Disposable eyewear should be provided or patient eyewear can be decontaminated between use.

Uses and Types of Protective Eyewear

Protective eyewear should be worn whenever there may be contamination of the eyes with aerosols, sprays, or splashes of body fluids or chemicals and whenever projectiles may be generated during any grinding, polishing, or buffing procedure with rotary instruments or equipment. Protective eyewear worn by the dental team should be thoroughly decontaminated before reuse with subsequent patients. Appropriate eye protection also should be used when using ultraviolet irradiation. Table 10-1 compares different types of eye protection in relation to the American National Standard for Occupational and Educational Eye and Face Protection, Z87.1-1989. The design, construction, testing, and use of eye and face protection devices should be in accordance with this standard developed by the American National Standards Institute (ANSI).

Limitations of Protective Eyewear

Goggles that may be used by themselves or over prescription glasses (Figure 10-3) give the greatest eye protection against front and side splashes and impacts. Although glasses give protection against front splashes and impacts, side protection is poor unless they have shields (Figure 10-4). The degree of impact protection from projectiles depends on the strength of the lenses as determined by the ANSI standard. Some protective eyeglasses have replaceable lenses (if scratching occurs), have antifogging properties, and are autoclavable. The OSHA bloodborne pathogens standard (see Chapter 8) indicates that appropriate protective eyewear, in relation to splashes or sprays of body fluids, provides protection to the front and the sides of the eyes.

If face shields are used, they should be chin-length, provide top protection, and be curved to provide side protection. Some faceshields are made of thin plastic and may not offer adequate protection against particles with a high impact velocity. Also, masks should be worn with faceshields to reduce inhalation of fluid aerosols and "dust" particles.

PROTECTIVE CLOTHING

Protective Value

Potentially infectious microorganisms may be present in the aerosols, sprays, splashes, and droplets from the oral fluids of patients. These not only contaminate unprotected eyes and mucous membranes of the mouth and nose but also contaminate other body sites of the dental team, including the forearms and chest area. Larger droplets also may settle on the lap while seated at chairside. Outer protective clothing can protect against this contamination, which otherwise may lead to infection through nonintact skin or at least to spread of the contamination from office to home or elsewhere on unprotected clothing. Changing of obviously contaminated protective clothing before providing care for the next patient is perceived as providing patient protection. Also, covering up microorganisms present on street clothes with protective clothing is perceived to provide some degree of patient protection. This prevents shedding of microorganisms from street clothes into the air near a patient who may have open tissue. Although it seems reasonable to use protective clothing for dental team and patient protection, little evidence is available on the extent to which this prevents disease spread.

Table 10-1 Comparison of Eye Protection Devices

TYPE	FRONT SPLASH PROTECTION	SIDE SPLASH PROTECTION	FRONT IMPACT PROTECTION	SIDE IMPACT PROTECTION	NECK AND FACE PROTECTION
Goggles	Excellent	Excellent	Excellent	Excellent	Poor
Glasses (no shields)	Good	Poor	Excellent	Poor	Poor
Glasses (with shields)	Good	Good	Excellent	Fair	Poor
Face shield*	Excellent	Good to Excellent	Variable (depends on thickness)	Variable (depends on thickness)	Variable (depends on type/length)

*Should include side and top protection.
Adapted from American National Standards Institute, Inc: *Occupational and Educational Eye and Face Protection: Z87.1—1989.* New York, NY, American National Standards Institute, 1989, p. 15–18; and Palenik CJ, Miller CH: Protecting your eyes: it's the law, *Trends & Techniq Contemp Dental Lab* 8:69–74, 1991.

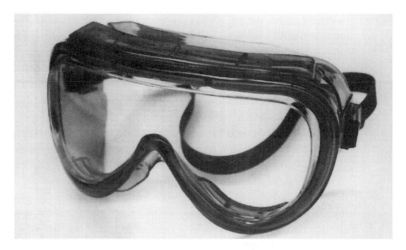

FIGURE 10-3   Goggles for eye protection. Other types not shown are available.

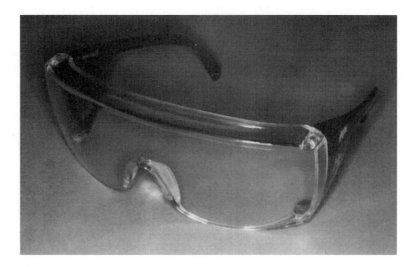

FIGURE 10-4   Protective eyeglasses with top and side shields. Other types not shown are available.

Uses and Types of Protective Clothing

Protective clothing should be worn whenever there is a chance for contamination of skin or other clothing with spray or splashes of saliva, blood, or other potentially infectious materials. Thus the same conditions at chairside that require use of masks and protective eyewear also require use of protective clothing. If this clothing becomes visibly soiled, it should be changed before caring for the next patient, and fresh protective clothing should be put on before surgery. Protective clothing should be removed when leaving clinical areas and should not be worn in lunch rooms or outside the office. The OSHA bloodborne pathogens standard also indicates that contaminated clothing and linens cannot be taken home by employees for laundering. Laundering is the responsibility of the employer through laundering in the office or by contracting with a commercial laundering service. Although not required by any law, dental team members also should consider having work shoes that are worn only in the office.

Protective clothing is the outer layer of clothing that protects/covers underlying work clothes, street clothes, undergarments, or skin. Examples include uniforms, clinic jackets, laboratory coats, aprons, and gowns. This clothing should protect against contamination of underlying clothes or skin, and materials with the greatest resistance to fluids provide the greatest protection. Few, if any, chairside dental procedures require fluid-proof clothing. Also, head covers and shoe covers are not mandated for use in dentistry but head covers may be appropriate to give maximum patient protection during surgery.

A convenient approach to office management of protective clothing involves use of disposable gowns with long sleeves and a high neck to cover regular work clothes (Figure 10-5). For routine dental procedures, these may be changed at least once a day (e.g., over the lunch hour) or more frequently if they become visibly soiled. Another approach is use of reusable protective clothing such as uniforms, lab coats, or other attire that may be put

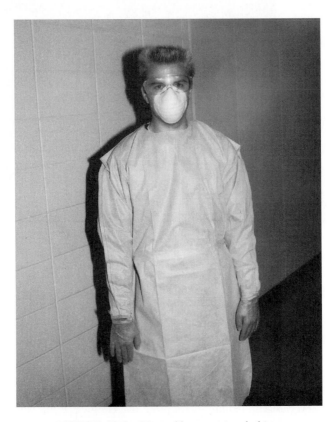

FIGURE 10-5   Disposable protective clothing.

on at the beginning of the day, but it must be changed for lunch, changed when it becomes visibly soiled, and removed before leaving the office. It is not wise to use protective clothing that is pulled on and removed over the head because removal may contaminate the face/head with the outside of the clothing. Reusable protective clothing is laundered in the office or sent to a laundry service.

PLACING AND REMOVING BARRIERS

All of the steps involved in chairside asepsis are presented in Chapter 17. However, procedures for putting on and taking off barriers will be further discussed here. Putting on and taking off barriers should be done in a sequence that limits further spread of microorganisms. This is true when preparing for routine and surgical procedures. For this discussion, it is assumed that the operatory has been cleaned and disinfected, surface covers placed, sterilized instrument packages or cassettes placed on the bracket table or cart, the patient has been seated, and the history and any discussions have been completed. The important point to remember about the sequence of putting on protective barriers is that gloves are put on last. This avoids contaminating the gloves before they are used in the patient's mouth.

The first step is to put on protective clothing (Box 10-6) and place the patient's bib. Unpackage the instruments and supply items without directly touching them. Next, put on mask and eyewear. Just before performing treatment, wash, rinse, and dry hands and put on gloves. Do not touch any contaminated items or surfaces with the gloves before they go into the patient's mouth.

After patient treatment, two key issues are considered when removing the now-contaminated protective barriers:

- Your gloves can contaminate anything they touch
- Your hands may become contaminated if you touch certain parts of the protective barriers with ungloved hands

One approach to removing contaminated barriers is also given in Box 10-6. If you are going to remove your contaminated protective clothing, do it first. To remove a disposable gown, pull it off over your gloved hands, turning it inside out, and immediately place it into a waste receptacle. When removing disposable or reusable protective clothing, do not touch underlying clothes or skin with the contaminated gloves. Next, remove gloves and wash your hands. When removing the gloves, do not touch your skin but rather pinch

---

Box 10-6   Putting On and Removing Barriers **Step-by-Step Procedures**

Putting On	Removing
1. Protective clothing	1. Disposable gown
2. Protective eyewear	2. Gloves
3. Mask	3. Protective eyewear
4. Gloves	4. Mask

the gloves in the wrist area on one hand, stretch it out away from the wrist, and slide it off toward the fingertips, but only slide it off about half way. Repeat this for the other hand, completely removing this glove and discarding it into the waste receptacle. Then go back to the first hand, place your ungloved thumb under the edge of the glove, which now has the noncontaminated side turned out. Stretch the glove out away from the hand, slide it completely off toward the fingertips, and place it into the waste receptacle. Remove eyeglasses by touching them only on the ear rests (which are usually not contaminated) and place them in an appropriate area from subsequent decontamination. Remove your mask by touching only the elastic bands around your head or ears or only the ties in back of your head. Immediately discard the mask into the waste receptacle. Wash, rinse, and dry your hands.

SELECTED READINGS

American Dental Association Councils on Scientific Affairs and Dental Practice, Instruments and Equipment, Dental Therapeutics, Dental Research and Dental Practice: Infection control recommendations for the dental office and the dental laboratory, *J Amer Dent Assoc* 127:672-680,1996.

American Dental Association. Belkin NL: Surgical gowns and drapes as aseptic barriers, *Am J Infect Control* 16:14-18, 1988.

Chen C-C, Willeke K: Aerosol penetration through surgical masks, *Am J Infect Control* 20:117-184, 1992.

Hamann CP: Natural rubber latex protein sensitivity in review, *Amer J Cont Derm* 4:1-21, 1993.

Hamann B, Hamann C, Taylor JS: Managing latex allergies in the dental office, *CDA Journal* 23:45-50, 1995.

Larson E, Kumudini M, Laughton BA: Influence of two handwashing frequencies in reduction in colonizing flora with three handwashing products used by health care personnel, *Am J Infect Control* 17:83-88, 1989.

Larson EL: APIC guideline for handwashing and hand antisepsis in health care settings, *Am J Infect Control* 23:251-269, 1995.

Manzella JP, McConville JH, Valenti W et al.: An outbreak of herpes simplex virus type I gingivostomatitis in a dental hygiene practice, *J Am Med Assoc* 252:2019-2222, 1984.

Miller CH: Barrier techniques for infection control, *Calif Dent Assoc J* 13:53-59, 1985.

Miller CH: Wide variety of barriers protect providers, patients, environment, *RDH* 12:14, 1992.

Smart ER, Macleod RI, Lawrence CM: Allergic reactions to rubber gloves in dental patients: report of three cases, *Br Dent J* 172:445-447, 1992.

Chapter 11

INSTRUMENT PROCESSING

Instrument processing is a collection of procedures that prepares contaminated instruments for reuse. The processing must be performed carefully so that disease agents from a previous patient, from a member of the dental team who handled the instruments, or from the environment will not be transferred by the instruments to the next patient. Processing also must be performed correctly to keep instrument damage to a minimum. The overall process consists of seven steps, outlined below. Although the steps are not particularly difficult to perform, each must be performed properly in a routine, disciplined manner to ensure the desired outcome of patient protection with minimal instrument damage.

STERILIZATION VERSUS DISINFECTION

Because killing of microorganisms is the ultimate goal of instrument processing, it is important to first have a general understanding of microbial killing methods before other steps in the process are described (Box 11-1).

Sterilization

Sterilization is a process intended to kill all microorganisms and is the highest level of microbial kill that can be achieved. Because it is not possible to routinely determine if a microbial killing process actually kills all microorganisms, a highly resistant microorganism is selected as the standard challenge. If the process kills this microorganism, it is considered to be a sterilization process. The bacterial endospore is selected as the standard challenge for sterilization because of its high resistance to killing by heat and chemicals (Figure 11-1). Endospores are more fully described in Chapter 2 and later in the section on Sterilization Monitoring. These spores are more difficult to kill than all of the common pathogenic microorganisms, including *Mycobacterium tuberculosis,* hepatitis viruses, HIV-1, fungal spores, herpesviruses, *Staphylococcus aureus,* and the thousands of other microorganisms. Thus a process cannot be called a sterilization process unless it is capable of killing high levels of bacterial endospores (is sporicidal). There are three types of sterilization processes used in dentistry: (1) heat sterilization, (2) gas sterilization, and (3) liquid chemical sterilization. Other types of sterilization procedures exist but they have not been applied to the field of dentistry or have not yet been made practical for use in the office. Heat sterilization involving steam, dry heat, and unsaturated chemical vapor is the most common type of sterilization used in offices today. The heat sterilizers operate at 250° F to 375° F, and their sterilization processes can be routinely monitored for effectiveness using bacterial endospores (called biologic monitoring).

Box 11-1   Instrument Processing

1. Holding (presoaking)
2. Precleaning
3. Corrosion control, drying, lubrication
4. Packaging
5. Sterilization
6. Sterilization monitoring
7. Handling processed instruments

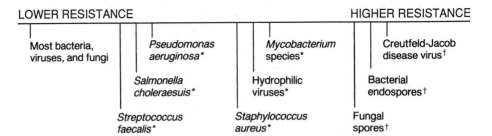

LOWER RESISTANCE   HIGHER RESISTANCE

Most bacteria, viruses, and fungi	*Pseudomonas aeruginosa**	*Mycobacterium species**	Creutfeld-Jacob disease virus[†]
	*Salmonella choleraesuis**	Hydrophilic viruses*	Bacterial endospores[†]
	*Streptococcus faecalis**	*Staphylococcus aureus**	Fungal spores[†]

FIGURE 11-1   Relative resistance of microorganisms to killing with chemicals and heat. *Higher resistance to killing with chemicals; [†]higher resistance to killing with both chemicals and heat.

Ethylene oxide gas sterilizers that operate at 72° F to 140° F (much lower than heat sterilizers) also can be monitored with bacterial endospores but this type of sterilization is not commonly used in dental offices because of the long exposure time required for sterilization, the high cost of gas sterilizers, and the required special handling of the ethylene oxide gas sterilant.

Liquid chemical sterilization is used on items that are damaged by heat sterilization. The liquid chemical sterilant used is 2.0% to 3.4% glutaraldehyde, and although it can be shown to be sporicidal in controlled laboratory testing, the microbial killing that occurs during actual use in the office cannot be routinely determined. Spore tests for biologic monitoring have not yet been developed for office-testing of liquid sterilants. The best that can be done is to chemically estimate the concentration of active glutaraldehyde remaining in the used solution. It slowly becomes inactive. More information about sterilization is given later in this chapter.

Disinfection

Disinfection is a less lethal process than sterilization and is intended to kill disease-producing microorganisms but not bacterial endospores. Disinfection usually refers to the use of liquid chemicals to kill microorganisms at room temperature on surfaces. If the chemical is not sporicidal but can kill other microorganisms, it is called a disinfectant. There are several types of disinfectants (e.g., synthetic phenolics, phenol, iodophors, alcohol-phenolics, sodium hypochlorite, quaternary ammonium compounds, alcohol, alcohol-quaternary ammonium compounds). Chemicals classified as disinfectants cannot be expected to achieve sterilization. Details on these disinfectants and their uses are given in Chapter 12 but an important point to understand here is that the level of microbial killing actually achieved by these disinfectants cannot be routinely determined during use in the office. Thus one never knows how well disinfectants are working.

Some liquid chemicals are sporicidal (sterilants) under some conditions and nonsporicidal (disinfectants) under other conditions. Glutaraldehyde (as discussed above) is a sterilant when used at 2.0% to 3.4% concentrations but only after a 10-hour contact time on precleaned items. When used at lower concentrations or for shorter times, it can achieve only disinfection. Also, as already mentioned, microbial killing by glutaraldehyde (or any other liquid chemical) cannot be determined in the office.

Sterility Assurance for Patient Protection

Universal sterilization means that all reusable instruments and handpieces are sterilized (rather than just disinfected) between use on patients. This provides the highest level of patient protection. If an item used in the patient's mouth cannot be sterilized or cannot withstand the conditions of sterilization, or cannot be prevented from becoming contaminated during use, it should not be used or should be discarded after use on one patient.

Maximum patient protection with universal sterilization can be achieved only by practicing *sterility assurance.* Since the sterility of each processed instrument cannot be routinely measured, one must depend on the reliability of the instrument processing procedures being performed. Thus sterility assurance is the correct performance of the proper instrument processing steps and monitoring of the sterilization step with biologic and chemical indicators. This assurance program is achieved by taking four steps:

- Select the proper procedure and confirm the correct way to perform that procedure
- Prepare a written step-by-step description of the correct procedure to be used as a reference in training and to document patient safety techniques used in the office
- Incorporate the procedure into the office training program to assure that new employees learn the correct procedure
- Monitor the performance of the procedure to assure its routine use and, when possible, measure the results of the procedure

The statement that "instruments have been sterilized" is true only if sterility assurance is practiced, showing by frequent biologic and chemical monitoring that the process used kills bacterial endospores.

INSTRUMENT PROCESSING PROCEDURES

Box 11-2 presents suggested step-by-step procedures for instrument processing. Contaminated instruments must be handled very carefully to avoid cuts and punctures from sharp items, any of which constitute an exposure. Always use personal protective equipment, including utility gloves, mask, and protective eyewear and clothing during these procedures.

Box 11-2   Instrument Processing **Step-by-Step Procedures**

1. Put on heavy utility gloves, protective eyewear, mask, and protective clothing
2. Gross debris may be removed from instruments by wiping at chairside but only if great care is taken to avoid sharp injuries
3. Place loose, contaminated instruments in ultrasonic cleaning basket and place basket in holding solution until ready to thoroughly clean. If using cassettes, remove and dispose of waste and rinse cassette/instruments with water
4. Remove basket of instruments from holding solution, rinse with minimum splashing, and place in ultrasonic cleaner, or place cassettes in cleaning rack and place rack in cleaner
5. Make sure cleaning unit has been filled to proper level with cleaning solution
6. Place cover on cleaning unit and operate for the time recommended by the cleaning unit manufacturer and/or cassette manufacturer. In general, these times are 4 to 6 minutes (loose instruments) or 16 minutes (cassettes)
7. Remove cover and lift out cleaning basket or cassette rack and rinse under tap water with a minimum of splashing. Rinse cassettes individually and thoroughly
8. Check instruments for broken tips and cleanliness, and dry loose instruments with a towel or let cassette drain. Replace or re-clean items as needed. Apply rust inhibitor as needed for nonstainless items to be processed in steam
9. Place instruments into functional sets or add desired items to cassettes, including the appropriate biological and chemical indicators. Use packaging material that is compatible with the method of sterilization. Seal the package or wrap the cassette and label for content identification and sterilization date. Make sure chemical indicators are present or visible on the outside of the packages
10. Sterilize following manufacturer's recommendations for loading, sterilizing time, and temperature drying
11. Observe external chemical indicators for proper reaction
12. Store or distribute packages to chairside, retrieve biological indicators for analysis, and observe internal chemical indicators
13. Maintain sterility assurance records on results, date, and conditions of sterilization for biological and chemical indicators

Prepared by CH Miller with personal communication from Kathryn Bernard.

Holding (Presoaking)

If instruments cannot be cleaned soon after use, place them in a holding solution to prevent drying of the saliva and blood. This can facilitate the actual cleaning. Some plastic/resin cassette manufacturers do not recommend presoaking, so follow their instructions for cleaning. Extended presoaking for more than a few hours is not recommended because this may enhance corrosion of some instruments. The holding solution may be the same detergent as that to be used for subsequent cleaning or it may be water or an enzyme solution. Place loose instruments in a perforated cleaning basket and then place the basket in the holding solution (Figure 11-2). Use of the basket reduces direct han-

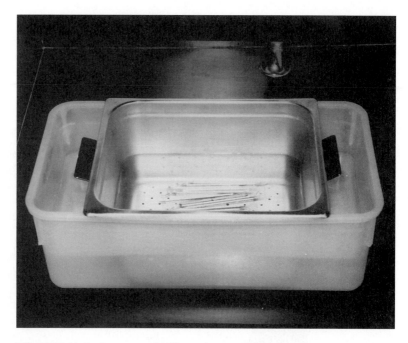

FIGURE 11-2 Instrument holding prior to precleaning. Instruments are placed in an ultrasonic cleaning basket and the basket is placed in a pan of the holding solution.

dling of instruments through the subsequent rinsing, cleaning, and rinsing steps. The presoaked instruments and the holding solution must be considered contaminated. The solution should be discarded at least once a day (or earlier if visibly soiled) while wearing protective equipment.

Precleaning

Precleaning is an essential step before any sterilization or disinfection procedure. It reduces the number of microorganisms present and removes blood, saliva, and other materials that may insulate microorganisms from the sterilizing agent. A "dirty" instrument may in some instances become sterile during subsequent processing but this cannot be confirmed. (Besides, a patient will never be convinced that a dirty instrument is safe for use, even if it really is sterile!)

Ultrasonic Cleaning

Ultrasonic cleaning, compared with scrubbing instruments by hand, reduces direct handling of the contaminated instruments and the chances for cuts and punctures. It is also an excellent cleaning mechanism, and staff can do other tasks while the instruments are being cleaned. The ultrasonic energy produces billions of tiny bubbles in the cleaning solution that collapse and create high turbulence at the surface of the instruments. This dislodges the debris and suspends it in the solution or it dissolves. Very few instruments cannot be ultrasonically cleaned. One exception is some high-speed handpieces, although others can withstand ultrasonics. Check the handpiece manufacturers' instructions for cleaning.

Ultrasonic cleaning units come in several sizes that are freestanding or can be built into countertops to accommodate any office or clinic that processes instruments that are loose or are in cassettes (Figure 11-3). Always use a cleaning basket or rack to suspend the items in the cleaning solution, and operate the unit with the cover in place following the manufacturer's directions.

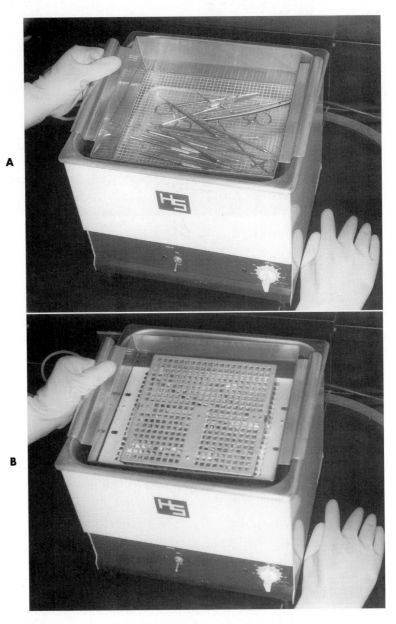

FIGURE 11-3 Ultrasonic cleaning of instruments. **A,** Loose instruments in a basket; **B,** instruments in cassettes that can be held in a basket or cleaning rack.

Use a cleaning solution that is recommended for use in ultrasonic cleaners and maintain the solution at the proper level in the cleaning chamber, ensuring that all items being cleaned are completely submerged. Cleaning solutions that also have antimicrobial activity will reduce the buildup of microorganisms in the solution as it is repeatedly used. However, common disinfectants should not be used in place of a detergent solution unless they are designed for this use. Instruments should be processed in the cleaner until they are visibly clean. This time may vary, depending on the instruments, the amount or type of material on the instruments, and the efficiency of the ultrasonic unit. This time ranges from about 4 to 15 minutes. Instruments in plastic/resin cassettes require longer cleaning times because the plastic/resin absorbs some of the ultrasonic energy.

After cleaning, remove the basket or cassette rack and thoroughly rinse the instruments under tap water with a minimum of splashing. The cleaned instruments and cassettes are still contaminated and must be handled with gloves. Discard the cleaning solution at least daily, earlier if it becomes visibly soiled. Rinse, disinfect, rinse, and dry the cleaning chamber at the end of the day while wearing protective equipment.

The functioning of an ultrasonic unit can be tested using the aluminum foil test. Cut a piece of lightweight aluminum foil about one inch shorter than the length of the chamber and one inch longer than the depth of the solution in the chamber. Insert the foil vertically into the filled chamber with the length of the foil running the length of the chamber and the bottom of the foil about one inch above the bottom. Do not let the foil touch the bottom of the tank. Operate the unit for 20 seconds. Remove the foil and observe for small indentations (pebbling) on the foil. This pebbling should be fairly evenly distributed over the entire foil. If there are areas greater than one half inch square having no pebbling, the unit may need servicing. Some ultrasonic unit manufacturers may use variations of this aluminum foil procedure described here, follow their specific directions.

Manual Scrubbing of Instruments

Scrubbing contaminated instruments by hand is dangerous even though it is a very effective method of removing debris, if performed properly. All surfaces of all instruments should be thoroughly brushed while the instruments are submerged in a cleaning solution to avoid spattering. It is also best to use a long-handled brush to keep the scrubbing hand as far away from the sharp instrument tips as possible. This is followed by thorough rinsing with a minimum of splashing.

Routine manual scrubbing of instruments is not recommended, however, because it requires maximum direct contact with the contaminated instruments, increasing the chances for cuts or punctures through the gloves. Also, there is no real need to hand scrub and ultrasonically clean all instruments if the ultrasonic cleaner is working properly; occasionally, however, an ultrasonically cleaned item may need additional hand cleaning to remove some cements.

Instrument Washers

Washers designed to clean medical and dental instruments are used in some large facilities (hospitals, dental schools) and in some smaller dental offices. These units automatically provide cleaning and rinsing and some (called washer-disinfectors) use very hot water and achieve disinfection of the instruments with cleaning. Instrument washers are FDA-regulated medical devices. Household dishwashers are not recommended for use on contaminated instruments because their manufacturers did not design them for this purpose and have not sought FDA assurances of safety and effectiveness.

CORROSION CONTROL, DRYING, AND LUBRICATION

Instruments or portions of instruments and burs made of carbon steel will rust during steam sterilization. Examples might be non–stainless steel cutting or scraping instruments such as scalers, hoes, hacketts, the cutting surfaces of orthodontic pliers, and the grasping surfaces of forceps. Although rust inhibitors (e.g., sodium nitrite) that can be sprayed on the instruments or used as a dip will reduce rusting of some of these items, the best approach is not to process such items through steam. Instead, thoroughly dry the instruments and use dry heat or unsaturated chemical vapor sterilization.

Instruments to be processed through a steam sterilizer should at least be shaken to remove excess water or dried more thoroughly if they will be packaged in paper or paper-plastic sterilization wrap. This will avoid accidental tearing of wet paper during packaging. Some hinged instruments may need to be lubricated to maintain proper functioning but as much excess lubricant as possible should be removed before heat processing.

Packaging

Proper instrument processing is more than just sterilizing instruments between patients. It is **delivering sterile instruments to chairside** for use on the next patient. To do this, the sterility of the instruments must be maintained after sterilization. Packaging instruments before processing through the sterilizer prevents them from becoming contaminated after sterilization during storage or when being distributed to chairside. Unpackaged instruments are completely exposed to the environment immediately after the sterilizer door is opened and can be contaminated by dust or aerosols in the air, by improper handling, or by contact with contaminated surfaces.

Packaging involves organizing the cleaned instruments in functional sets and wrapping them or placing them in sterilization pouches, bags, trays, or cassettes. Biologic and chemical indicators (described later) are added during the packaging procedures.

General Packaging Procedures

Only use packaging material or open containers that have been designed for use in sterilizers, and use the appropriate sterilization packaging materials for the sterilization method being used (Box 11-3). Other wrap, plastic bags, containers, or paper may melt, prevent the sterilizing agent from penetrating to the instruments inside, or may release unwanted chemicals into the sterilizer chamber. Sterilization pouches, wraps, or bags should never be sealed with metal closures, including staples or anything that can puncture the material and breech sterility.

Closed containers such as trays or pans with solid tops and bottoms, capped glass vials, or wrap such as aluminum foil should never be used to package items for sterilization in steam or unsaturated chemical vapor sterilizers. The steam or hot chemical vapor will not penetrate these containers or materials to reach the items inside. These may be appropriate for sterilization in dry heat, however, if sufficient exposure time is used. Sharps containers and biohazard bags containing regulated waste that will be sterilized before disposal must be left open during the sterilization process and then closed after removal from the sterilizer (see Chapter 16). If they are closed, the steam or chemical vapor will not reach the items inside the containers or bags. Not all sharps containers and biohazard bags can withstand the high temperature in heat sterilization.

STERILIZATION METHOD	PACKAGING MATERIAL	PRECAUTIONS

Box 11-3   Types and Use of Sterilization Packaging Materials

STERILIZATION METHOD	PACKAGING MATERIAL	PRECAUTIONS
Steam autoclave*	Paper wrap Nylon "plastic" tubing Paper/plastic peel pouches Thin cloth Wrapped perforated cassettes	No closed containers Thick cloth may absorb too much steam Some plastic containers melt Use only material approved for steam
Dry heat sterilizers	Paper wrap Appropriate nylon "plastic" tubing Closed containers† Wrapped perforated cassettes Aluminum foil‡	Some paper may char Some plastic containers melt Only use material approved for dry heat
Unsaturated chemical sterilizer	Paper wrap Paper/plastic peel pouches Wrapped perforated cassettes	No closed containers Cloth absorbs too much chemical vapor Some plastic containers melt Use only material approved for chemical vapor

*"Flash" (or "unwrapped") sterilization cycles that operate at higher temperatures for shorter times indicate that the items being processed not be packaged.
†Biologic indicators (spore tests) should be used to confirm that sterilizing conditions are achieved within any closed containers used.
‡Aluminum foil will easily tear or be punctured.

Penetration of steam, hot chemical vapor, or heated air through a particular type of packaging material or container can be tested by placing spore strips inside and processing through the sterilizer to make sure the spores are killed. This is not recommended for testing filled sharps containers unless very special care is taken to avoid injuries when placing and retrieving the spore strips.

Wrapping or Bagging

Functional sets of instruments can be placed on a small sterilizable tray and the entire tray wrapped with sterilization wrap. Figure 11-4 diagrams the wrapping procedure. Seal the wrap with tape that will withstand the heat process (e.g., "autoclave tape").

Functional sets also may be placed in "see-through" paper/plastic pouches that have clear "plastic" film on one side and heavy sterilization paper on the other side. These are available in many different sizes, can be used in steam or unsaturated chemical vapor sterilizers, and have chemical indicators (discussed later) printed directly on the paper side of the pouch. Some pouches are self-sealing; others need to be heat-sealed or sealed with

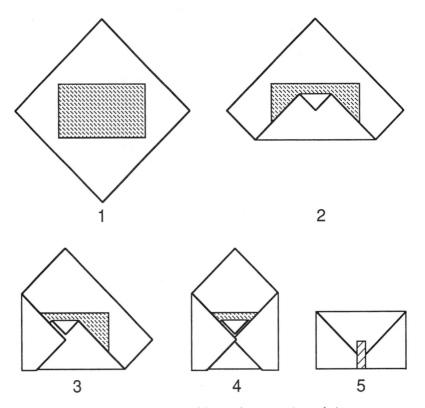

FIGURE 11-4 Diagram of the envelope wrapping technique.

tape. The pouches are easily opened after sterilization by peeling the plastic away from the paper (Figure 11-5). A nylon type of clear "plastic" tubing comes on a roll and may be cut to varying lengths, filled with instruments, and heat-sealed or taped. One type can be used in steam and another type can be used in dry heat sterilizers (Figure 11-6). Paper bags are available but care must be taken because sharp and pointed instruments can easily puncture the paper, and paper becomes wet during steam sterilization and will tear if handled before drying. Expel as much air as possible out of bags and pouches before sterilization.

Using Cassettes

Numerous styles of cassettes are available that contain functional sets of instruments during use at chairside and during the ultrasonic precleaning, rinsing, and sterilizing processes (Figure 11-7). Using cassettes reduces direct handling of contaminated instruments and keeps the instruments together through the entire processing. After ultrasonic cleaning, rinsing, and drying, sterilizable supply-type items may be added to the cassette, and the cassette is wrapped, sterilized, and stored or used immediately. Using an instrument cassette system requires planning to ensure that the proper size ultrasonic cleaner and sterilizer are available for processing. Cassettes are available in stainless steel, aluminum, and plastic/resin material that can withstand steam, chemical vapor, and dry heat sterilization. Follow the cassette manufacturer's recommendations for ultrasonic cleaning, wrapping or bagging, and sterilization.

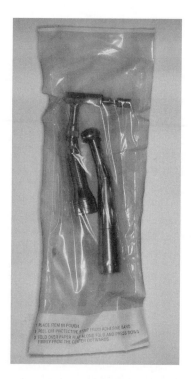

FIGURE 11–5   Instrument packaging using a self-sealing, paper/plastic peal pouch.

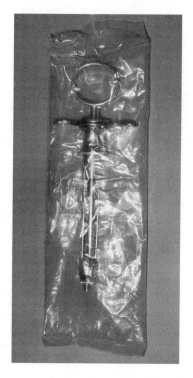

FIGURE 11–6   Instrument packaging using nylon plastic tubing that is heat-sealed.

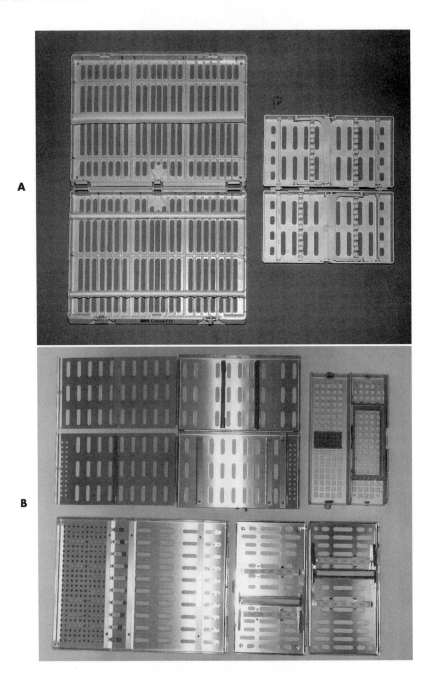

FIGURE 11-7 Examples of cassettes used to package functional sets of instruments through ultrasonic cleaning, rinsing, drying, packaging, sterilizing, and for direct use at chairside. **A,** Resin cassettes; **B,** metal cassettes.

Unwrapped Instruments

Sterilizing unpackaged instruments is the least satisfactory approach to patient protection because it allows for unnecessary contamination before the instruments are actually used on the next patient. If for some reason unwrapped instruments are sterilized (e.g., flash sterilization of an item in short supply that was dropped on the floor during patient care), they must subsequently be handled with very special care to reduce post-sterilization contamination as much as possible. This includes handling the instruments with sterilized tongs or clean/sterile gloves, protecting them from dust or aerosols in the air, and preventing contact with any contaminated surface by using clean/sterile wrap or covers. A carefully written protocol for minimizing the risk of post-sterilization contamination of unpackaged instruments should be prepared and strictly followed.

Sterilization

Precleaned, packaged instruments are ready for processing through a heat sterilizer. A comparison of the three most common types of sterilizers used in dental offices is given in Table 11-1. Appendix G gives recommended methods for sterilizing many different dental instruments and materials.

Steam Sterilization

Steam sterilization involves heating water to generate steam in a closed chamber, producing a moist heat that rapidly kills microorganisms. Because the steam is formed in a closed system, the steam completely fills (saturates) the sterilizer chamber, pushing the cooler air out of an escape valve, which then closes and allows a build-up of pressure. It is the heat, however, not the pressure, that actually kills the microorganisms. In the absence of air in a closed system, the steam creates higher temperatures than steam coming from an open pan of boiling water (at 212° F or 100° C), which allows the steam to be mixed with cooler air above the pan. Manufacturers set their sterilizers to reach maximum steam temperatures of approximately 250° F (121.1° C) or 273° F (134° C) with respective pressures of 103 or 206 kilopascals (kPa), which is the same as 15 or 30 pounds per square inch (psi).

Types of Steam Sterilizers. Although all steam sterilizers operate in a similar fashion, different models and brands have different features, including chamber size and mechanisms of air removal, steam generation, drying, temperature displays, and recording devices.

Small office sterilizers. The typical dental office steam sterilizer usually operates through four cycles: the heat-up cycle, the sterilizing cycle, the depressurization cycle, and the drying cycle. After the water is added, the chamber is loaded, the door is closed, the unit is turned on, and the heat-up cycle begins to generate the steam. The steam pushes out the air in the chamber (called gravity air removal), and when the set temperature is reached, the sterilizing cycle begins. The temperature is maintained for the set time, usually ranging from 3 to 30 minutes. Typical preset sterilizing cycles are:

- 250° F (121° C) for 30 minutes
- 250° F (121° C) for 15 minutes
- 273° F (134° C) for 10 minutes
- 273° F (134° C) for 3 minutes

Table 11-1 Comparison of Heat Sterilization Methods Using Small Office Sterilizers

METHOD	STANDARD STERILIZING CONDITIONS*	ADVANTAGES	PRECAUTIONS	SPORE-TESTING
Steam Autoclave Standard cycles	20-30 min at 250°F	Time efficient Good penetration Sterilizes water-based liquids in standard cycles†	Do not use closed containers Damage to plastic and rubber Nonstainless steel metal items corrode Use of hard water may leave deposits Items may be wet after cycle Unwrapped items quickly contaminate after processing	*Bacillus stearothermophilus* strips or vials
"Flash" cycles	3-10 min at 273°F			
Unsaturated Chemical Vapor	20 min at 270°F	Time efficient No corrosion Items dry quickly after cycle	Do not use closed containers Damage to plastic and rubber Must use special solution Predry instruments Provide adequate ventilation Cannot sterilize liquids Cloth wraps may absorb chemicals Unwrapped items quickly contaminate after processing	*Bacillus stearothermophilus* strips

Dry Heat				
Oven-type sterilizer (static-air)	60–120 min at 320°F	No corrosion Can use closed containers‡ Low cost Items are dry after cycle	Long sterilization time Damage to plastic and rubber Predry instruments Do not open door during cycle Cannot sterilize liquids Unwrapped items quickly contaminate after processing	*Bacillus subtilis* strips
Rapid heat transfer (forced-air)	12 min at 375°F (wrapped) 6 min at 375°F (unwrapped)	No corrosion Short cycle Items are dry after cycle	Damage to some plastic and rubber Predry instruments Do not open door during cycle Cannot sterilize liquids Unwrapped items quickly contaminate after processing	*Bacillus subtilis* strips

Adapted from Miller CH: Take the safe approach to disease prevention. RHD 9:35, 1989; and Miller CH: Sterilization and disinfection: what every dentist should know, *JADA* 123:26, 1992.

*These conditions do not include warm-up or cool down time and they may vary depending on the nature and volume of the load and brand of the sterilizer. Sterilizing conditions actually achieved in the office should be defined by results of spore-testing.

†It is best to use purchased sterile irrigating fluids with certified sterility for clinical use.

‡Processing in closed containers should be carefully checked by spore-testing.

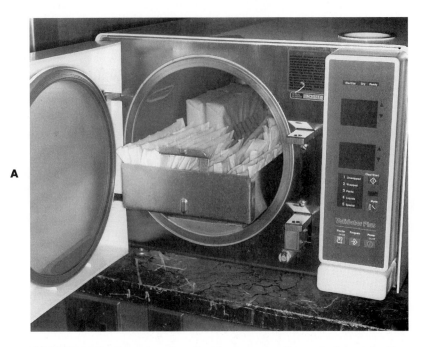

A

FIGURE 11-8   Examples of small, office steam sterilizers. **A,** A model with a 10-inch diameter chamber.

At the end of the sterilizing cycle, the depressurization cycle begins and the steam is slowly released, with a decrease in temperature and pressure. At the end of this cycle, all of the items inside are wet and the drying cycle can be initiated. This cycle maintains heat inside the chamber to evaporate the remaining water but the chamber is opened to the air so the water vapor can escape and the items can become dry. Some sterilizers have an automatic drying cycle that can be up to an hour long. With others, the door is simply opened about one-half inch for a time to let the moisture escape.

Small office steam sterilizers usually have chambers of 8 to 12 inches in diameter or have a small cassette containing the instruments that is inserted into the sterilizer, serving as the sterilizer chamber. Some units also have printout devices that record the time and temperature of each sterilizing cycle to help maintain sterility assurance records (Figure 11-8).

Hospital-type sterilizers.   Steam sterilizers used in hospitals, dental schools, and some large clinics have much larger chambers and are connected directly to a steam line, which eliminates the need to generate its own steam, or are connected to a water line that allows them to generate their own steam (Figure 11-9). Most of these sterilizers have a vacuum system for air removal from the chamber so that when the steam enters, it has a better chance of coming into direct contact with everything in the chamber, since no air is around the items that can insulate them from the hot steam. These units also have a post-sterilization vacuum cycle that removes the steam and water after the sterilizing cycle to give dry instrument packs. No matter what type of sterilizer you are using, be sure to follow all of the manufacturer's directions for routine maintenance, loading, monitoring, and safe operation.

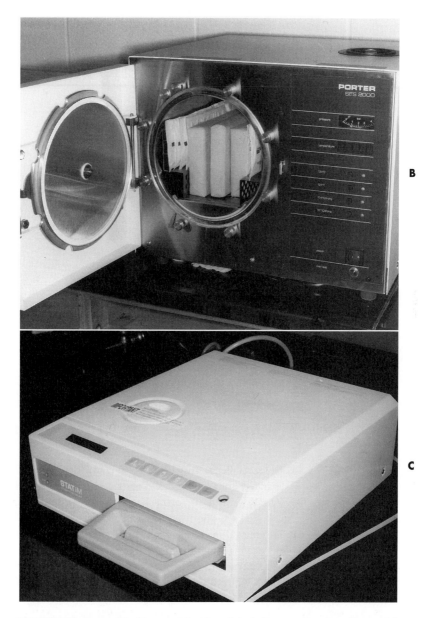

FIGURE 11-8, cont'd   B, a model with an 8-inch diameter chamber; **C,** a model with a removable chamber.

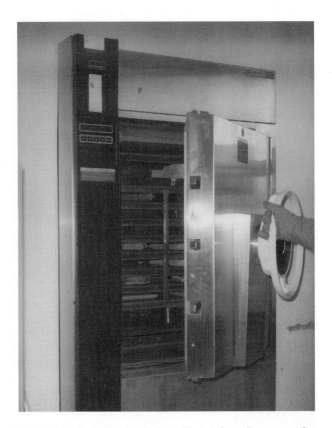

FIGURE 11-9   Example of a large, "hospital type" steam sterilizer.

Loading.   Load the sterilizer as instructed by the manufacturer and keep packs, pouches, or cassettes separated from each other so the steam has access to all package surfaces. Some sterilizers come with racks for packages that keep them separated and on their edge. Do not stack packages, pouches, or cassettes flat in layers; this will impede steam circulation and air removal in the chamber. Place them on their edges.

Sterilizing.   Follow the manufacturer's instructions for the time and temperature of exposure. Remember, the sterilizing cycle does not begin until the chamber reaches a temperature of 250° F (121° C) or 273° F (134° C). The exposure times of about 3 to 30 minutes at these temperatures are set to include extra time to ensure microbial killing (safety factor). Thus, when the shorter times are used, safety factors are reduced. This is of particular concern with "flash" sterilization cycles that operate in the range of 3 minutes at the higher temperature. These "flash" cycles were originally designed for use only in emergency situations, for example, when an expensive instrument in short supply is dropped on the floor while caring for a patient and it has to be cleaned and resterilized quickly for continued use. Not only is the time shortened in a "flash" cycle but the item to be sterilized is not wrapped or packaged in any way so that it can have immediate contact with the steam in this very short cycle. Because the item is not wrapped, it is open to immediate recontamination when it is removed from the sterilizer. Thus "flash" sterilization of instruments should not be used routinely as a substitute for purchasing additional

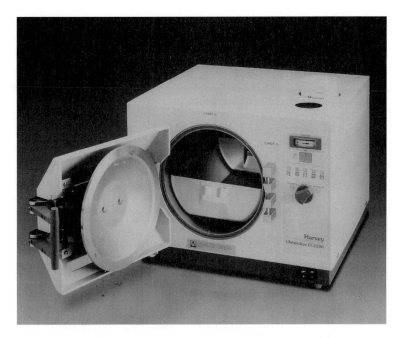

FIGURE 11-10 The unsaturated chemical vapor sterilizer.

instruments or simply to reduce instrument processing time because this weakens sterility assurance that might jeopardize patient protection.

Unsaturated Chemical Vapor Sterilization

Unsaturated chemical vapor sterilization involves heating a special chemical solution in a closed chamber, producing hot chemical vapors that kill microorganisms. The chemical solution contains 0.23% formaldehyde and 72.38% ethanol plus acetone, ketone, water, and other alcohols. Protect the skin and eyes from contact with the solution and do not breathe its vapors.

The unsaturated chemical vapor sterilizer is called the Harvey Chemiclave (Figure 11-10). It operates through four cycles: the heat-up/vaporization cycle, the sterilization cycle, the depressurization cycle, and an optional purge cycle. After the special chemical solution is added, the chamber is loaded, the door is closed, and the unit turned on. The heat-up cycle causes the chemical solution to vaporize, yielding a pressure of approximately 172 kPa (25 psi), and when the temperature reaches about 270° F (132° C), the sterilizing cycle begins. The temperature is maintained for 20 minutes, and the chamber is depressurized, with a decrease in temperature.

A positive feature of chemical vapor sterilization is that corrosion of carbon steel instruments is eliminated or greatly reduced. The amount of water in the chemical solution used is below the level that causes corrosion. This is why it is extremely important to dry the instruments before processing in this sterilizer. Residual water remaining on wet instruments could override the rust-free process. Because the chemical solution used rapidly vaporizes in heat, items processed through this sterilizer are essentially dry at the end of the depressurization cycle.

Follow the manufacturer's directions for packaging, loading, and operating, and wear gloves and protective eyewear when handling the special chemical solution. As with the steam sterilizer, it is very important to leave space around the packages being processed through the chemical vapor sterilizer to ensure adequate contact with the chemical vapors. This is best achieved by placing packages or cassettes on their edges. Also, closed containers are not to be used but paper/plastic peel pouches, bags, or paper sterilization wrap indicated for use in the Chemiclave are appropriate for packaging. Do not use as packaging or attempt to sterilize linens, textiles, fabrics, or other absorbent material such as paper towels. These may absorb the chemicals and reduce vaporization.

Operate the sterilizer in a room that has at least normal ventilation. A purge system that collects chemicals from the vapors in the chamber at the end of the process can be purchased as an attachment to the sterilizer. This greatly reduces the smell from the chemicals when the door is opened. In California, the chamber vapors are to be vented outside the office.

Dry Heat Sterilization

Dry heat sterilization involves heating air with transfer of heat energy from the air to the instruments. This form of killing requires higher temperatures than steam or unsaturated chemical vapor sterilization. Dry heat sterilizers operate at approximately 320° F to 375° F (160° C to 190° C), depending on the type of sterilizer. The main advantage of dry heat sterilization is that carbon steel items do not corrode as they do during steam sterilization.

Static-Air Type of Dry Heat Sterilizers.   This type of dry heat sterilizer is sometimes referred to as the oven type of dry heat sterilizer. The heating coils in the bottom of these sterilizers cause the hot air to rise inside the chamber through natural convection (Figure 11-11). Heat energy from the static air is transferred to the instruments, and sterilization is reported to occur after 1 to 2 hours at 320° F (160° C). Because sterilization time may vary depending on the nature of the load, it is very important to spore-test these units (as is true for all sterilizers) to determine the proper exposure time under the conditions of actual use.

The heat-up time for this type of sterilizer may be 15 to 30 minutes from a cold start. Thus the sterilization cycle is not started until the proper temperature (e.g., 320° F or 160° C) is reached. The instruments then are held at this "sterilizing temperature" for the proper time. Because many of these units do not have automatic timers, sufficient time for heat-up must be included in the timer setting. After the sterilizing temperature is reached, the chamber door must not be opened (e.g., to add forgotten items) until the scheduled time. If opened during the cycle, the temperature drops severely and the cycle must be started again from time zero. Follow the sterilizer manufacturer's directions carefully for loading and operating these sterilizers. Again, do not layer or stack items in the chamber but place them on their edges.

The type of packaging or wrapping material used must be able to withstand the high temperatures in dry heat sterilization. Some wraps appropriate for steam or chemical vapor sterilization may melt in dry heat units. Closed containers can be used in dry heat sterilizers if sterilization inside the containers is routinely confirmed by spore testing. Although the static-air type of dry heat sterilizer requires longer sterilization times than the forced-air type described below, it is the least expensive.

Forced-Air Type of Dry Heat Sterilizer.   This type of dry heat sterilizer is sometimes referred to as a rapid heat transfer sterilizer. It circulates the heated air throughout the chamber at a high velocity (Figure 11-12). This permits a more rapid transfer of heat energy from the air to the instruments, reducing the time needed for sterilization.

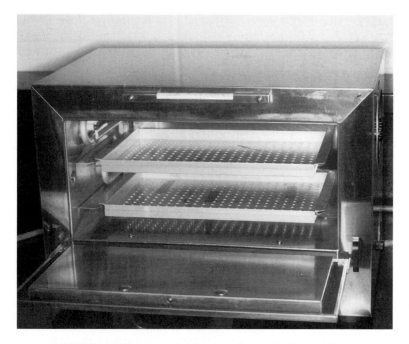

FIGURE 11-11   Example of a static-air type dry heat sterilizer.

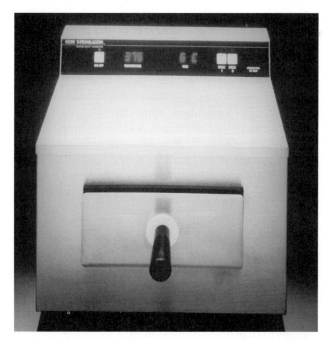

FIGURE 11-12   Example of a forced-air rapid heat transfer dry heat sterilizer.

One type of forced-air unit is a continuous heating type. The instruments are placed into a preheated chamber and, when the factory-set temperature of 375° F (190° C) is reached, the selected exposure time for the sterilizing cycle automatically begins. The instruments are removed from the chamber at the end of the exposure period and allowed to cool. A second type of forced-air dry heat sterilizer begins from a cold (room temperature) start. After the chamber is loaded and the unit activated, the sterilizing cycle automatically begins when the factory-set temperature is reached and continues for the selected exposure time. At the end of the exposure period, the heating elements automatically turn off and air is circulated in the chamber to cool the instruments.

Exposure time after the sterilizing temperature has been reached in these forced-air units ranges from 12 minutes for packaged items to 6 minutes for unpackaged items. As with the static-air dry heat sterilizers, important procedures to achieve successful sterilization are: keep the chamber door closed, use proper packaging material and routine spore testing, and follow manufacturer's directions for loading and operating forced-air dry heat sterilizers.

Sterilization Monitoring

The goal of sterilization is the complete killing of all forms of microbial life on the items being processed. The only way to determine if all items processed through a sterilizer are truly sterile is to test each item for all living microorganisms. This is impossible because such tested items then could not be used for patient care. Thus there are no procedures or products that can be used to absolutely prove sterility of the items. Therefore a degree of risk that a nonsterile item exists in a processed load is always present. The object is to keep this risk as low as possible by using properly designed sterilization equipment in a carefully controlled manner. With such efforts, it is possible to achieve a 99.9999%, or better, probability of success, which means the possibility of the presence of a nonsterile item is only 1 in 1,000,000. Sterilization monitoring is part of the overall controlled sterilization process needed to achieve this high level of sterility.

Heat sterilization failures result when direct contact between the sterilizing agent and all surfaces of items being processed does not occur for the appropriate length of time. Several things can cause sterilization failures, including improper instrument cleaning and packaging, and improper use and functioning of the sterilizer (Table 11-2). In many instances, these failures will not be detected unless proper sterilization monitoring is performed. There are three forms of sterilization monitoring, all of which must be used to achieve sterility assurance: biologic, chemical, and physical monitoring.

Biologic Monitoring

Biologic monitoring provides the main guarantee of sterilization. It involves processing highly resistant bacterial spores (see Figure 11-1) through the sterilizer and then culturing the spores to determine if they have been killed.

Types of Biologic Indicators.   Biologic indicators (BI) contain the bacterial endospores used for monitoring. The spores used are *Bacillus stearothermophilus* (for testing steam or chemical vapor sterilization) or *Bacillus subtilis* (for testing dry heat or ethylene oxide gas sterilization). There are no BIs available to routinely test liquid chemical sterilants or disinfectants during use in the office.

Table 11-2 Some Causes of Sterilization Failure

CAUSES	POTENTIAL PROBLEM
Improper Cleaning of Instruments	Debris may insulate organsims from direct contact with the sterilizing agent
Improper Packaging	
Wrong packaging material for method of sterilization	Prevents penetration of the sterilizing agent; packaging material may melt
Excessive packaging material	Retards penetration of the sterilizing agent
Cloth wrap in chemical vapor sterilizer	Cloth may absorb chemicals, preventing sufficient vaporization needed for sterilization
Closed container in steam or chemical vapor sterilizer	Prevents direct contact with the sterilizing agent
Improper Loading of Sterilizer	
Overloading	Increases heat-up time and will retard penetration of the sterilizing agent to the center of the sterilizer load
No separation between packages or cassettes even without overloading	May prevent or retard thorough contact of sterilizing agent with all items in the chamber
Improper Timing	
Incorrect operation of the sterilizer	Insufficient time at proper temperature to achieve kill
Timing for sterilization started before proper temperature is reached in units with nonautomatic timers	Insufficient time at proper temperature to achieve kill
Dry heat sterilizer door opened during sterilizing cycle without starting cycle over	Insufficient time at proper temperature to achieve kill
Sterilizer timer malfunction	Insufficient time at proper temperature to achieve kill
Improper Temperature	
Incorrect operation of the sterilizer	Insufficient heat for proper time to achieve kill
Sterilizer malfunction	Insufficient heat for proper time to achieve kill
Improper Method of Sterilization	
Solutions or water processed in a chemical vapor sterilizer	Sterilizing agent will not penetrate the solution
Solutions or water processed in a dry heat sterilizer	Will boil over and evaporate
Processing of heat-sensitive item (e.g., some plastics)	Items will melt or be distorted

BIs are packaged in different forms (Figure 11-13). Spore strips are paper strips about one-inch long that contain one type of spore or may contain both types of spores (dual species BIs) that can be used to test all four types of sterilizers. Spore strips are enclosed in a protective glassine envelope, and after processing through the sterilizer the internal spore strip is aseptically removed and placed in a tube of appropriate culture medium that is incubated for 7 days at 55° C (for *B. stearothermophilus*) or at 37° C (for *B. subtilis*). If live spores are still present, they will grow and produce cloudiness and/or change the color of the growth medium, indicating sterilization failure. Spore strips can be used to monitor all forms of heat sterilization.

Another form of BI is called a self-contained vial and contains a spore strip or disk with an ampule of growth medium in a plastic vial with a vented cap to permit entrance of the sterilizing agent into the vial (see Figure 11-13). After processing through the sterilizer, the vial is squeezed or the cap is pushed down to break the internal ampule, mixing the growth medium with the spores. The vial is then incubated at 55° C, and if live spores are still present they will grow and change the color of the growth medium, indicating sterilization failure. Self-contained vials currently available can be used to monitor steam sterilization.

Use of Biologic Indicators.   In hospital-type steam sterilizers, BIs are placed inside of a standardized test pack of towels, processed through the sterilizer, and analyzed. Test packs are still under development for use with small office-type steam, chemical vapor, and dry heat sterilizers. Until such test packs are developed and verified, routine biologic monitoring of small office-type sterilizers should involve placement of the BI inside one of each type of package (pouch, bags, pack, cassette) processed through the sterilizer. A control BI that is not processed through the sterilizer but is otherwise handled the same way as the test BI must be analyzed along with the test BI that is processed through the sterilizer. The control BI should yield growth of the spores, confirming that if live spores are present, they can grow and be detected.

The Centers for Disease Control and Prevention, the American Dental Association, the OSAP Research Foundation, and the Association for the Advancement of Medical Instrumentation recommend at least weekly spore testing of each sterilizer in the office. Some states have passed laws requiring routine spore-testing of dental office sterilizers, including Ohio, Indiana, Oregon, Washington, Florida, and California. Nonroutine use of biologic monitoring is also important, as described in Table 11-3.

Analysis of Biologic Indicators.   Proper analysis of a microbiologic test such as use of a BI involves confirming that the test organisms were alive before the test (by using a control BI that is not processed through the sterilizer) and by confirming that organisms that grow after the test BI has been processed through the sterilizer are indeed the actual test microorganisms and not just a contaminant from hands or the air that accidentally entered the growth medium before incubation. Thus control BIs should always yield growth of the spores, and growth from test BIs should be gram-positive bacilli when a sample of the growth medium is smeared on a glass slide, gram-stained, and observed at a magnification of about 1,000 times under the microscope. These techniques, with use of a growth medium that has been verified as being sterile to begin with and able to support growth of the test spores, confirm the reliability of each biologic monitoring test. The equipment and supplies necessary to perform these verification techniques are not commonly found in dental offices. Also, self-contained vials do not easily lend themselves to microbiologic analysis of a positive test BI through sampling of the growth medium inside the capped vial.

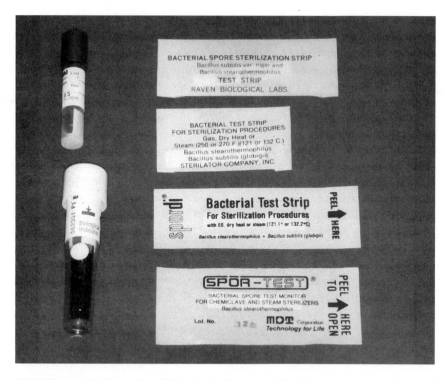

FIGURE 11-13 Examples of biological indicators. *(Left)* Self-contained spore vials used in steam sterilizers; *(right)* spore strips in protective glassine envelopes used in steam, unsaturated chemical vapor, or dry heat sterilizers.

Table 11-3   Spore Testing of Small Office Sterilizers

WHEN	WHY
Once per week	To verify proper use and functioning
Whenever a new type of packaging material or tray is used	To ensure that the sterilizing agent is getting inside to the surface of the instruments
After training of new sterilization personnel	To verify proper use of the sterilizer
During initial uses of a new sterilizer	To make sure unfamiliar operating instructions are being followed
First run after repair of a sterilizer	To make sure that the sterilizer is functioning properly
With every implantable device and hold device until results of test are known	Extra precaution for sterilization of item to be implanted into tissues
After any other change in the sterilizing procedure	To make sure change does not prevent sterilization

Reprinted with permission from Miller CH, Palenik CJ: Sterilization, disinfection and aespsis in dentistry. In *Sterilization, Disinfection and Preservation* (Block SS, editor), Philadelphia, 1991, Lea & Febiger.

Management of Biologic Monitoring.   There are two acceptable approaches to biologic monitoring: in-office monitoring, and mail-in monitoring (Box 11-4).

In-office monitoring.   This approach to biologic monitoring involves purchasing the appropriate supplies and equipment, analyzing the BI in the office, and preparing appropriate records. Steam sterilizers can be monitored in the office by purchasing a self-contained vial-type of BI of *B. stearothermophilus* and a 55° C incubator available from the BI supplier. Care must be taken to handle the BIs aseptically and to perform the incubation and analysis as described in the manufacturer's directions. Records of the testing should include the date of the test, type of sterilizer, time and temperature of the sterilizing conditions, type of packaging material (packs, pouches, cassettes), location in the sterilizer, results of the test and of the control BI, and name of whomever conducted the test. Microbiologic confirmation of growth in the self-contained vial should not be attempted in the office. Self-contained plastic vial BIs are not currently available for in-office testing of chemical vapor or dry heat sterilizers. Spore strip types of BIs can be used to test these as well as the steam sterilizer but this requires the purchase of separate tubes of growth medium plus the incubator and even greater care to avoid contamination of the growth medium used for analysis.

Mail-in monitoring.   A convenient approach to biologic monitoring is for an office to subscribe to a mail-in sterilization monitoring service available from private companies

---

> ### *Box 11-4*   Biologic Monitoring **Step-by-Step Procedures**
>
> 1. Use BIs containing *Bacillus stearothermophilus* spores for monitoring steam and chemical vapor sterilizers and *Bacillus subtilis* for monitoring dry heat or ethylene oxide gas sterilizers
> 2. Insert BI inside of a pack, pouch, or cassette and complete the packaging procedure. If a spore strip BI is used, do not remove the strip from the blue glassine envelope. If appropriate, identify the pack, pouch, or cassette containing the BI
> 3. Place the pack, pouch, or cassette in the center of the load and process as part of a normal load through a normal sterilizer cycle
> 4. Record the date of the test, type of sterilizer, temperature and time of the sterilization cycle, nature of the package containing the BI, and the name of the sterilizer operator
> 5. Retrieve the test BIs and, with the control BI, mail back to the sterilization monitoring service. If analyzed in the office, follow the BI manufacturer's directions carefully and monitor the temperature of the incubator
> 6. Receive and maintain records of results from the monitoring service or record the proper results for the test and control BIs analyzed in the office
> 7. If a positive BI occurs (sterilization failure), repeat the test under carefully controlled conditions, and do not use instruments processed through that sterilizer until the nature of the problem had been identified and corrected

or through some dental schools. These services can monitor any type of sterilizer and provide the office with the appropriate BIs (usually spore strips) and instructions for their use. After processing through the sterilizer, the BIs are mailed back to the service where they are analyzed, and a report of the results is sent to the office for recordkeeping. If a sterilization failure is detected, the service usually notifies the office by phone. The most complete mail-in services provide a control BI and two test BIs for each test. Some also provide newsletters on asepsis, a certificate of participation, and a phone number to call with questions about spore testing or any aspect of office infection control. Mail-in services should perform microbiologic confirmation of results and use a growth medium that has been verified for sterility and growth promotion.

What to Do After a Sterilization Failure. The desired outcome of biologic monitoring is the killing of test spores. Failure to kill the spores (i.e., having a positive spore test) is a significant event that requires immediate action so that patient safety is not compromised. However, before this action program can be put into place, the office has to develop confidence in the biologic monitoring procedure used so that when a positive spore test result is obtained, the validity of the test itself is not questioned. Confidence in the spore testing procedures can be obtained by using the same four steps described above to achieve sterility assurance (see p. 137). Ask the following questions and act accordingly to ensure the correctness of the spore testing procedure:

- Were the proper BIs used and were they stored properly as described on their labels?
- Did all of the BIs used in the testing have the same manufacturer's lot number?
- Were the BIs used before their expiration date?
- Were the BIs handled properly before and after processing through the sterilizer?
- Were all the BIs mailed back to the service together or analyzed in the office together?
- Were the BIs incubated for the correct time at the correct temperature?
- Did the unprocessed control BI from the same lot number show growth (yield a positive result) after culturing?
- If a mail-in service is used did the service confirm the positive result by microbiologic means?

When a spore test is positive, indicating a sterilization failure, follow the steps given in Box 11-5.

Chemical Monitoring

Chemical monitoring uses heat-sensitive chemicals (rather than live spores as in biologic monitoring) to assess the physical conditions during the sterilization process. Chemical monitoring involves the use of indicators that change color or physical form when exposed to certain temperatures. Examples include autoclave tape; special markings on pouches and bags; chemical indicator strips; tabs, packets, or tubes of colored liquid (Figure 11-14).

There are two types of chemical indicators. The rapid-change indicator changes color rapidly after a certain temperature has been reached (e.g., autoclave tape and special markings on pouches and bags). The rapid-change indicator is used as an external indicator on the outside of every pack, pouch, or cassette to indicate that the item has at least been processed through a heat sterilizer. This identifies items that have been heat-processed and items that have not, for otherwise they may look identical. This prevents the accidental clinical use of unprocessed items. The rapid-change indicators do not indicate that steril-

---

Box 11-5   Following Up on a Sterilization Failure **Step-by-Step Procedures**

1. **Take the sterilizer out of service**
   Immediately stop using the sterilizer for patient care items until the cause of failure is determined and appropriate changes are made. Items processed in the sterilizer since the last spore test may not have been sterilized and, if still un-used, need to be collected, re-packaged, and re-processed through a properly operating sterilizer. A second properly monitored sterilizer in the office may be used or a loaner from the sales/repair company may be obtained so that pa-tient flow is not interrupted.

2. **Review sterilization procedures**
   Review all past chemical monitoring records since the last negative spore test. Review the proper sterilizer loading and operating procedures and determine if procedures were actually followed by the instrument processing staff. Were there any changes in the packaging or loading procedures? Was sufficient fluid added to the sterilizer before the cycle? Were the times and temperatures set correctly? Was there anything different about the cycle that yielded a failure? Was a new staff person involved with instrument processing?

3. **Retest and observe the cycle**
   If problems were detected in Step 2, make the necessary changes. Retest the sterilizer using the same cycle and approximate load that yielded the sterilization failure. Place a chemical indicator next to the BI on the inside of a package. Ob-serve the sterilizer gauges, lights, dials, and/or digital readouts during this repeat cycle to determine if they indicate the proper sterilizing conditions.

4. **Determine the fate of the sterilizer**
   If the spore test results are negative and if the chemical indicator had changed to an appropriate color, the sterilizer may be placed back into service. If the spore test is positive and you have confirmed that the packaging, loading, and operating procedures were performed correctly, contact your sterilizer service representative for repair or replacement.

5. **Test repair or replacement sterilizer**
   Before a repaired or a new sterilizer is placed into service, it should be spore tested under normal operating conditions and achieve a negative result.

---

ization has been achieved or even that a complete sterilization cycle has occurred. A ster-ilizer could heat up to the proper temperature, causing a change in the chemical indica-tor, and then immediately malfunction, preventing sterilization, but the indicator would have already changed color. Thus the rapid-change indicator demonstrates only that an item has been exposed to a certain temperature for some length of time.

The second type of chemical indicator is called a slow-change or integrated indicator that changes color or form slowly, responding to a combination of time and temperature or time, temperature, and the presence of steam. These indicators are used on the inside of every pack, pouch, or cassette to assess if the instruments have been exposed to steril-izing conditions. Use of chemical indicators is summarized in Box 11-6.

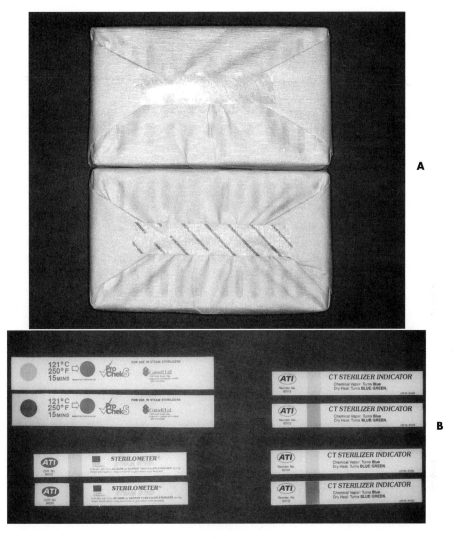

FIGURE 11-14   Examples of chemicals indicators. **A,** *(Top)* Autoclave tape before being heat-processed, *(bottom)* autoclave tape after being heat-processed; **B,** other chemical indicators. The top of each pair shows appearance before heat-processing and the bottom shows the color change after heat-processing.

Physical Monitoring

Physical monitoring of the sterilization process involves observing the gauges and displays on the sterilizer and recording the sterilizing temperature, pressure, and exposure time. Although correct readings do not guarantee sterilization, incorrect readings give the first indication that a problem has likely occurred. Many small office sterilizers now have recording devices that print out these parameters, providing a physical monitoring record for each run. It must be remembered that sterilizer gauges and displays indicate the conditions in the sterilizer chamber rather than conditions within the packs, pouches, or cas-

---

Box 11-6   Chemical Monitoring ****Step-by-Step Procedures****

---

1. Place the appropriate slow-change integrated chemical indicator on the inside of every pack, pouch, or cassette to be processed through steam or the static-air dry heat sterilizer. These indicators are currently not available for the chemical vapor sterilizer or the forced-air rapid heat transfer dry heat sterilizers; thus use an appropriate rapid-change indicator inside of packages being processed through these types of sterilizers.
2. Place a rapid-change indicator on the outside of every pack, pouch, or cassette. Some pouches have a chemical indicator already printed on the pouch. If the internal indicator can be seen through the packaging material, an external indicator is not necessary
3. After packs, pouches or cassettes have been processed through the sterilizer, observe the external indicators. If the appropriate color change has not occured, do not use the processed items. Immediately spore test the sterilizer process to verify and ultimately correct any problem with the use or functioning of the sterilizer. Do not use the sterilizer until the problem has been corrected. If the indicator has appropriately changed, distribute the packages for clinical use.
4. After opening a processed pack, pouch, or cassette, immediately observe the internal indicator. If the appropriate change has not occurred, do not use the items, and verify and correct any problem with the use or functioning of the sterilizer as described in step 3. If the approipriate change has occurred, use the instruments as long as the periodic spore testing has routinely verified the sterilization process.

---

settes being processed. Thus physical monitoring may not detect problems resulting from overloading, improper packaging material, or use of closed containers.

The Complete Monitoring Program

Appropriate sterilization monitoring involves use of a chemical indicator on the inside and outside of each pack, pouch, and cassette, physical monitoring of each cycle, and biologic monitoring of each type of pack, pouch, or cassette at least once a week. Records of all three types of monitoring should be maintained to document sterility assurance. Such information may be requested by those who may investigate the infection control practices in the office, and it can be used to demonstrate the use of safe practices to curious patients. Physical monitoring alone will not detect all of the potential problems that may cause sterilization failure. Spore testing provides the main guarantee of sterilization but it is performed only periodically and takes two to seven days before the results are available. Use of internal chemical indicators in every pack, pouch, and cassette provides an immediate indication as to whether the sterilizing agent has penetrated the packaging material and actually reached the instruments inside. If the internal chemical indicator displays the appropriate color or form, and physical and biologic monitoring has not indicated any problems, the instruments are considered safe to use. Use of external chemical indicators on every pack, pouch, and cassette helps manage and maintain clear separation of processed and nonprocessed packs, pouches, and cassettes, eliminating the possibility of using nonsterilized instruments.

Handling Processed Instruments

Instrument sterility should be maintained until the sterilized packs, pouches, or cassettes are opened for use at chairside. Thus handling processed items properly is a very important part of the sterility assurance program for the office.

Drying and Cooling

Packs, pouches, or cassettes processed through small-office steam sterilizers may be wet and must be allowed to dry before handling. This is particularly true when paper or paper/biofilm pouches are used because the wet paper may "draw" microorganisms through the wrap or be easily torn when handled. Most steam sterilizer manufacturers provide drying instructions, and some may even have a programmed drying cycle, as described earlier.

Hospital-type steam sterilizers usually have a post-sterilization vacuum cycle that removes the moisture by evacuating the chamber. Chemical vapor and dry heat sterilizers yield dry packs after the sterilization cycle.

Cooling of warm packs should be done slowly to avoid the formation of condensation on the instruments. Do not place warm packs under air-conditioning or cool-air vents or transfer them to cold surfaces. Using a fan or blower in the sterilizing room to dry or cool down instruments is not recommended; this causes undue circulation of potentially contaminated room-air around the packs.

If unpackaged instruments are processed through the sterilizer (e.g., in an emergency "flash" sterilization cycle), they must be immediately covered or otherwise protected from the air and from coming into contact with contaminated surfaces before presentation at chairside.

Storage

Handling of sterile packages should be kept to a minimum, and those that are dropped on the floor, torn, compressed, or become wet must be considered as contaminated. Also, action must be taken to prevent the mingling of sterile packs with nonsterile packs. External chemical indicators serve as the primary control measure to identify items that have already been processed through the sterilizer.

Storage of sterile packs for more than a few days at the most is uncommon in dentistry because short turn-around time reduces the total number (and expense) of instrument sets needed. Nevertheless, proper sterility assurance dictates the need for protection of sterile instruments from recontamination regardless of the time between sterilization and reuse at chairside.

Store sterile packages in dry, enclosed, low-dust areas protected from obvious sources of contamination. Store them away from sinks and sewer and water pipes and a few inches away from ceilings, floors, and outside walls. This prevents packages from becoming wet with splashed water, floor-cleaning products, and condensation on pipes or walls. Also, store the packages away from heat sources that may make the packaging material brittle and more susceptible to tearing or puncture.

Shelf life of sterile packages is the period of time during which sterility is assumed to be maintained. If sterile packages become wet or are torn or punctured, sterility is compromised. Unwrapped instruments have a zero shelf life. Since shelf life primarily depends on maintaining the integrity of the packaging material, there is no exact time for which all instrument packages may be safely stored. Thus shelf life is mainly a function of how carefully the packages are handled and stored. This concept is referred to as *event-related storage*. The "oldest" sterile packs should be used first, as long as the packaging material is intact. This is referred to as the "first in - first out" system of stock rotation. A maximum storage time might be considered as one month, at which time all unused items are unpackaged, re-packaged with new packaging material, and re-processed through the sterilizer.

Distribution

Instruments from sterile packs or pouches can be placed on sterile, disposable, or at least cleaned and disinfected trays at chairside. Sterilized instrument cassettes are distributed to and opened at chairside. Placing unwrapped or wrapped instruments in drawers or cabinets for direct use at chairside during patient care is not recommended. The drawers or cabinets and their contents are too easily contaminated from retrieval of items with saliva-coated fingers and from contaminated aerosols. This type of storage/distribution system at chairside for instruments or supplies is fraught with great potential for cross-contamination.

Opening Instrument Packages

For routine dentistry, instrument packages at chairside should be checked for tears or punctures and, if intact, opened without touching the instruments inside. As described in Chapter 10, Protective Barriers, open the packages with clean, ungloved hands after the patient is seated and then put on gloves just before first contact with the patient's mouth. Alternatively, the packages may be opened with ungloved hands and the instruments immediately covered with a sterile drape before the patient is seated. If instrument packages are opened with gloved hands, the gloves will become contaminated with any microorganisms on the outside of the packaging. If instruments must be manipulated just before patient treatment begins (e.g., arranging bagged instruments on the bracket table), handle them with sterile tongs. Prearranging instruments on trays or in cassettes before placing them into the sterilizer eliminates the need to manipulate the instruments after sterilization. The trays or cassettes hold the instruments at chairside.

For surgery, the instruments are commonly double wrapped to enhance sterility maintenance. Any contamination of the packaging during storage and transport to the surgical operatory can be removed by removing the outer packaging. When the outer packaging is removed, the protected inner packaging may be touched/opened with gloved hands.

DESIGN OF THE INSTRUMENT PROCESSING AREA

Three goals should be accomplished when designing or organizing an instrument processing area in a dental office:

- Locate in a low-contamination environment
- Physical design is based on work flow
- Separate "clean" instruments from "dirty" instruments ("contaminated" from "sterile")

General Location and Utilities

The area should be centrally located, if possible, for easy access from all operatories but it should be away from traffic flow. That is, it should be a facility dedicated only to instrument processing, be physically separated from the operatories and dental laboratory, and not be part of a common walkway. It should not have a door that opens to the outside nor should it have open windows because these enhance entrance of dust. It should have good ventilation to control the heat generated by the sterilizers, and there should be good access to the room air filters for frequent changing. The size of the facility must accommodate all the equipment and supplies needed to perform instrument processing, such as those listed in Table 11-4. Utilities should include multiple outlets and proper lighting, water, and an air line and vacuum line for lubricating and flushing high-speed handpieces. The cabinetry should include chemical- and heat-resistant countertops wide enough for sterilizers and other equipment, a deep sink with hands-free controls for instrument rinsing, closed storage areas, and (if space permits) a separate handwashing sink. Accessories should include a hands-free soap dispenser and foot-operated or other hands-free trash receptacle. The flooring should be an uncarpeted seamless hard surface.

Work Flow Design

Just about any room or group of adjacent rooms can be used for instrument processing if there is enough space; the utilities, flooring, and ventilation are appropriate; and the placement of the equipment in the room or rooms is based on the work flow pattern. One approach to the general layout of the instrument processing area is to have a long narrow room with doors at each end and a linear work flow proceeding from one end to the other. A U-shaped work flow pattern in a room with a single door is diagramed in Figure 11-15.

A key aspect in design of the processing area is to separate the three main areas of activity:

- Decontamination area
- Packaging area
- Sterilizing area

Ideally there should be a physical separation involving three adjoining rooms but practically there is seldom such space in a dental office. Usually a single room is involved and the separation is by space designation, using signs rather than walls or partitions. Proper placement of signs (e.g., "Contaminated Items Only," "Cleaned Items Only," "Sterile Items Only," "Decontamination Area," "Clean Packaging Area," "Sterilization Area") with training on the exact meaning of the signs used can work quite well in preventing the intermingling of contaminated and sterile items.

As shown in Table 11-4, the *decontamination area* contains the items needed for personal protection, waste disposal, and instrument and handpieces cleaning and rinsing. The *packaging area* contains the materials and space for rust inhibition, wrapping and bagging, adding spore tests and chemical indicators, and adding replacement instruments, burs, and supplies. The *sterilizing area* contains the sterilizers and related supplies, incubators for analyzing spore tests in the office, and can contain enclosed storage for sterile items and disposable (single use) items.

If carts are used for distribution and collection of instruments to and from the opera-

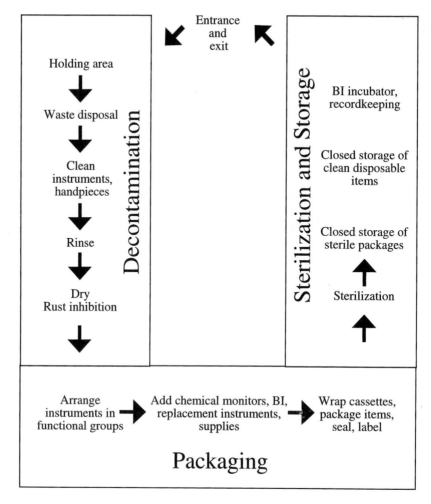

FIGURE 11-15   Diagram of a U-shaped sterilization room work flow pattern. Work flow proceeds through the area from decontamination to packaging to sterilization and storage.

tories, the carts also should be identified for "Contaminated" or "Sterile" items and be properly cleaned and disinfected or covered with barriers between uses.

INSTRUMENT SHARPENING

Instrument sharpening is difficult to manage from an infection control point of view. Sharpening of contaminated instruments presents a risk for disease spread through accidental cuts or punctures. Thus the greatest safety is achieved by cleaning, sterilizing, sharpening, and resterilizing the instruments. If instruments (e.g., scalers) may need to be resharpened while being used on a patient, it is best (and much more safe) to provide several

Table 11-4 Equipment and Supplies Used in the Instrument Processing Facility

ITEM	USE
Decontamination Area	
Gloves, mask, eyewear, clothing	Prevent exposure to contaminated materials
Sharps container	Receives any sharps not discarded in the operatory
Tongs	Picks up sharps
Biohazard bags	Receives non-sharp solid regulated waste
Trash receptacle	Receives nonregulated waste
Instrument cleaner	Ultrasonically cleans or washes instrument
Instrument detergent	Use in instrument cleaner
Cleaners/lubricants	Clean/lubricate handpieces
Air line and vacuum line	Flush materials out of handpieces into vacuum line
Sink with hands-free faucets	Handwashing and instrument rinsing
Disinfectant and towels	Disinfect countertops and ultrasonic cleaner chamber
Instrument scrub brush	Clean occasional item still soiled after mechanical cleaning
Handwashing dispenser and detergent	Wash hands
Drainer	Dry instruments /cassettes after cleaning and rinsing
Signs identifying decontamination area	Prevent intermingling of sterile and contaminated items
Packaging Area	
Rust inhibitor	Retards corrosion of non-stainless steel items in steam
Replacement instruments and burs	Replace damaged items in instrument set-ups
Instruments cassettes	Hold instruments during processing and use
Gauze pads	Place in cassettes or packages before heat processing
Biological indicators (spore tests)	Monitor the use and functioning of the sterilizers
Chemical indicators	Monitor the sterilization process
Instrument packaging materials	Protect instruments from contamination after sterilization
Heat sealer	Seal nylon "plastic" instrument packaging tubing
Heat-resistant (e.g., autoclave) tape	Seal wrapped cassettes or other instrument packages
Signs identifying packaging area	Prevent intermingling of sterile and contaminated items

Continued

Table 11-4   Equipment and Supplies Used in the Instrument Processing Facility—cont'd

ITEM	USE
Sterilizing Area	
Sterilizer(s)	Heat process cleaned and packaged instruments
Distilled water or special solution	Use with sterilizer(s)
Liquid sterilant (e.g., glutaraldehyde)	Kill microorganisms on items that cannot be heat processed
Covered container for liquid sterilant	Use with liquid sterilant
Glutaraldehyde monitor	Estimates the potency of the glutaraldehyde sterilant
Handpiece lubricant	Lubricates sterilized handpieces
Air line and vacuum line	Flush excess lubricant from handpieces into vacuum line
Incubator	Cultures spore tests for in-office analysis
Enclosed storage	Store sterile instruments and clean disposable items
Signs identifying sterilizing area	Prevent intermingling of sterile and contaminated items

scalers in each instrument set-up than to sharpen contaminated scalers. If sharpening at chairside must be done, cleaned and sterilized sharpening stones should be provided for each patient. Take great care when sharpening a contaminated instrument.

INSTRUMENT PROTECTION

Instrument processing can cause damage to instruments but several steps can be taken to keep this at a minimum (Box 11-7).

Stainless steel instruments are least affected by corrosion from moisture and heat but some clinicians prefer instruments with carbon steel rather than stainless steel cutting surfaces that may retain a sharp edge longer. Unfortunately, carbon steel items corrode and lose sharpness during steam sterilization. For example, tungsten carbide burs lose about 64% of their cutting efficiency after steam sterilization. Use of dip or spray rust inhibitors usually reduces corrosion but with repeated steam sterilization cycles the items will be damaged. Carbon steel items are best sterilized in a noncorrosion producing environment such as dry heat or unsaturated chemical vapor sterilizer. Every effort should be made to rinse away or remove biologic debris, disinfecting or sterilizing solutions, chloride salts, and highly alkaline detergents before heat processing instruments. These substances may cause pitting or staining of metal surfaces that can be aggravated with heat. It is best not to package items of widely dissimilar metals together during heat processing because of a potential for electrolytic damage to instrument surfaces. However, this is difficult to accomplish on a practical basis due to the wide variety of instruments needed for single procedures.

Box 11-7   Tips for Protecting Dental Instruments

---

1. Clean as soon as possible after use to remove corrosive materials, such as blood and salts
2. Keep instruments from knocking against each other as much as possible during the cleaning process
3. Do not store for long periods of time in water or chloride solutions
4. Use only cleaning solutions that are recommended for dental or medical instruments
5. Rinse well after cleaning
6. Use distilled or deionized water in steam sterilizers to avoid water spotting of instruments and damage to the sterilizer
7. Use rust inhibitors for carbon-steel items to be processed through steam, **or** process these items through a dry heat or unsaturated chemical vapor sterilizer to prevent corrosion
8. Dry items before processing through dry heat or chemical vapor sterilizers

---

HANDPIECE ASEPSIS

High-speed handpieces, reusable prophy angles, contra angles, nose cones, and slow-speed handpiece motors should be cleaned and sterilized by heat processing between patients. It is possible that patient material may enter the internal portions of handpieces and their attachments during use. Likewise, these materials may exit into the mouth of the next patient if this equipment has not been properly decontaminated. Thus decontamination procedures must address the outside and the inside of handpieces and their attachments. Guidelines for processing handpieces are presented in Box 11-8.

Although some dental units contain anti-retraction valves in their water lines that prevent retraction of fluids back into the high-speed water-spray handpieces and air/water syringe when they are turned off, these valves periodically fail. Thus the high-speed handpiece and air/water syringe should be flushed for about 25 seconds at the completion of each appointment. The functioning of the antiretraction valves also should be checked at least every month.

Follow the handpiece manufacturer's directions for cleaning, lubricating, and heat processing very carefully—this is essential to achieve maximum longevity of the working parts. As with any decontamination process, personal protective equipment such as gloves, mask, protective eyewear or face shield, and protective clothing should be worn during these procedures. Also, when flushing out cleaner or lubricant, spray into a vacuum line or container to avoid spread of potentially contaminated aerosols.

STERILIZATION OF HEAT-LABILE ITEMS

Although most reusable instruments can withstand heat processing, a few plastic-type items such as certain rubber dam frames, shade guides, rulers, and x-ray collimating devices will be damaged by the heat. Thus a liquid germicide such as 2.0% to 3.4% glutaraldehyde must be used for sterilizing these items. Sterilization in glutaraldehyde requires a 10-hour contact time, anything less than 10 hours is disinfection, not sterilization. Use of a glu-

---

Box 11-8   Handpiece Asepsis **Step-by-Step Procedures**

Follow very carefully the handpiece manufacturer's directions for cleaning, lubricating and sterilizing

1. Leave the handpiece attached to the hose after treatment, and wipe away visible debris from the handpiece. For high-speed handpieces, operate the air/water system for 20 to 30 seconds to flush the water and air lines into the vacuum line or a sink, container, or absorbent material

2. Remove the handpiece from the hose and clean the outside thoroughly, rinse and dry. Do not soak unless recommended by the manufacturer. Use ultrasonic cleaning only when recommended by the handpiece manufacturer

3. Clean/lubricate internal portions as directed by the manufacturer. Reattach to the air/water system and blow out excess cleaner/lubricant into a vaccum line or sink, container, or absorbent material. Depending on the handpiece, some must be lubricated before, after, or before and after sterilization, or not at all. Use separate cans of lubricant for pre- and post-sterilization lubrication. Most handpiece brands should be operated only with a bur or blank in place. Check manufacturer's instructions

4. Wipe away excess lubricant from the outside. If using fiber optic handpieces, clean away lubricant from the fiber optic connecting interface as directed by the manufacturer

5. Follow the handpiece manufacturer's instructions for the type of heat sterilizer (e.g., steam autoclave, chemical vapor) and maximum temperature that can be used. Package the handpiece in the proper bag for the type of sterilizer being used and heat process following the sterilizer operating instructions

6. Following heat processing, allow time for the handpiece to dry and cool and keep it packaged until ready to prepare it for patient use

7. If post-sterilization lubrication is required, handle the heat-processed handpiece aseptically. Open the bag, spray the lubricant into the handpiece (use a separate can reserved only for post-sterilization lubrication), attach to the hose, and blow out excess lubricant

Adapted from Miller CH: Cleaning, sterilization and disinfection: the basics of microbial killing for infection control, *J Amer Dent Assoc* 124:1-9, 1993, with additional information provided by Dr. John Young (personal communication).

taraldehyde to disinfect heat-tolerant instruments is not recommended. Step-by-step procedures for use of a liquid sterilant are given in Box 11-9. Additional information on glutaraldehydes is given in Appendix F.

OTHER METHODS OF STERILIZATION

The use of ethylene oxide gas is a recognized method of sterilization. The advantage is that the method operates at low temperatures, permitting sterilization of plastic and rubber items that melt in heat sterilizers. Disadvantages are that this method requires from 4 to 12 hours for sterilization, depending on the sterilizer model, at least 16 hours of post-sterilization aeration to remove gas molecules that have bound to plastic and rubber sur-

---

Box 11-9 Use of a Liquid Sterilant for Heat-labile Items **Step-by-Step Procedures**

1. Make sure a material safety data sheet for the liquid sterilant (e.g., glutaraldehyde) is on file in the office and that employees have been properly trained on how to handle the product
2. Use gloves, mask, protective eyewear, and protective clothing when preparing, using and discarding the solution
3. Follow the manufacturer's directions for preparing/activating, using and disposing of the solution
4. Prepare the solution for use as a sterilant, and label the containers with the appropriate date to indicate the length of the shelf life
5. Use a cover on the use-container, and label this container with the name of the chemical, the date to indicate the length of the use-life, and any other information that relates to the office hazard communication program for the safe use of chemicals
6. Use the solution to sterilize only items that are not heat-tolerant and are not intended to penetrate tissue but can be submerged
7. Preclean, rinse, and dry all items to be processed
8. Place the items in a perforated tray or pan, and place the pan in the solution and cover the container. Alternatively, place the items in the solution using tongs and avoid splashing
9. Make sure items being sterilized are completely submerged for the entire contact time needed for sterilization as indicated on the product label
10. Rinse processed items thoroughly with water and dry
11. Handle processed items with aseptic techniques (e.g., sterile tongs)
12. Place items in clean packaging material NOTE: Sterility is best maintained by rinsing with sterile water, drying, and placing in a sterile container
13. Periodically test the glutaraldehyde concentration of the use solution with a chemical test kit (contact the glutaraldehyde manufacturer/distributor for the proper test kit). Replace the use solution when indicated based on label instructions, concentration test results and/or when the level of the solution is low, or the solution becomes visibly dirty
14. When replacing the use-solution, discard all of the solution in the use-container, clean with a detergent, rinse with water, dry, and fill the container with fresh solution

---

faces, ineffectiveness on wet items, and the potential toxicity of ethylene oxide if not handled properly.

A more recently developed low temperature sterilizer involves vaporized hydrogen peroxide. Unfortunately, these units are still relatively expensive for use in dental offices.

Bead "sterilizers" provide a form of dry heat processing. These small, flower-pot–shaped units contain an electric heater that heats up glass beads (or sand or salt) to temperatures in the 425° F range. The tips of instruments, endodontic files, and broaches are then immersed into the hot beads for 25 to 30 seconds. However, the temperature varies at different levels in the beads, and biologic indicators are not available for monitoring these units. Thus bead "sterilizers" should not be used as a means of "sterilizing" instruments for reuse on another patient.

Hot oil "sterilizers" are not commonly used today but consist of a pan of mineral oil and a heater. As with bead "sterilizers," uneven temperatures occur in the oil and there is no method for routinely verifying effectiveness. Thus the hot oil bath should not be used as a means of "sterilizing" instruments for reuse on another patient.

SELECTED READINGS

American Dental Association, Councils on Scientific Affairs and Dental Practice: Infection control recommendations for the dental office and the dental laboratory, *J Amer Dent Assoc* 127:972, 1996.

Gardner JF, Peel, (editors): *Introduction to sterilization and disinfection,* New York, 1986, Churchill Livingstone.

Miller CH, Hardwick LM: Ultrasonic cleaning of dental instruments in cassettes, *Gen Dent* 36:31-36, 1988.

Miller CH, Palenik CJ: Sterilization, disinfection and asepsis in dentistry. In Block SS, editor: *Sterilization, disinfection and preservation,* ed 4, Philadelphia, 1991, Lea & Febiger.

Miller CH: Sterilization and disinfection: what every dentist needs to know, *J Amer Dent Assoc* 123:46-54, 1992.

Miller CH; Cleaning, sterilization and disinfection: the basics of microbial killing for infection control, *J Amer Dent Assoc* 124:48-56, 1993.

Miller CH, Riggen SD, Sheldrake MA, Neeb JM: Presence of microorganisms in used ultrasonic cleaning solutions, *Am J Dent* 6:27-31, 1993.

Miller CH: Update on heat sterilization and sterilization monitoring, *Compendium Dent Cont Ed* 14:304-316, 1993.

Chapter 12

SURFACE AND EQUIPMENT ASEPSIS

During patient care, many operatory and other surfaces may become contaminated with patient materials. Members of the dental team may touch surfaces with saliva-coated fingers, or droplets of the patient's oral fluids generated during care may settle on nearby surfaces. If surfaces are contaminated and are to be involved in the care of the next patient, proper surface asepsis must be practiced to prevent patient-to-patient spread of microorganisms. Examples of such surfaces are given in Box 12-1.

Different microorganisms may survive on environmental surfaces for different periods, as determined in laboratory studies. For example, *Mycobacterium tuberculosis* may survive for weeks, whereas the herpes simplex virus dies in a matter of seconds to minutes. Various conditions influence the survival time of microorganisms in the environment, including humidity, temperature, the presence of nutrients and blood or saliva, and the general surface properties of the microorganism. It is impossible to accurately predict how long any microorganism may actually survive on a dental office surface because of these unknown variables. Thus if a surface becomes contaminated with saliva, blood, or other potentially infectious material, the safest approach is to assume that it indeed contains live microorganisms that must be removed or killed before the surface is involved in the treatment of the next patient.

There are two general approaches to surface asepsis. One is to prevent the surface or item from becoming contaminated by use of a surface cover, and the other is to preclean and disinfect the surface after contamination and before reuse. There are advantages and disadvantages to both approaches and usually an office will use a combination of both (Table 12-1).

SURFACE COVERS

The best way to manage surface asepsis from an infection control point of view is to prevent contamination of the surface so it will not have to be precleaned and disinfected before reuse.

Types of Surface Covers

Contamination can be prevented by proper placement of a surface cover before there is an opportunity for contamination. Surface covers should be impervious to fluids to keep microorganisms in saliva, blood, or other liquids from soaking through to contact the surface. Examples of appropriate material for surface covers include clear plastic wrap, bags, or tubes, and plastic-backed paper. Some plastics are designed specifically for use as surface covers in the office in that they have the shape of the item to be covered (e.g., air/wa-

---

Box 12-1   Examples of Surfaces Susceptible to Contamination During Patient Care Activities

Headrest on chair*
Chair control buttons*
Light handles*
Light switch*
Bracket table
Handpiece control switches*
Handpiece hoses*
Evacuator hoses*
Evacuator control*
Air/water syringe handle*
Air/water syringe hoses*

Drawer handles
Countertops
X-ray unit handle and cone
X-ray unit controls*
X-ray view box switch*
Dental team chair backs
Supply containers and bottles
Light curing handle and tip*
Mirror handles
Faucet handles*
Shade guides

---

*Usually more easily covered than precleaned and disinfected, although all surfaces lend themselves to covering.

Table 12-1   Surface Covers Versus Precleaning and Disinfection

ADVANTAGES	DISADVANTAGES
Surface Covers	
Prevents contamination	A variety of appropriate sizes and types may be needed
Protects surfaces that are difficult to preclean adequately	Adds non-biodegradable plastic to the environment upon disposal
May be less time-consuming to perform	May be esthetically unattractive
Reduces handling and storing of disinfecting chemicals	May be more expensive than precleaning and disinfection
Precleaning and Disinfection	
Requires purchase of fewer items to accomplish surface asepsis	Very time-consuming when performed properly
May be less expensive than using surface covers	Must use barriers to protect against contact with the chemicals
Does not change the esthetic appearance of the office	Cannot verify if the microbes have been removed or killed
Does not add plastic to the environment	Some surfaces cannot be adequately precleaned
	Some chemicals may damage some surfaces
	Use of the chemicals requires proper material safety data sheets to be on file in office
	Use-containers must be properly labeled
	Some disinfectants must be prepared fresh daily
	Chemicals are added to the environment upon disposal

ter syringe handle covers, hose covers, pen covers). Some sheets of plastic also have a slightly sticky substance on one side so they will be held on the surface. Other plastics (e.g., some food wraps) have a natural "clinging" ability on contact with a smooth surface. Some plastic bags are available with drawstrings that will hold them around an item to be protected. To reduce costs, thin rather than thick plastic sheets or bags can be used as long as they are not punctured by the surface being covered. Patient bibs are made of plastic-backed paper and also can be used to cover flat operatory surfaces, although thin plastic sheets may be less expensive.

Use of Surface Covers

Dental units come in several shapes and sizes with different positioning of the handpiece control system and light and other accessories. Thus the sizes and shapes of surfaces to be covered vary from one office to the next but general procedures for use of surface covers are the same (Box 12-2).

Clear plastic bags are available in various sizes and are easy to use. For example, if a chair has control buttons on the side, one bag can be used to cover the headrest and the buttons (Figure 12-1). Wraparound backs of chairs used by the dental team may be touched during patient care and can be covered with a large plastic bag (Figure 12-2). On units with a bracket table, one bag may be used to cover the handpiece control unit and the bracket table (Figure 12-3). Hoses and connectors can be covered with plastic tubing that is se-

---

Box 12-2 Use of Surface Covers ****Step-by-Step Procedures****

1. Apply appropriate surface covers before the surfaces have a chance to become contaminated with patient material
2. If the surfaces to be covered have been previously contaminated with patient materials, preclean and disinfect the surface and then remove gloves and wash hands before applying the surface covers
3. Place each surface cover so that it protects the entire surface and will not come off when the surface is touched
4. Wear gloves during removal of surface covers after patient care or other activities are completed
5. Carefully remove each cover without touching the underlying surface
6. If a surface is touched during removal of the cover, preclean and disinfect the surface
7. Discard used covers into the regular trash unless local laws consider these items as regulated waste, then dispose of them as indicated by the law*
8. Remove and discard contaminated gloves, wash hands, and apply fresh surface covers for care of the next patient

---

*In most states, non–sharp contaminated waste such as surface covers is not considered as regulated waste unless an item is soaked or caked with blood or saliva that would be released if the item was compressed.

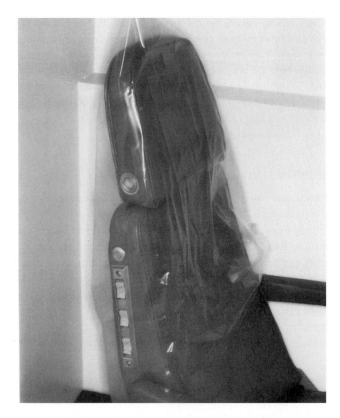

FIGURE 12-1   Surface cover for headrest and chair buttons.

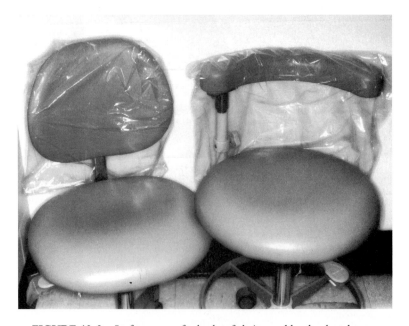

FIGURE 12-2   Surface covers for backs of chairs used by the dental team.

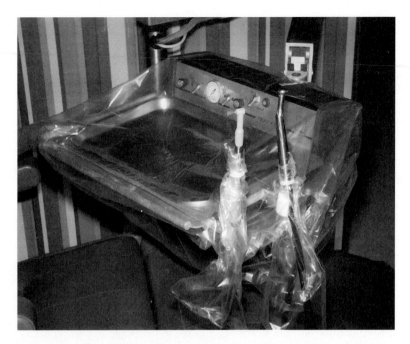

FIGURE 12-3   Surface cover for a control unit and instrument tray holder.

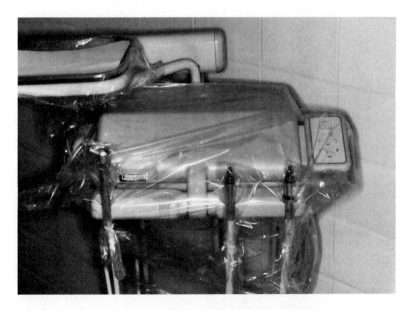

FIGURE 12-4   Surface covers for separate control unit and instrument tray holder.

cured with tape or a rubber band at the connector, or a narrow, long plastic bag may be forced over the connector end (Figure 12-5). Light handles and light switches are commonly touched during patient care and can be covered with plastic wrap or bags, depending on their shape (Figure 12-6). Some lights have removable handles that can be cleaned and heat sterilized before reuse. Covering the air/water syringe handle with plas-

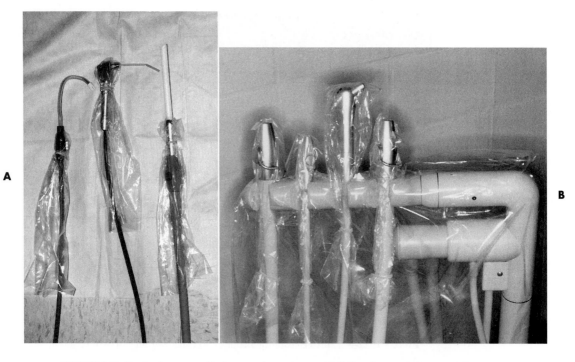

FIGURE 12-5 Surface covers for hoses and connectors. **A,** Saliva ejector connector, air/water syringe handle, and high volume evacuation connector; **B,** various connectors on holders.

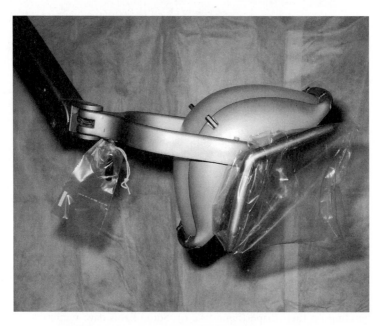

FIGURE 12-6 Surface covers for a light handle and switch.

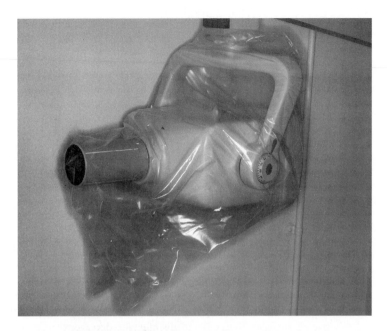

FIGURE 12-7 Surface covers for an x-ray machine.

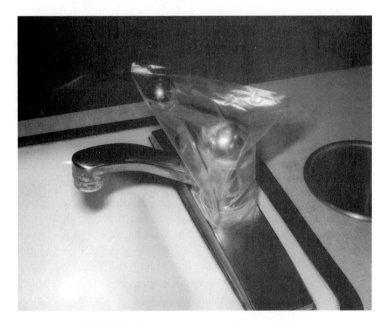

FIGURE 12-8 Surface covers for a sink faucet.

tic wrap to prevent contamination is better than trying to properly preclean and disinfect around the buttons that tend to retain debris (see Figure 12-5). The heads of x-ray units and the control panels can be covered (Figure 12-7), and if the water at sinks is not controlled by elbow-levers, foot pedals, or automatic devices, faucet handles can be covered with plastic bags (Figure 12-8).

PRECLEANING AND DISINFECTION

This approach to surface asepsis best lends itself to surfaces that are smooth and easily accessible for facilitating good contact with the decontaminating chemicals. General procedures for precleaning and disinfecting surfaces are described in Box 12-3.

Precleaning

Surfaces to be disinfected must first be precleaned. This reduces the number of contaminating microorganisms and the blood or saliva present (referred to as bioburden) and facilitates action of the disinfecting chemical. Precleaning is a very important step that must not be slighted. The organic material in blood and saliva will insulate microorganisms from contact with a disinfecting chemical and also may inactivate a portion of the active chemical in the disinfectant.

During the precleaning process, regular soap and water may be used but it is best to use a surface cleaner/disinfectant that contains detergents for both the precleaning step and the disinfecting step. This (along with wearing heavy utility gloves, a mask, protective eyewear, and protective clothing that provide protection during the procedure) starts the killing process during the cleaning step and reduces the chances of spreading the contamination to adjacent surfaces. Water-based disinfectant-detergents (e.g., some synthetic phenolics, iodophors, and quat-alcohols) solubilize organic materials like blood and saliva and facilitate their removal. Also, these same products can be used in the disinfection step described later.

Spray the cleaner on the surface or apply the cleaner with a saturated paper towel or gauze pad (Figure 12-9). Do not store towels or pads in the cleaner (unless supplied in that state by a manufacturer) but wet them immediately before use. After the cleaner is applied, vigorously wipe the surface with a paper towel or gauze pad. In some instances, a surface may require scrubbing with a brush for proper cleaning. If this cannot be performed at the sink, be careful not to splatter the contamination and make sure gloves, a mask, protective eyewear, and protective clothing are in place.

Disinfection

As described in Box 12-3, the precleaned surface is now ready for disinfection (see Figure 12-9). Spray the disinfectant on the precleaned surface and let it remain moist for the longest contact-time indicated on the disinfectant label (usually 10 minutes). If moisture remains, wipe it away with a towel. If a disinfected item will be used in a patient's mouth, rinse away the disinfectant with water and dry. The disinfection procedure is intended to kill disease-producing microorganisms that remain on the surface after precleaning. Unfortunately, the effectiveness of disinfecting surfaces cannot be determined. Thus it is very important to perform the procedures carefully and use the disinfectant as described on the product label.

Characteristics of Disinfectants

Labels on antimicrobial products can be confusing but it is very important to read these labels carefully before using the product. These labels commonly include the type of antimicrobial agent such as:

- *Antiseptic* (for use in killing microorganisms on the skin or other body surfaces)

Box 12-3   Precleaning and Disinfecting Surfaces **Step-by-Step Procedures**

1. Put on utility gloves, mask, protective eyewear, and protective clothing to prevent contact with contaminants and chemicals through touching or splashing
2. Choose a product that is compatable with the surfaces to be cleaned and disinfected. Many manufacturers of dental equipment have determined which surface disinfectants are most appropriate for their products (e.g., dental chairs and unit accessories) from a material compatibility point of view
3. Confirm that the precleaning-disinfecting product(s) have been prepared correctly (if diluted) and are fresh (if necessary). Read and follow the product label directions
4. Preclean the surface. Spray the surface with the cleaning agent and vigorously wipe with paper towels. Holding paper towels behind appropriate surfaces during the procedure will reduce overspray. Alternatively, saturate a paper towel or gauze pad with the cleaning agent and vigorously wipe the surface. Use a brush for surfaces that do not become visibly clean from wiping. If cleaning large areas or multiple surfaces or large spills, use several towels or pads for cleaning so as not to transfer contamination to other surfaces
5. Disinfect the precleaned surface. Spray the disinfecting agent over the entire surfase using towels to reduce overspray (or apply with a saturated pad). Let the surface remain moist for the longest contact time indicated on the product label (usually 10 minutes). Vertical surfaces may dry more quickly
6. If the surface is still wet when ready for patient care, wipe dry. If the surface will come into direct contact with the patient's skin or mouth, rinse off residual disinfectant with water

---

- *Disinfectant* (for use in killing microorganisms on environmental/inanimate surfaces or objects)
- *Sterilant* (for killing all microorganisms on environmental/inanimate surfaces or objects)

The label also lists the general types of microorganisms that can be killed when the product is used as directed, such as:

- *virucidal* (kills at least some viruses)
- *bactericidal* (kills at least some bacteria)
- *fungicidal* (kills at least some fungi)
- *tuberculocidal* (kills the tuberculosis bacterium)
- *sporicidal* (kills bacterial spores, which means it is a sterilant)
- hospital disinfectant (at least kills the three bacteria *Staphylococcus aureus, Salmonella choleraesuis, Pseudomonas aeruginosa*)

The label also lists:

- specific microorganisms (genus and species) shown to be killed in laboratory testing (along with the necessary contact time)
- directions for use of the product, including the need for precleaning
- precautionary statements on handling the product
- storage and disposal information

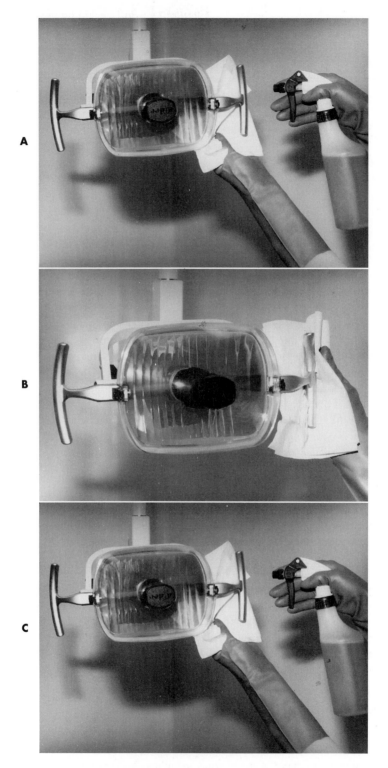

FIGURE 12-9 Surface precleaning and disinfecting by the spray-wipe-spray technique. Precleaning consists of, **A,** spraying with a detergent-disinfectant and, **B,** wiping the surface to clean it. Disinfection is, **C,** reapplying the detergent-disinfectant followed by the appropriate contact time.

- list of the active (antimicrobial) ingredients
- name and address of the manufacturer/distributor; volume of the container; and Environmental Protection Agency (EPA) registration number

There is no perfect disinfectant that will rapidly kill all types of disease-producing microorganisms, have no toxic properties, be unaffected by organic materials, be odorless, not cause any damage to any surface, and be economical. Nevertheless, there are several classes of disinfecting chemicals that have gained wide use in dentistry and medicine. These classes are identified by the type of antimicrobial agents present in the product, which are listed on the product label as "active ingredients" (Table 12-2). Examples of disinfectant products are given in Appendix F.

Since *Mycobacterium tuberculosis* is more difficult to kill than most other microorganisms, disinfectants with tuberculocidal activity are considered as "strong" disinfectants (See Chapter 11, Figure 11-1, *Mycobacterium* species). Stronger disinfectants are active against non-enveloped hydrophilic viruses also, as described in Table 12-3. Use of a water-based disinfectant is reported to provide better cleaning of biologic material such as blood than use of an alcohol-based disinfectant. For dental infection control, a water-based surface disinfectant that is EPA-registered and tuberculocidal (such as iodophors, phenolics, or chlorines) is appropriate if used as directed by the manufacturer and careful precleaning is performed. Manufacturers of disinfectants must submit testing data on the antimicrobial activity and safety of their products to the EPA. If the data are consistent with claims stated on the product labeling, the EPA registers the product. Also, the U.S. Food and Drug Aministration must grant marketing clearance to liquid chemical sterilants labeled for use on medical devices such as dental instruments.

Chlorine Compounds

Chlorine compounds have been used for many years to disinfect drinking water, swimming pool water, and various inanimate surfaces. These agents kill a wide variety of microorganisms and are tuberculocidal. Sodium hypochlorite (which is the main chemical in bleach) is an example of a chlorine compound that is used to disinfect surfaces. It should be noted that commercial bleach (which contains about 5.25% sodium hypochlorite) is a good surface disinfectant at a 1:10 dilution with water, even though it is not an EPA-registered disinfectant. However an EPA-registered disinfectant containing sodium hypochlorite is available. Sodium hypochlorite can damage fabrics and metal surfaces (particularly aluminum), and its activity is reduced in the presence of organic material. If diluted commercial bleach is used as a disinfectant, it should be prepared fresh daily. Gloves, protective eyewear, a mask, and protective clothing should be worn when using any disinfectant.

Iodophors

Iodine and iodine-alcohol mixtures (known as tinctures of iodine) are well known killing agents but have some undesirable properties of corrosiveness, staining, irritation of tissues, and allergenicity. When iodine is complexed with certain organic materials, the compound is referred to as an iodophor (see Table 12-2). Iodophors retain the broad spectrum antimicrobial activity (including tuberculocidal activity) of iodine but they are less corrosive, less irritating to tissues, and have reduced staining activity. Detergents are added to iodophor preparations used as surface disinfectants to enhance the cleaning ability of the solution. Iodophor disinfectants are purchased as concentrated solutions and must be di-

Table 12-2   Active Ingredients in Surface Disinfectants

TYPE OF DISINFECTANT	EXAMPLE OF ACTIVE INGREDIENT(S) LISTED ON PRODUCT LABEL
Chlorines*	Sodium hypochlorite
	Chlorine dioxide
Iodophors*	Butoxypolypropoxypolyethoxyethanol-iodine complex
Water-based phenolics*	
Tri-phenolics	o-Phenylphenol, o-benzyl-p-chlorophenol, and tertiary amylphenol
Dual phenolics	o-Phenylphenol and o-benzyl-p-chlorophenol
Alcohol-based phenolics*	Ethyl or isopropyl alcohol plus
	o-phenylphenol or o-phenylphenol and tertiary amylphenol
Alcohols*	Isopropyl alcohol
Quaternary ammonium compounds (quats)†	
First generation	Benzalkonium chloride
Second generation	Alkyldimethylethylbenzyl ammonium chloride or alkyl-dimethyl-3,4-dichloro-benzyl ammonium chloride
Third generation	Combination of 1st and 2nd generation
Fourth generation	Dioctyldemethyl ammonium bromide or dide-cyldemethyl ammonium bromide
Fifth generation	Combination of 1st and 4th generation
Alcohol-quaternary ammonium compound*	A benzyl ammonium chloride plus isopropyl alcohol

*Tuberculocidal.
†Not tuberculocidal.

luted correctly before use. The diluted solution that is used should be prepared fresh daily unless the manufacturer's label indicates otherwise. Since activity may be reduced by hard water, iodophor disinfectants should be diluted with distilled or deionized water. Iodophors may still be slightly corrosive to some metals and may cause slight staining with repeated use on light-colored surfaces. However, this stain can usually be removed by wiping with alcohol. Gloves, protective eyewear, a mask, and protective clothing should be worn when using any disinfectant.

Alcohols

Isopropyl alcohol (isopropanol, sometimes referred to as rubbing alcohol) and ethyl alcohol (ethanol) have been used as antiseptics and disinfectants for many years because they are relatively non-irritating to the skin; although, alcohol does "sting" when placed on

Table 12-3   Types of Viruses Used in Testing Disinfectant

CLASS	VIRUS	SOLUBILITY
Non-enveloped viruses	Polio virus type I	Hydrophilic*
	Coxsackievirus B_1, B_2	Hydrophilic
	ECHO type 6	Hydrophilic
	Rhinovirus type 17	Hydrophilic
	Adenovirus type 2 or 7	Intermediate†
	Reovirus	Intermediate
	Rotavirus	Intermediate
	V-40 virus	Intermediate
Enveloped viruses	Herpes simplex 1	Lipophilic‡
	Influenza A_2	Lipophilic
	Vaccinia	Lipophilic
	HIV	Lipophilic

*Hydrophilic viruses do not have an envelope and this makes them more difficult to kill with disinfecting chemicals and makes them more soluble in water.
†Intermediate viruses do not have an envelope but their susceptibility to killing by disinfecting chemicals is intermediate between lipophilic and hydrophilic viruses and they are more soluble in lipid materials than other non-enveloped viruses.
‡Lipophilic viruses have a lipid envelope that makes them easier to inactivate with disinfecting chemicals and makes them more soluble in lipid materials then in water.

mucosa (e.g., eye, mouth, nostrils). Although alcohols at 50% to 70% concentration rapidly kill many microorganisms and are tuberculocidal, they evaporate rapidly when sprayed or wiped on surfaces. To counteract this drawback, extenders that retard evaporation of the alcohol after it is placed on a surface have been added to some isopropanol preparations sold as surface disinfectants. Nevertheless, alcohol has other properties that make it less desirable than other agents as a disinfectant. These include a reduction in activity by organic material, corrosiveness, and destruction of some plastic surfaces. Also, alcohols do not solubilize protein material in blood or saliva very well and have been reported to be poor cleaners. Alcohols dry out the skin because they tend to dissolve fat and oil that serve as natural skin moisteners. The "waterless" alcohol-containing handwashing agents (used when handwashing facilities are not readily available) also contain special skin moisteners to reduce these drying effects. While other agents are more appropriate than alcohol as surface cleaners/disinfectants, alcohol is an important component of some disinfectant preparations (see Table 12-2).

Synthetic Phenolics

Phenol (also known as carbolic acid) has the distinction of being the first widely recognized disinfectant used in hospitals. Lord Joseph Lister suggested the use of phenol as an antiseptic during surgical procedures and as an environmental surface disinfectant more than 100 years ago. While it clearly reduced post-operative infections, it was very toxic to tissues, and its use on humans was stopped. Several phenol-related (phenolic) compounds have since been synthesized and used for microbial killing. Thus these compounds are referred to as synthetic phenolics with some use today as active ingredients in surface disinfectants (see Table 12-2), and in mouthrinses and handwashing agents.

The synthetic phenolic disinfectants are tuberculocidal and may contain one, two, or three phenolics, as well as detergents to facilitate cleaning. Some also contain alcohol. Some preparations must be diluted before use and should be prepared fresh daily unless otherwise stated on the product label. Some preparations are packaged in aerosol cans and others are contained in pump-spray bottles. Some preparations may leave a film on the disinfected surface, degrade plastic surfaces with prolonged contact, or may etch glass surfaces. Gloves, protective eyewear, a mask, and protective clothing should be worn when using any disinfectant.

Quaternary Ammonium Compounds

Alcohol-Free Quats.   Quaternary ammonium compounds are also called quats. They are cationic detergents with some antimicrobial activity. A wide variety of quats have been developed over the years, and each time a new type of quat is developed it is referred to as the "next generation"(see Table 12-2). All of the alcohol-free quat disinfectants have a low level of antimicrobial activity and none are tuberculocidal. They also may be inactivated by organic materials and soaps. Although they may be appropriate for disinfection of floors and walls, they are less desirable for items more directly involved in patient treatment. Because of these drawbacks, the American Dental Association recommended in 1978 that quaternary ammonium compounds (free of alcohol) not be used in dentistry.

Quat-Alcohols.   The addition of alcohol to quaternary ammonium compounds enhances their antimicrobial activity. These disinfectants are tuberculocidal and are appropriate for use in dentistry.

ASEPTIC DISTRIBUTION OF DENTAL SUPPLIES

Numerous supplies are used for patient care, and their storage and distribution present a major challenge to infection control. Examples of such items include cotton balls and rolls, gauze pads, floss, articulating paper, retraction cord, orthodontic wire, and tubes or bottles of dental materials, to mention only a few. The major problems relate to surface asepsis and how these supplies are obtained for use at chairside without cross-contamination.

Aseptic Retrieval

If supply items are stored in bulk, such as a container of cotton rolls, an aseptic retrieval system must be used (rather than saliva-coated gloved fingers) to avoid contamination of unused items in the container. Providing sterile forceps (to retrieve the supply item) with the instruments needed for each patient is one approach to this problem. Storing supplies (or instruments) in drawers at chairside lends itself to cross-contamination of the drawer handle (if not covered or precleaned and disinfected) or of bulk items inside (if aseptic retrieval is not used).

Unit Dosing

Supply containers, bottles, and tubes of materials used at chairside on more than one patient (multidose containers) may be protected with a surface cover for each patient or in some instances may be precleaned and disinfected between patients. Many types of disposable supplies can be unit dosed. This means that the supplies are distributed or packaged in small numbers sufficient for care of just one patient and placed at chairside before care begins. For example, a package may contain four cotton rolls, three cotton balls, two gauze pads, articulating paper, etc., or whatever is anticipated for a single patient. Whatever is not used with a patient is discarded. Some supply items are unit dosed by the manufacturers, saving office staff time. Although unit dosing can solve some cross-contamination problems, unfortunately it can be somewhat expensive and wasteful if not organized properly.

SELECTED READINGS

Miller CH: Infection control, *Dent Clin North Am* 40:437-456, 1996.

Miller CH: Sterilization and disinfection, *J Am Dent Assoc* 123:46-54, 1992.

Miller CH, Palenik CJ: Sterilization, disinfection and asepsis in dentistry. In Block SS, editor: *Sterilization, disinfection and preservation,* ed 4, Philadelphia, 1991, Lea & Febiger.

Miller CH: Disinfection of surfaces and equipment, *Dent Assist* 8:21-27, 1988.

Molinari JA, Gleason MJ, Cottone JA et al.: Cleaning and disinfectant properties of dental surface disinfectants, *J Am Dent Assoc* 117:179-182, 1988.

Molinari JA, Runnells RR: Role of disinfectants in infection control, *Dent Clin North Am* 35:323-337, 1991.

Chapter 13

DENTAL UNIT WATER ASEPSIS

The goal of infection control in dentistry is to reduce or eliminate exposures of patients and the dental team to microorganisms. Examples of how this is accomplished have been discussed in other chapters; here we describe contamination of the patient and the dental team with microorganisms present in dental unit water and what may be done to control the quality of dental unit water.

DENTAL UNIT WATER

Water enters the dental office from municipal supplies or from wells. As in our homes, it is then routed to various sites, including sink faucets, toilets, water-heaters, air-conditioners, humidifiers, washers, and, in dental offices, dental units. At the dental unit it enters plastic waterlines, which pass through a multichannel control box that allows the water to be distributed to the hoses that feed various attachments such as high speed handpieces, air/water syringe, and, sometimes, an ultrasonic scaler. The waterlines in dental units have a very small bore, and in the standard 4-hole handpiece hose, it is one of the two smaller lines (Figure 13-1). Thus the water that enters the dental unit is the same water that supplies the entire office.

PRESENCE OF MICROORGANISMS IN DENTAL UNIT WATER

The water that enters the dental unit usually contains just a very few microorganisms (e.g., 0-100) per milliliter (mL). However, water exiting the handpiece and other hoses frequently contains over 100,000 microorganisms per mL. Table 13-1 lists the results of some studies conducted in the U.S. that have measured the concentration of bacteria in dental unit water. Maximum reported recoveries from dental unit water in the U.S. have been 1.2 million and 10 million per mL. Dental unit water contamination apparently occurs worldwide, with reports describing various levels of bacteria from England, Germany, Austria, Denmark, New Zealand, and Canada.

TYPES AND IMPORTANCE OF MICROORGANISMS IN DENTAL UNIT WATER

Waterborne and human oral microorganisms have been found in dental unit water, indicating that both the incoming community water and patient's mouths are sources of these microorganisms (Table 13-2). Most of the microorganisms detected are of very low pathogenicity, or are opportunistic pathogens causing harmful infections only under special

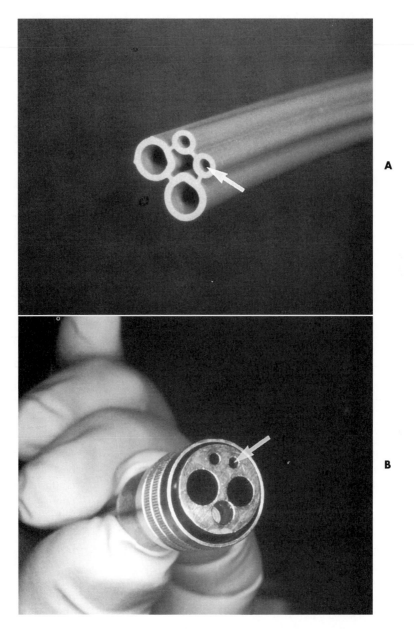

FIGURE 13-1 Dental unit waterline. **A,** The 4-hole high-speed handpiece hose; **B,** the connector at the end of the hose to which a high-speed handpiece is attached. (*Arrows* indicate the waterlines.)

Table 13-1   Presence of Bacteria in Dental Unit Water

LOCATION	SOURCE	cfu/mL (MEAN)
San Francisco*	10 dental units from 3 offices	180,000
	Tap water from same offices	15
Washington,	54 air/water syringe hoses	165,000
California,	22 high speed handpiece hoses	739,000
Oregon[†]	10 faucets	<30
	4 water coolers	<30
	11 rivers and streams	28,200
Indianapolis[‡]	5 dental units	148,000
New Orleans[§]	6 dental units	188,333
Baltimore[||]	8 dental units	110,000

*Abel LC et al.: *J Dent Res* 50:1567-1569, 1971.
[†]Santiago JI et al.: *Gen Dent* 42:528-544, 1994.
[‡]Unpublished data from the author, 1996.
[§]Mayo JA et al.: *Clin Prev Dent* 12:13-20, 1990.
[||]Williams HN, Brockington AM: *Quint Interntl* 26:31-36, 1995.

Table 13-2   Microbes Isolated From Dental Unit Water

MICROORGANISM	PROBABLE SOURCE	PATHOGENICITY
Bacteria		
Achromobacter xyloxidans	Water	Low
Acinetobacter sp.	Water	Opportunistic
Actinomyces sp.	Mouth	Low
Alcaligenes denitrificans	Water	Opportunistic
Bacillus sp.	Water	Low
Bacillus subtilis	Water	Low
Bacteroides sp.	Mouth	Low
Flavobacterium sp.	Water	Low
Fusobacterium sp.	Mouth	Low
Klebsiella pneumoniae	Water	Low
Lactobacillus sp.	Mouth	Low
Legionella pneumophila	Water	Opportunistic
Legionella sp.	Water	Opportunistic
Methylobacterium mesophilica	Water	Low
Micrococcus luteus	Water	Low
Moraxella sp.	Water	Low
Norcardia sp.	Mouth	Low

Table 13-2 Microbes Isolated From Dental Unit Water—cont'd

MICROORGANISM	PROBABLE SOURCE	PATHOGENICITY
Bacteria cont'd		
Ochromobacterium sp.	Water	Low
Mycobacterium gordonae	Water	Low
Pasteurella hemolytica	Water	Low
Pasteurella sp.	Water	Low
Peptostreptococcus sp.	Mouth	Low
Pseudomonas aeruginosa	Water	Opportunistic
Pseudomonas cepacia	Water	Opportunistic
Pseudomonas posimobilis	Water	Opportunistic
Pseudomonas sp.	Water	Opportunistic
Serratia marcescens	Water	Opportunistic
Streptococcus sp.	Mouth	Low
Staphylococcus aureus	Mouth	Intermediate
Staphylococcus sp.	Mouth	Low
Veillonella alkalescens	Mouth	Low
Xanthomonas sp.	Water	Low
Fungi		
Alternaria sp.	Water	Low
Cephalosporium sp.	Water	Low
Cladosporium sp.	Water	Low
Penicillium sp.	Water	Low
Scopulariopsis sp.	Water	Low
Protozoa		
Acanthamoebae sp.	Water	Low
Naeglaria sp.	Water	Low

Adapted from: Miller CH: Dental unit waterline contamination. *Operatory Infection Control Updates*(1):1-8, 1994, with permission from Dental Learning Systems Co., Inc.

conditions or in immunocompromised persons. Microorganisms of main concern are species of *Pseudomonas, Legionella, and Mycobacterium.*

Pseudomonas

Pseudomonas aeruginosa and *P. cepacia* are common inhabitants of our environment, existing in soil and natural waters. Many strains can survive and even multiply in water of very low nutrient content such as distilled water. Thus it is not unusual to find *Pseudomonas* species in almost any type of domestic water supply, storage tanks, and drain line. *P. cepacia* is an important respiratory pathogen in patients with cystic fibrosis. *P. aeruginosa* is usually opportunistic in causing urinary tract infections, wound infections, pneumonia, and septicemia in burn patients, and, it along with *P. cepacia,* usually has a higher degree of resistance than many bacteria to killing by disinfecting chemicals and by antibiotics. The only scientific report that directly implicates any microorganism from dental unit water as a health risk has involved *Pseudomonas.* The report from England implicated *P. aeruginosa* from dental unit water as the cause of oral infections in two medically compromised dental patients.

Legionella

Legionella pneumophila and other species are gram-negative bacteria that naturally occur in water and may gain some protection against the chlorine present in domestic water because they can exist inside certain free-living amoeba also present in the water. *L. pneumophila* is the causative agent of a type of pneumonia called legionnaires' disease, which was first recognized in 1976 when 182 attendees at an American Legion convention in Philadelphia became infected with this bacterium that was present in water in the convention hotel. The bacterium is usually transmitted by inhalation of aerosolized or contaminated water by aspiration of organisms that have colonized the oropharnyx. Specific examples of how *L. pneumophila* may have been transmitted to humans from various sources of water involve cooling towers, heat-exchange apparatuses, a mist machine spraying produce in a grocery store, humidifiers, shower heads, hot water faucets, tap water used to clean medical equipment, and whirlpools in hospitals. However, the route of spread has not been identified for all cases detected. *L. pneumophila* also may cause a nonpulmonary infection called Pontiac fever, and, rarely, wound infections follow irrigation with *Legionella*-contaminated water. While *L. pneumophila* is the principal pathogen in this genus, 30 other species of *Legionella* exist and may cause up to 20% to 30% of all *Legionella* infections.

L. pneumophila or other *Legionella* species have been detected in dental unit water. *L. pneumophila* was found in the water from about 10% of 42 units in 35 practices in Austria, from three of five units in a hospital dental clinic in London, from 4% of 194 dental units at levels above 100 cfu/mL in a London teaching hospital, and from several dental units at the University of Dresden in Germany. In the U.S., *L. pneumophila* has been detected in dental unit water in an Ohio dental school clinic and in 8% of the water samples taken from 28 dental facilities in California, Massachusetts, Michigan, Minnesota, Oregon, and Washington. In the latter study, *L. pneumophila* was never detected at concentrations above 1,000 cfu/mL, but other species of *Legionella* were found in 68% of the water samples tested and at levels of at least 10,000 cfu/mL in 19% of the samples.

While *L. pneumophila* and other *Legionella* species may be present in some dental unit waters in the U.S., there is no documentation that dental unit water has ever caused legionnaires' disease in patients or in dental team members. However, a comment about unpublished data in a report about *Legionella* in dental unit water infers that a dentist in California who died of legionellosis may have contacted the causative agent from his dental unit water. Indirect evidence that dental team members may have occupational exposure to legionellae comes from two studies that showed higher rates of seroconversion with antibodies to legionellae in dental personnel than in non-dental personnel. One of the studies also showed that seroconversion rates increased as the years of experience in dentistry increased. This information suggests that dental workers are at least exposed to *Legionella.*

Mycobacterium

Nontuberculus mycobacteria (e.g., *Mycobacterium chelonae*) have been detected in some domestic water supplies. They are somewhat resistant to chemical killing, and have caused infections in dialysis patients and have been detected in the water used to process dialyzers. There is also a case report of an intraoral infection with *M. chelonae* but the source of this bacterium was not known.

Other Bacteria

Acinetobacter, Alcaligenes, Klebsiella, and *Serratia* (see Table 13-2) are all gram-negative bacteria that are opportunistic pathogens that may cause harmful infections in compromised hosts. No specific documentation exists that these bacteria from dental unit water have caused any infections in patients or in dental team members. The oral bacteria of *Bacteroides, Fusobacterium, Lactobacillus, Peptostreptococcus,* and *Streptococcus* are involved in causing dental caries or periodontal diseases and have opportunistic pathogenicity if allowed to accumulate on tooth surfaces in plaque.

BIOFILM IN DENTAL UNIT WATERLINES

General Nature of Biofilm

Water entering dental units usually has a very low number of microorganisms present but the water that passes out of the dental unit through handpieces, scalers, and air/water syringes is highly contaminated. Thus the incoming water becomes highly contaminated when inside the dental unit. This contamination comes from *biofilm* attached to the inside of the dental unit waterlines.

Microorganisms exist in dental unit waterlines in two types of communities. One bacterial community exists in the water itself and is referred to as the *planktonic* (free floating) microorganisms. The other exists in a sessile form attached to the inside walls of the waterlines called biofilm.

Biofilm is defined as a mass of microorganisms attached to a surface exposed to moisture. Biofilms are very common; they form just about anywhere there is a moist nonsterile environment. This includes the surfaces associated with natural water environments in streams, lakes, and oceans and those associated with "domestic/industrial" water environments such as waterlines, sewer systems, drain lines, wells, septic tanks, sewage treatment facilities, water storage containers, humidifiers, spray heads, etc. Biofilms also form on biomedical materials implanted in or associated with the human body, including many types of catheters, sutures, wound drainage tubes, endotracheal tubes, mechanical heart valves, and intrauterine contraceptive devices (IUDs)

The best example of biofilm in dentistry is dental plaque. Thus there is a type of "plaque" that develops inside of dental unit waterlines that causes a permanent infection of the water delivery system.

Mechanisms of Biofilm Formation

Biofilm forms when bacterial cells adhere to a surface using cell surface polymers. Many of these polymers are highly hydrated exopolysaccharides, referred to as glycocalyx polymers, that give the biofilm a "slimy" nature. As the attached cells multiply within the glycocalyx, the new cells remain embedded and form microcolonies on the surface. Continued multiplication results in the joining of microcolonies, and this with the continual recruitment of additional bacteria from the planktonic phase can result in a covering of the surface.

Biofilm forms on the inside of the dental unit waterlines as the water is flowing through the unit. Several factors allow this to occur (Box 13-1). The water in the dental unit waterlines moves at normal line pressures, which is more slowly than one might imagine. It is not pressurized into the form of the handpiece spray until the water and air mix inside the handpiece. Intermittent stagnation of the water inside the units commonly occurs between patients, overnight, and over the weekends. This facilitates attachment of bacteria from the planktonic community. The dynamics of fluid flowing through a line are such that maximum flow rate occurs in the center of the stream of fluid and the minimum flow occurs near the surfaces of the wall of the tubing. Thus the water is moving more slowly near the surface of the walls, facilitating attachment of bacteria. Another key factor in waterline biofilm formation is that most waterborne bacteria have developed the ability to more efficiently attach to surfaces than most non-waterborne bacteria. This allows these bacteria to become stabilized on a surface and let the nutrients in the water come to them.

Rate of Biofilm Formation

The rate at which biofilm forms depends on the factors mentioned above. As we all know, the biofilm on our teeth (dental plaque) begins to reform immediately after we brush

---

Box 13-1   Factors that Influence the Formation of Dental Unit Waterline Biofilm

1. Water stagnation
     Water in the tubing is not under high pressure
     Water flow rate in the lines is low near the walls of the tubing
     Small diameter tubing creates large surface to volume ratio
2. Even though bacteria are usually at low levels in the incoming water, they are continually present, providing the pioneer bacteria for biofilm formation
3. Some bacteria in air or in patient materials may enter the dental unit waterline system through contamination of waterline openings or retraction through the handpiece or air/water syringe
4. Waterborne bacteria entering the system have special abilities to attach to surfaces, facilitating biofilm formation
5. Incoming water brings a continuous source of nutrient to the bacteria in the developing biofilm
6. Bacteria that attach to tubing walls or to other attached bacteria multiply to increase the mass of the biofilm
7. As water flows by the biofilm, it picks up bacteria from the biofilm and carries it through handpiece, air/water syringes, scalers, and cup fillers

them. By the end of the day most people can even see this plaque. Dental unit waterline biofilm forms more slowly but begins in a new dental unit within hours. A continuous biofilm is visible under the scanning electron microscope within 3 to 6 months after the new unit is placed into operation.

Figure 13-2 shows what mature biofilm in dental handpiece waterlines looks like under the scanning electron microscope (SEM). This particular waterline was used in a dental unit for at least five years. Figure 13-3 shows SEM photomicrographs of biofilm that formed in an air/water syringe waterline of a new dental unit that was in operation for just 5.3 months.

Biofilm can serve as a continuous source of contamination of the flowing water as cells or "chunks" dislodge naturally or from physical stress placed on the line. The fact that biofilm serves as a source of microorganisms in the exiting water has been demonstrated. When waterlines containing biofilm were flushed to remove planktonic bacteria and the lines filled with sterile water, the sterile water became heavily contaminated after a few hours.

Although humans can't live without water, we commonly think of it as having little nutritional value. However, tap water contains low concentrations of inorganic and organic material that can serve as a source of nutrients for microorganisms. In fact biofilm in waterlines serves as a great mechanism by which bacteria can gain continuous access to the low levels of nutrients in a "never-ending" flow of water. Also, the waterborne bacteria are conditioned to an existence in low nutrient environments. For example, strains of *Pseudomonas aeruginosa* and *P. cepacia* have been shown to multiply to high levels in water taken from distilled water reservoirs and commercially prepared distilled water.

THE NEED TO IMPROVE DENTAL UNIT WATER QUALITY

There is no evidence for the occurrence of any widespread public health problem from exposure to dental unit water. On the other hand, the source of the microorganisms causing low levels of infectious diseases in the community are not always identified, and the presence of potential pathogens in dental unit water is of concern. Also, the goal of infection control is to eliminate or reduce exposure to microorganisms. Since infectious diseases may occur when humans and microorganisms come into contact with each other, all health care providers have a responsibility to reduce this possible contact, particularly when it may occur between patients and microorganisms in a health care facility. Using dental unit water that is heavily contaminated with microorganisms of any kind for dental treatment is contrary to the goals of infection control.

Thus improving the quality of dental unit water as means become available is a natural part of maintaining the high quality of patient care and staff protection for which dentistry is well noted.

CURRENT INFECTION CONTROL RECOMMENDATIONS

Centers For Disease Control and Prevention

Current recommendations from the Centers for Disease Control and Prevention (CDC) relate to microorganisms in dental unit water as follows:

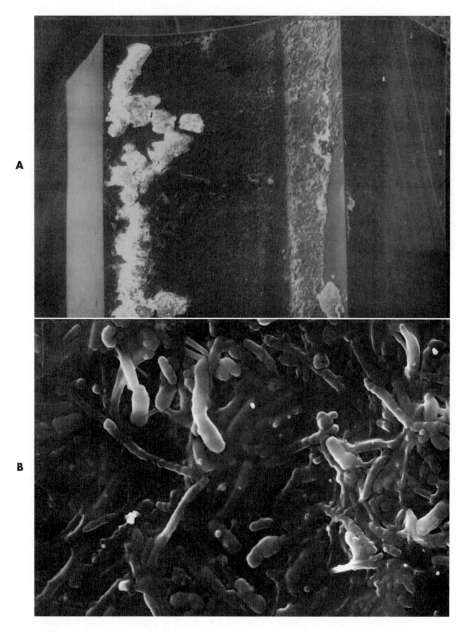

FIGURE 13-2   Scanning electron micrographs of the inside of a small section of high-speed dental handpiece waterline. A one-half inch long section of handpiece hose attached to a dental unit was removed and the waterline separated from the other three lines. The waterline section was cut longitudinally with a clean sterile scalpel to expose the inner lumen. The waterline section was then fixed in 5% glutaraldehyde in cacodylate buffer containing 0.15% ruthenium red. After rinsing with buffer, the section was treated with 4% osmium tetraoxide for 2 hours at room temperature, rinsed again, dehydrated in increasing concentrations of ethanol, incubated for 2 hours in hemamethyl-disilizane, dried for 3 days, exposed to colloidal graphite, and sputter-coated with gold-palladium. **A,** Low-power magnification (80 X) with cut edges of the waterline on the right and left sides and the lumen with biofilm in the middle; **B,** high-power magnification (6,000 X) of the same sample showing biofilm in the lumen. (From Miller CH: Infection control, *Dent Clin No Amer* 40 (No. 2): 437-456, 1996, with permission).

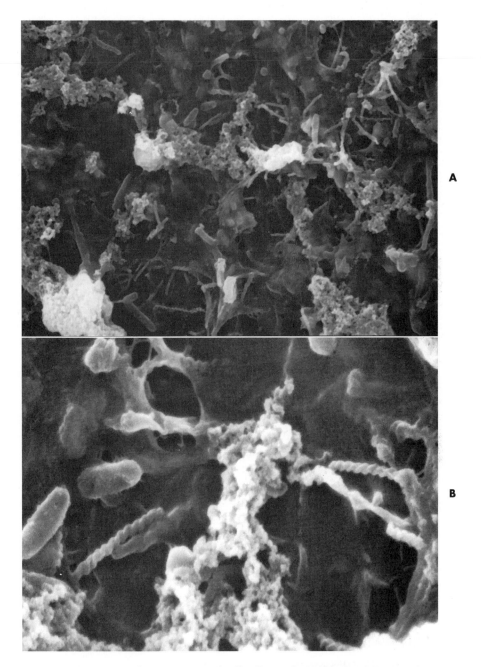

FIGURE 13-3   Scanning electron micrograph of biofilm on the inside of an air/water syringe waterline. The samples were prepared as described in the legend of Figure 13-2. **A,** Original magnification of 1,500; **B,** original magnification of 6,000.

"High-speed handpieces should be flushed to discharge water and air for a minimum of 20-30 seconds after use on each patient. This procedure is intended to aid in physically flushing out patient material that may have entered the turbine and air or water lines. Use of an enclosed container or high-velocity evacuation should be considered to minimize the spread of spray, spatter, and aerosols generated during discharge procedures. Additionally, there is evidence that overnight or weekend microbial accumulation in water lines can be reduced substantially by removing the handpiece and allowing water lines to run and discharge water for several minutes at the beginning of each clinic day. Sterile saline or sterile water should be used as a coolant/irrigator when surgical procedures involving the cutting of bone are performed."

American Dental Association

In 1995, the American Dental Association (ADA) board of Trustees approved the following statement prepared by the ADA Council on Scientific Affairs:

"The Council recommends an ambitious and aggressive course to encourage industry and the research community to improve the design of dental equipment so that by the year 2000, water delivered to patients during nonsurgical dental procedures consistently contains no more than 200 colony forming units per milliliter (cfu/mL) of aerobic mesophilic heterotrophic bacteria at any point in time in the unfiltered output of the dental unit; this is equivalent to an existing quality assurance standard for dialysate fluid that ensures the fluid delivery systems in hemodialysis units have not been colonized by indigenous waterborne organisms. Manufacturers of dental equipment are encouraged to develop accessory components that can be retrofitted to dental units currently in use, whatever the water source (public or independent), to aid in achieving this goal. Further, the ADA should urge industry to ensure that all dental units manufactured and marketed in the USA in the future have the capability of being equipped with a separate water reservoir independent of the public water supply. In this way, dentists will not only have better control over the quality of the source water used in patient care, but also will be able to avoid interruptions in dental care when "boil water" notices are issued by local health authorities. At the present time commercially available options for improving dental unit water quality are limited and will involve some additional expense. They include the use of independent water reservoirs, chemical treatment regimens, daily draining and air purging regimens, and point of use filters."

DENTAL UNIT WATER AND INFECTION CONTROL

Using the Proper Water

The CDC guidelines should be followed by not using dental unit water as an irrigant for surgery involving the exposure of bone. Such surgeries may involve the use of sterile water delivery systems as mentioned in the next section or hand irrigation using sterile water in a sterile disposable syringe. Specialties, including oral surgery, endodontics, and periodontics may have other recommendations concerning the use of irrigants.

Flushing Waterlines

Waterlines and handpieces should be flushed in the mornings and between patients as recommended by the CDC (see above). Although this will not remove biofilms from the lines (biofilm forms while water is moving through the lines), it may temporarily reduce the microbial count in the water and will help clean the handpiece waterlines of materials that may have entered from the patient's mouth. Flushing also brings into the dental unit a fresh supply of chlorinated water from the main waterlines.

Minimizing Sprays and Spatter

The routine use of high-volume evacuation with the high-speed handpiece, ultrasonic scaler, and air/water syringe reduces exposure of the dental team to aerosol and spatter from the patient's oral fluids and from contamination with the water spray from handpiece, scaler, and syringe. This evacuation also may somewhat reduce exposure of the patient to these waterborne microorganisms.

Barriers for the Patient and Dental Team

The rubber dam serves as a protective barrier for the patient from dental unit water. The dam does not totally eliminate exposure but greatly reduces direct contact. The dam also greatly reduces the aerosolizing and spattering of patient microorganisms onto the dental team but does not reduce exposure of the dental team to dental unit water. On the other hand protective barriers of eyewear, masks, and faceshields do serve as barriers for the dental team against microorganisms coming from the patients' mouths and from the aerosols and sprays of dental unit water.

APPROACHES TO IMPROVE DENTAL UNIT WATER QUALITY

Developing approaches to improve the quality of water used for patient treatment is a rapidly advancing field and breakthroughs could occur at any time. Basic considerations when designing approaches to improve dental water quality are given in Box 13-2. Approaches that are being considered include separate water delivery systems, disinfection of the dental unit waterlines, air-purging of the waterlines, using special waterlines, chemical treatment and ultraviolet irradiation of the water itself, and filtration; but they all still need long-term scientific validation (Box 13-3).

Improving Quality of Incoming Water
Sterile Water Delivery Systems

Systems are currently available and cleared by the FDA that completely bypass the dental unit and deliver sterile water through sterile lines to the patient. These are used in some surgical procedures but would be very expensive to use for routine dentistry.

Box 13-2   Considerations When Designing Improvements in Dental Water Quality

---

1. The quality of municipal water as it enters the dental unit cannot be guaranteed
2. Biofilm will develop in any reusable water delivery system that is not maintained
3. Any water that passes through lines containing biofilm will become heavily contaminated
4. Development of approaches should include early testing in a dental unit to help assure later success
5. Several different approaches may be needed simultaneously
6. Water or biofilm treatment chemicals must be compatible with the dental unit and be easily removed from the system by flushing or be non-toxic at the residual levels remaining in the waterlines
7. Use of chemicals to treat water or biofilm must be consistent with the uses indicated by the manufacturer of the chemical
8. Manufacturers of devices for the control of microbial quality of dental unit water must be cleared by FDA before the products can be marketed for that use

---

Box 13-3   Main Approaches to Improve Dental Water Quality

---

1. Improve quality of the incoming water
    Provide sterile water through a sterile delivery system
    Chemically treat and/or filter incoming water
    Use a separate independent water delivery system
2. Prevent or control formation of biofilm
    Disinfect inside of the unit waterlines
    Air-purge waterlines
    Use special waterlines
3. Improve water quality as it leaves the dental unit
    Use a microbial filter

Water Treatment Systems

Water treatment systems treat dental unit water before it is used on the patient. One dental unit manufacturer has a FDA cleared unit that adds a low level of an antimicrobial solution (contains hydrogen peroxide and silver) to the incoming water to disinfect the water as it passes through the unit waterlines. Periodically, the concentrated antimicrobial solution is allowed to stand in the lines for disinfection and control of biofilm formation. This disinfection is followed by water flushing to remove residual chemicals before patient treatment is resumed. Another manufacturer has a combined filtration and chemical treatment (iodination) of the water before it enters the dental unit.

Independent Water Reservoir

The independent water reservoir system uses a separate container of water instead of the plumbed municipal water. A separate bottle is filled with treatment water and then the bottle is pressurized with air from the unit to push the water through the dental unit waterlines. One independent water reservoir system that has FDA clearance recommends using clean water in the reservoir, removing water from the unit waterlines every night by air-purging the lines, disinfecting the dental unit waterlines weekly for 10 minutes with a 0.5% solution of diluted sodium hypochlorite (e.g., a 1:10 dilution of commercial bleach) followed by air-purging and thorough flushing of the lines with water to remove residual bleach before patient treatment is resumed. Most offices with independent water reservoirs on their dental units use distilled water as the patient treatment water. This system provides high quality treatment water if it is faithfully maintained.

Prevent Biofilm Formation in Dental Unit Waterlines

Even though independent water systems or "disinfected water" may be used as described above, it is still necessary to disinfect the inside of the dental unit waterlines (also described above) to hopefully assure that biofilm will not develop in the non-sterile lines. Air-purging the waterlines to remove the water at the end of the day facilitates drying of the biofilm and death of some of the associated microorganisms. Another consideration is development of waterline in which biofilm will not form.

Filter Outgoing Water

Placing a microbial filter in the waterline just before the water enters the handpiece or air/water syringe can greatly improve the quality of the treatment water. An FDA-cleared dental unit waterline filter is currently available. Some of the concerns for this approach are knowing when to change the filter, positioning of the filter in the line to avoid cross-contamination from any retraction of patient materials through the handpiece or air/water syringe, and the need to disinfect any part of the waterline downstream from the filter. Even though filtering the output water does not address the biofilm problem, a filter at the end of the line may be an important safety measure to use in conjunction with other water quality improvement approaches.

BOIL WATER NOTICES

Water treatment facilities in our cities and towns are charged with providing safe drinking water to the public. Occasionally problems will occur in the water treatment plant or with the water distribution system that brings the treated water to our home and offices. One of the most common problems is a break in a water main that allows ground water (contaminated with various microorganisms) to leak into the water distribution system and expose all sites downstream of the leak. Other problems are power failures or mechanical failures at the treatment plant that interrupt purification systems. When this occurs, the water company or health authorities issue a "boil water" notice indicating that the water should not be consumed or should be boiled before use. Such water also should not be used for patient care treatment. If a dental unit has an independent water system and does not use municipal water, there is no problem except with the office tap water. If there is no independent water system, dental unit water should not be used. This means that syringe irrigation is used with non-municipal water when water is needed for treatment or that no patients are seen until the water problem is solved.

A dental office involved in a "boil water" notice needs to contact the manufacturer of their dental units and determine exactly how to disinfect and/or flush the inside of the unit waterlines after the "all clear" notice is given.

SELECTED READINGS

Abel LC, Miller RL et al.: Studies on dental aerobiology: IV. Bacterial contamination of water delivered by dental units, *J Dent Res* 50(6):1567-9, 1971.

Atlas RM, Williams JF et al.: *Legionella* contamination of dental-unit waters, *Appl Environ Microbiol* 61:1208-13, 1995.

Bagga BSR, Murphy RA et al.: Contamination of dental unit cooling water with oral microorganisms and its prevention, *J Amer Dent Assoc* 109:712-16, 1984.

CDC: Recommended infection control practices for dentistry-1993, *MMWR* 41(RR-8):1-12, 1993.

Challacombe SJ, Fernandes LL: Detecting *Legionella pneumophila* in water systems: a comparison of various dental units, *J Amer Dent Assoc* 126:603-8, 1995.

Cochran MA, Miller CH et al.: The efficacy of the dental dam as a barrier to the spread of microorganisms during dental treatment, *J Amer Dent Assoc* 119:141-144, 1989.

Costerton WJ, Cheng K-J et al.: Bacterial biofilms in nature and disease, *Ann Rev Microbiol* 41:435-64, 1987.

Fotos PG, Westphal HN et al.: Prevalence of *Legionella*-specific IgG and IgM antibody in a dental clinic population, *J Dent Res* 64:1382-85, 1985.

Gross A, Divine MJ, Cutright DE: Microbial contamination of dental units and ultrasonic scalers, *Periodontol* 47:670-3, 1976.

Martin MV: The significance of the bacterial contamination of the dental unit water systems, *Br Dent J* 163:15204, 1987.

Mayo JA, Oertling KM et al.: Bacterial biofilm: a source of contamination in dental air-water syringes, *Clin Prev Dent* 12(2):13-20, 1990.

Miller CH: Microorganisms in dental unit water, *Calif Dent Assoc J* 24:47-52, 1996.

Reinthaler FF, Mascher F: *Legionella pneumophila* in dental units, *Zbl Bakt Hyg B* 183:86-8, 1986.

Reinthaler FF, Mascher F, Stunzer D: Serological examination for antibodies against *Legionella* species in dental personnel, *J Dent Res* 67:942-43, 1988.

Williams JF, Johnston AM et al.: Microbial contamination of dental unit waterlines, *J Amer Dent Assoc* 124:59-65, 1993.

Williams HN, Kelley J et al.: Assessing microbial contamination in clean water dental units and compliance with disinfection protocol, *J Amer Dent Assoc* 125:1205-11, 1993.

Chapter 14

ASEPTIC TECHNIQUES

Some infection control techniques do not fall under the major infection control categories discussed in previous chapters. Collectively, they are referred to as *aseptic techniques* because they prevent or reduce the spread of microorganisms from one site to another, such as from patient to dental team, from patient to operatory surfaces, or from one operatory surface to another.

TOUCH AS FEW SURFACES AS POSSIBLE

Gloves used for patient care are contaminated, and that contamination will be transferred to any surface touched. Thus touch as few surfaces as possible with saliva- or blood-coated fingers. If surfaces are touched, they should be protected with surface covers or precleaned and disinfected (see Chapter 12 on Surface and Equipment Asepsis). Make every effort to dispense all items needed at chairside before patient care begins. This reduces the need for leaving chairside with contaminated gloves, mask, and protective clothing, which may spread contamination to other parts of the office. As mentioned in Chapter 10, Protective Barriers, it is best to remove contaminated gloves or use an overglove before leaving chairside during patient care. Place gloves on or carefully remove and discard overgloves when returning to chairside. Another alternative is to have an uninvolved person retrieve items needed unexpectedly during patient care, which is particularly important during some types of surgery (e.g., implant surgery).

Do not rub your eyes, skin, nose, or touch your hair with contaminated, gloved hands.

MINIMIZE DENTAL AEROSOLS AND SPATTER

Dental aerosols and spatter are generated during use of handpieces, ultrasonic scalers, and the air/water syringe. Dental aerosols are small invisible particles of saliva that may contain a few microorganisms and may be inhaled or remain airborne for extended periods. Spatter consists of larger droplets propelled from the patient's mouth that settle rapidly or impact onto nearby operatory surfaces or the face, neck, chest, and arms of the dental team member providing care to the patient.

HIGH-VOLUME EVACUATION

High-volume evacuation (HVE) during use of rotary equipment and the air/water syringe greatly reduces the escape of salivary aerosols and spatter from the patient's mouth. This reduces contamination of the dental team and nearby surfaces. The HVE system should be cleaned at the end of the day by evacuating a detergent or water-based detergent-disinfectant through the system. Sodium hypochlorite should not be used because this may induce corrosion of metal parts in the system. The trap in the system should be removed and cleaned periodically. A safer approach, however, is to use a disposable trap. These traps may contain scrap amalgam that should be disposed of as hazardous material. Gloves, masks, protective eyewear, and protective clothing must be worn when cleaning or replacing these traps to avoid contact with patient materials in the lines from splashing and direct contact.

USE OF THE RUBBER DAM

Reduction in microorganisms escaping a patient's mouth in aerosols or spatter can approach 100% with proper use of the rubber dam, depending on the type and site of the intraoral procedure. Simultaneous use of HVE and the rubber dam provide the best approach to minimizing dental aerosols and spatter (Figure 14-1). A sealant is also available for placement at the rubber dam-tooth interface to further reduce leakage of saliva into the operative site.

Because the rubber dam reduces the amount of saliva present at the operative site, there is less saliva available for retraction into waterspray handpieces or air/water syringes if antiretraction valves in the dental unit fail.

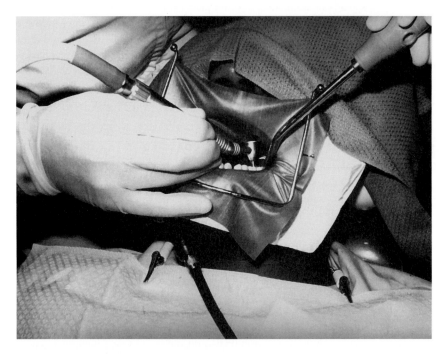

FIGURE 14-1   High volume evacuation and the rubber dam.

Even though the rubber dam and HVE greatly reduce the salivary aerosols and spatter, gloves, mask, protective eyewear, and protective clothing still must be used when employing these aseptic techniques. The rubber dam may not give a perfect seal, and microorganisms that may be present in biofilms on the inside of the dental unit waterlines may be released into the flowing water and aerosolized and sprayed into the face, neck, chest, and arms of the care provider.

Preprocedure Mouth Rinse

The application of antiseptics to skin or mucous membranes before surgery or injections has been practiced for many years. The goal of such application is to reduce the number of microorganisms on the surface to prevent their entry to underlying tissues, which could cause bacteremia, septicemia, or local harmful infections.

The use of an antimicrobial mouth rinse by the patient before dental procedures is based on a similar principle of reducing the number of oral microorganisms. This reduction also reduces the number of microorganisms that may escape a patient's mouth during dental care through aerosols, spatter, or direct contact. Thus fewer microorganisms contaminate the dental team and operatory surfaces. Although studies have not yet shown that the aseptic technique of *preprocedure mouth rinsing* actually prevents diseases in dental team members, studies have shown that a mouth rinse with a long-lasting antimicrobial agent such as chlorhexidine gluconate can reduce the level of oral microorganisms for up to 5 hours. Use of mouth rinses without a long-lasting antimicrobial activity likely would allow the oral microorganisms to return to their original levels before most dental procedures are completed, thus having little infection control value.

Although a preprocedure mouth rinse can be used before any dental procedure, it may be most beneficial before a prophylaxis using a prophylaxis cup or ultrasonic scaler. During these procedures, a rubber dam cannot be used to minimize aerosol and spatter generation, and unless a hygienist has an assistant, HVE is not commonly used. The mouth rinsing may be the only approach to minimizing contamination from aerosols and spatter.

USE OF DISPOSABLES

A disposable item is manufactured for a single use or for use on only one patient. Such items are manufactured from plastics or less expensive metals that are usually not heat tolerant or are not designed to be adequately cleaned. Thus an item that is labeled as disposable must be properly disposed of after use, and no attempt should be made to preclean and sterilize or disinfect it for reuse on another patient.

From an infection control point of view, a single-use (disposable) item has major advantages over a reusable item. It absolutely prevents the transfer of microorganisms from one patient to another because the contaminated item is discarded and not reused on another patient. Another advantage is that the reusable counterpart may be very difficult to adequately clean and sterilize (e.g., the lumen of a needle or the inside of the air/water syringe tip), thus increasing the risk of patient-to-patient cross-contamination. The disposable item eliminates this risk.

Disadvantages of disposables depend on the nature of the individual items, but may include less efficient operation than the reusable counterpart, increased expense, and

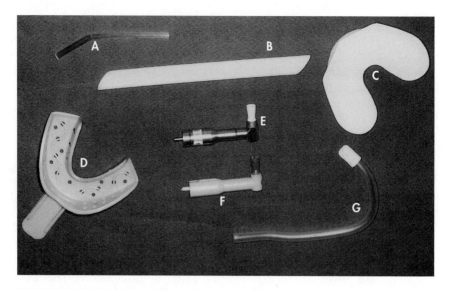

FIGURE 14-2   Examples of disposable items. **A,** Air/water syringe tip; **B,** high volume evacuator tip; **C,** fluoride gel tray; **D,** impression tray; **E,** prophy cup on nondisposable prophy angle; **F,** prophy angle and cup; **G,** saliva ejector tip.

adding nonbiodegradable materials to the environment on disposal. Determining cost-effectiveness in using disposables or reusables must include the cost of the items and also the labor dollars required to decontaminate the reusable items.

More and more disposable items are becoming available to dentistry and include injection needles, anesthetic carpules, air/water syringe tips, HVE tips, saliva ejector tips, curing light probes, certain hand instruments, prophylaxis angles, prophylaxis cups, high-speed handpieces, light handle attachments, impression trays, scalpel blades, and some burs (Figure 14-2). Other disposable items include patient care gloves, masks, gowns, some face shields, surface covers, patient bibs, sharps containers, biohazard bags, specimen containers, and vacuum line traps.

OTHER ASEPTIC TECHNIQUES

Use of a sterile retrieval system to prevent contamination of supply items was discussed in Chapter 12, as was unit dosing. Also, only items needed for the care of a single patient should be on the bracket table, portable unit, or countertops in the operatory. All other items should be stored elsewhere until needed to prevent their contamination.

Dusting of surfaces or sweeping floors in patient-care areas can distribute microorganism-laden dust particles to other surfaces unless performed with a wet cloth or wet mop. A smooth-surface floor rather than carpeting is more appropriate for patient-care areas because of its cleanability and lesser likelihood of accumulating dust and dirt. Dust covers might be considered for operatory and sterilizing room surfaces over the weekend or during vacation periods.

Several aseptic techniques relate to instrument processing, as mentioned in Chapter 11. The sterilizing room should be separated into "clean" and "dirty" areas to avoid mingling of sterile and nonsterile instruments. Chemical indicators on instrument packaging also help differentiate between items that have and have not been heat processed. Also, sterile packages should be handled and stored away from sinks in a dry area.

During high-speed handpiece processing, a cleaner/lubricant is sprayed into the drive-air line, and excess lubricant is flushed out by connecting the dental-unit air system on an air-line installed in the sterilizing room. Air-flushing must be performed so that the aerosol is not released into the air environment by flushing directly into the vacuum system or into a sink with water or a container with absorbent material that will "catch" the spray.

SELECTED READINGS

Cochran MA, Miller CH, Sheldrake MA: The efficacy of the dental dam as a barrier to the spread of microorganisms during dental treatment, *J Am Dent Assoc* 119:141-144, 1989.

Council on Dental Materials, Instruments and Equipment, American Dental Association: Dental units and water retraction, *J Am Dent Assoc* 116:417-420, 1988.

Miller, CH: Using effective aseptic procedures, *RDH* 11:20-21, 1991.

Miller RL, Micik RE, Abel C et al.: Studies on dental aerobiology: II. Microbial splatter discharged from the oral cavity of dental patients, *J Dent Res* 50:621-625, 1971.

Molinari JA, Molinari GE: Is mouthrinsing before dental procedures worthwhile? *J Am Dent Assoc* 123:75-80, 1992.

Chapter 15

LABORATORY AND RADIOGRAPHIC ASEPSIS

LABORATORY ASEPSIS

Any instrument or piece of equipment used in the oral cavity or on orally soiled prosthetic devices or impressions is a potential source of cross-infection. It is impossible to determine all infectious patients from medical histories or patient conversations. Therefore the only valid posture is to assume (and act as if) all patients are capable of transmitting highly infectious diseases. The same sets of criteria and techniques must be used in all cases.

If contaminated items were to enter the laboratory environment, infectious materials could be spread to prostheses and appliances of other patients. Unsuspecting laboratory personnel also could be placed at increased risk for cross-infection.

Protective Barriers

All items coming from the oral cavity must be sterilized or disinfected before being worked on in the laboratory and before being returned to the patients. Asepsis procedures vary for each type of dental material. General recommendations for procedures and materials can be made. Laboratory infection control also involves, depending on need, the wearing of personal protective barriers such as gloves, safety eyewear, gowns, and masks.

For a successful laboratory infection control program, two major criteria must be met. These are 1) the use of proper methods and materials for handling and decontaminating soiled items and 2) the establishment of a coordinated infection control program between dental offices and laboratories. This will help dental practitioners and dental technologists create and maintain mutually effective infection control programs.

Microbially Soiled Prostheses

Any prosthesis coming from the oral cavity is a potential source of infection (Table 15-1; also see Chapters 6 and 7). Most prostheses and appliances cannot withstand standard heat sterilization procedures. An alternative technique for most prostheses is disinfection by immersion after a thorough cleaning. There are a limited number of liquid chemicals capable of sterilization. The most commonly used agent in dentistry is glutaraldehyde. Fortunately, sterilization of prosthetic devices is rarely required. Disinfection is the choice in most circumstances.

Gloves and protective outerwear must be worn when handling orally soiled prostheses until they have been properly disinfected. Also, masks and protective eyewear must be in place whenever handling hazardous chemicals. All disinfectants must be considered hazardous. Therefore personal protective barriers and adequate ventilation must always

Table 15-1 Oral Pathogens of Concern*

MICROORGANISMS	BODY SOURCE	ESTIMATED SURVIVAL TIME (AT 21° C)
Epstein-Barr virus	Saliva	Seconds
Treponema pallidum	Lesion contact	Seconds
Mycoplamsa pneumonia	Saliva and secretions	Seconds to minutes
Cytomegalovirus	Saliva and blood	Seconds to minutes
Neisseria gonorrhoea	Exudate contact	Seconds to minutes
Human immunodeficiency virus, type 1	Blood	Seconds to minutes
Herpes simplex viruses, types 1 and 2	Saliva and secretions	Minutes
Respiratory viruses	Secretions and saliva	Hours
Varicella-zoster virus	Secretions and vesicles	Hours
Mumps virus	Saliva and secretions	Hours
Streptococcus pyogenes	Saliva and secretions	Hours to days
Staphylococcus aureus	Exudates, skin, and saliva	Days
Mycobacterium tuberculosis	Saliva and sputum	Days to weeks
Hepatitis B virus	Saliva and blood	Weeks
Hepatitis C virus	Saliva and blood	Weeks
Hepatitis A virus	Saliva, feces, and blood	Weeks to months

*Modified from Willett NP, White RR, Rosen S: *Essential dental microbiology,* Norwalk, Connecticut, 1991, Appleton & Lange.

be employed. Eye/face protection is mandatory whenever using rotary or air blasting cleaning equipment.

The best way to decontaminate soiled prostheses is through chairside disinfection immediately after removal. Prostheses are first rinsed well with tap water and then placed into glass/plastic containers or into "zippered" plastic bags containing appropriate disinfecting solutions. See Table 15-2 for specific recommendations. After at least 15 minutes, the prostheses are removed and rinsed well again with tap water. If glutaraldehydes are used, the prostheses should be rinsed in a container under running water for at least ten minutes. The prostheses are now ready to be transported to the office or commercial laboratory.

Some heavily soiled (e.g., with calculus or adhesive) prostheses require cleaning or scrubbing before disinfection. The most efficient (and safest) procedure is to place the prostheses into "zippered" plastic bags containing ultrasonic detergent and then to place the assembly into an ultrasonic cleaner (Figure 15-1). Glass or plastic beakers or containers can be used also. The bags are suspended by being pinned in place by the cleaner's lid. The goal is to position the bag near the middle of the cleaning solution. Poorer cleaning occurs near the top and bottom of the solution pool. If further hand scrubbing or cleaning is required, personal barriers must remain in place. Air-powdered blasters, such as shell blasters, should be used only on cleaned and disinfected prostheses.

Table 15-2   Recommendations for Disinfecting Prosthetic Devices and Appliances[*]

PROSTHETIC DEVICE[‡]	DISINFECTANTS[†]		
	GLUTARALDEHYDES	IODOPHORS	SODIUM HYPOCHLORITE
Complete dentures (plastic/porcelain)	No	Yes	Yes
Removable partials (metal/plastic)	No	Yes	Yes/No[§]
Fixed prostheses (metal/plastic/porcelain)	Yes	No	Yes/No[§]
Stone casts	No	Yes	Yes
Wax rims, bites[‖]	No	Yes	No

[*]Modified from ADA Council on Scientific Affairs and ADA Council on Dental Practice: infection control recommendations for the dental office and the dental laboratory, *Journal of the American Dental Association* 127:672-80, 1996, and Merchant VA: Infection control in the dental laboratory environment. In Cottone JA, Terezhalmy GT, Molinari JA: *Practical infection control in dentistry,* ed 2, Baltimore, 1996, Williams and Wilkins.

[†]Solutions must be prepared according to manufacturers' recommendations for surface or immersion disinfection. Routine immersion time is 15-30 minutes. Combination synthetic phenolics are not included in this listing. These solutions cannot be reused and cost significantly more than bleach or iodophors. Thus their practical use is limited to spraying.

[‡]Incompatibilities between fabrication materials and surface disinfectants are known to exist. Physical/chemical variability of a given type of material or solution per manufacturer limits the strength of general recommendations. Experimentation is required when handling new formulations.

[§]Use a 1:10 dilution of bleach. Bleach and some metals are somewhat incompatible, thus limit exposure to solutions to a maximum of ten minutes.

[‖]Use the "spray-wipe-spray" methods commonly used for environmental disinfection.

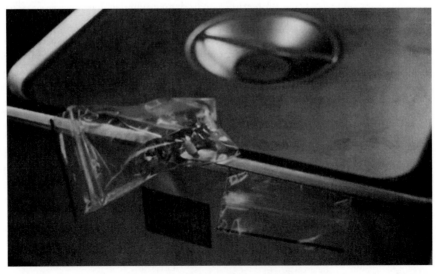

FIGURE 15-1   Ultrasonic cleaning of a heavily soiled prosthesis in a zippered plastic bag containing a disinfectant solution.

Only solutions that have proven reuse abilities (e.g., glutaraldehydes) can be used on subsequent cases. Disinfectants such as dilute bleach, iodophors, or phenolic compounds are single-use items. If used for immersion disinfection, they must be discarded after each use.

The same procedures must be used when the prostheses are being returned from the dental laboratory. Prostheses that have been properly disinfected (treated and rinsed) can be returned to the client office in a deodorizing solution such as a mouth rinse. Because of the increased risk for adverse tissue response (both to the patient and the office staff), prostheses should never be sent out or returned in disinfectant solutions, especially glutaraldehydes.

Dental Impressions

Dental impressions easily become contaminated with patient blood and saliva. Such fluids can contain overt viral and bacterial pathogens (see Table 15-1). Some of these microorganisms can exist for extended periods outside of their human hosts. Transfer of microorganisms from contaminated impressions to dental casts has been demonstrated. More recent information indicates that oral bacteria can remain viable in set gypsum materials for periods of up to seven days. Improper handling of orally soiled impressions, therefore, offers a definite opportunity for cross-infection.

Gloves, protective eyewear, and other outerwear must be worn whenever handling orally soiled impressions until they have been properly disinfected. Personal barriers and adequate ventilation must always be employed when hazardous materials such as disinfectants are being used.

The best way to decontaminate soiled impressions is through chairside disinfection immediately after removal. Currently, more commercial dental laboratories disinfect impressions than do dental offices. Many impressions, especially the elastomeric types, can be repeatedly disinfected. The hydrocolloids and polyethers are more sensitive and should be treated only once. Disinfection of impressions can be coordinated in several ways. An office and its referral laboratory could establish a written protocol. In some locations, dental component societies and laboratory organizations have formally established procedural standards.

Impressions should be rinsed with tap water after removal and then shaken to remove adherent water. Studies indicate that rinsing thoroughly serves an important function in the preliminary removal of adhering microorganisms. Rinsed impressions are placed into glass beakers, plastic containers, or "zippered" plastic bags containing appropriate disinfecting solutions (Figure 15-2). Specific recommendations are presented in Table 15-3. It is best to limit exposure to any disinfectant solution. All chemicals must be kept in well-sealed containers. Any contact, especially with skin and mucous membranes, must be avoided (see Chapter 12 for acceptable products). After 15 minutes, the impressions are removed, rinsed well with tap water, and shaken. The impressions are now ready for pouring.

Some types of impressions (e.g., polyethers) are sensitive to immersion. Exposure should be limited to ten minutes. Careful selection of disinfectant is required. As an alternative, these impressions can be sprayed thoroughly and wrapped with paper towels moistened well with the same disinfectant solution. After 15 minutes, the impressions are removed, rinsed well, shaken, and ready to be poured.

Spraying has several advantages. It is the treatment of choice for some types of dental materials. It uses less solution, and often the same disinfectant can be used for general disinfection of environmental surfaces. Spraying is probably not as effective as immersion, however,

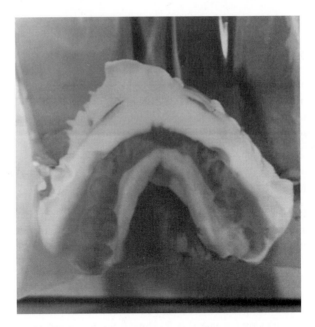

FIGURE 15-2   Disinfection of an impression within a zippered plastic bag.

Table 15-3   Recommendations for Disinfecting Impression Materials[*]

| | DISINFECTANTS[†] | | |
IMPRESSION MATERIAL[‡]	GLUTARALDEHYDES	IODOPHORS	SODIUM HYPOCHLORITE
Alginate	No	Yes	Yes
Polysulfides	Yes	Yes	Yes
Silicones	Yes	Yes	Yes
Polyethers	No	Yes[§]	Yes[§]
Reversable hydrocolloids	No	Yes	Yes
Compound	No	Yes	Yes

[*]Modified from ADA Council on Scientific Affairs and ADA Council on Dental Practice: infection control recommendations for the dental office and the dental laboratory, *Journal of the American Dental Association* 127:672-80, 1996, and Merchant VA: Infection control in the dental laboratory environment. In Cottone JA, Terezhalmy GT, Molinari JA: *Practical infection control in dentistry,* ed 2, Baltimore, 1996, Williams and Wilkins.

[†]Solutions must be prepared according to manufacturers' recommendations for surface or immersion disinfection. Routine immersion time is 15-30 minutes. Combination synthetic phenolics are not included in this listing. These solutions cannot be reused and cost significantly more than bleach or iodophors. Thus their practical use is limited to spraying.

[‡]Incompatibilities between fabrication materials and surface disinfectants are known to exist. Physical/chemical variability of a given type of material or solution per manufacturer limits the strength of general recommendations. Experimentation is required when handling new formulations

[§]Polyethers are unusually sensitive to immersion. Disinfection by spraying is the method of choice. See text for details.

because constant contact of disinfectant with all surfaces of the impression cannot be assured. When given a choice, immersion always should be selected. Also, spraying releases disinfectant into the air, thus increasing the chances of personnel exposure. Most disinfectants can be used for spraying. An exception is the glutaraldehyde, which should never be sprayed.

Disinfection of impression materials is an area of continuing research. Some impression types are harmed by disinfection in certain types of chemical solutions. Other types of disinfectants, however, can be used safely on the same impression materials. Variation in response within a type of impression material (e.g., alginate) by manufacturing source has been noted. A small amount of in-house experimentation is highly recommended.

Another way to reduce the chances of cross-infection related to the handling of impressions is the use of disinfectant-containing materials. Most of these are alginates supplemented with chlorhexidine or quaternary ammonia compounds. There is a small set of data that indicate that these materials can reduce the number of oral microorganisms on and within an impression. The attractive aspect is that some disinfection occurs during setting and does not require an additional procedure. However, such products still need to be disinfected by immersion before pouring.

Grinding, Polishing, and Blasting

Laboratory work on impressions, appliances, and prostheses should be performed only on disinfected items. Bringing untreated materials into the laboratory establishes the potential for cross-infection.

Operating a dental lathe provides an opportunity for the spread of infection and for injury. The rotary action of the wheels, stones, and bands generates aerosols, splatter, and projectiles. Whenever the lathe is being used, protective eyewear must be in place, the front Plexiglas shield must be down, and the ventilation system must be operating properly. The use of a mask is highly recommended. The air suction motor should be capable of producing an air velocity of at least 200 feet/minute. Maximum containment of aerosols and splatter can be achieved when a metal enclosure with hand holes is fixed to the front of the lathe's hood. All attachments, such as stones, rag wheels, and bands, can be sterilized or disinfected between uses or thrown away. The lathe unit must be disinfected twice a day.

Fresh pumice and pan liners should be used for each case (Figure 15-3). The modest cost of the materials and the proven significant microbial contamination in reused pumice prohibits repeated use.

Polishing appliances and prostheses before delivery is a necessary activity. Polishing exposes the operator to potential cross-infections and physical injury. However, if the item being polished has been aseptically prepared, the risks of infection are reduced to a minimum. To avoid the potential spread of microorganisms, all polishing agents (e.g., rouge) should be obtained in small quantities from larger reservoirs. Unused materials should never be returned to the central stock; they should be thrown away. Most polishing attachments (e.g., brushes, wheels, and cups) are single-use, disposable items. Reusable items should be sterilized between uses, if possible, or at least be disinfected.

Intermediate Cases

Complete and partial dentures undergo an intermediate wax try-in stage. Crowns, splinted bridges, and partial denture frameworks are often "test seated" before cementation or sol-

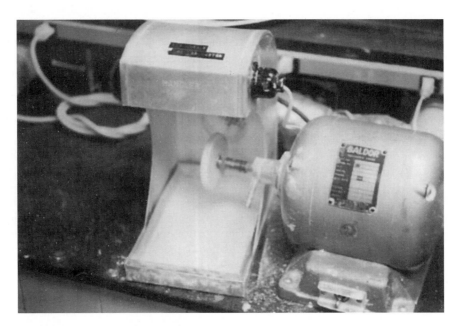

FIGURE 15-3   Polishing with a rag wheel and pumice. Lathe is lined with a single use plastic liner.

dering. These devices, like wax try-in step dentures, can become soiled with oral fluids. Before returning the items to the laboratory for further processing, they must be disinfected. The procedures in most cases are the same as those described for completed projects (see Table 15-2).

Returning Completed Cases

Appliances and prostheses being returned to the patient are not free of microbial contamination. These organisms could come from other cases, as well as from the operator's body, if aseptic procedures are not rigorously followed. Many patients have open oral lesions or are sufficiently traumatized during treatment so as to facilitate easier microbial penetration. Also, a growing number of patients have impaired immune defense systems or are on chemotherapy programs that render them more susceptible to infectious diseases. The best location for disinfection procedures is chairside.

Other Thoughts

All laboratory infection control activities are designed to accomplish a single goal—breaking the chain of disease transmission. If the person-to-person flow of infection can be interrupted, the safety of the work environment will be improved. Also, the chances of patient acquisition of disease during treatment would be greatly reduced.

Infection control processes can be effective only when performed consistently well. For dental laboratory asepsis to be successful, offices and laboratories must perform essential tasks. Redundancies in the system should be identified and minimized. An overall increase in efficiency could be realized when offices and laboratories formally and properly coordinate their efforts.

RADIOGRAPHIC ASEPSIS

Proper infection control methods and materials for dental radiology differ little from those used for procedures more likely to result in blood exposure, such as periodontal therapy, surgical procedures, and many restorative treatments.

Consistent use of the most effective and efficient types of personal protective equipment, such as gloves, masks, gowns, and eyeglasses decreases the chances of exposure to infectious agents. Appropriate environmental covers, cleaning, and disinfection must also be performed. For dental radiology, only a limited number of items require sterilization.

Correct materials must be used in conjunction with a well-written office infection control procedures manual and correct and regularly scheduled training sessions. A consistently appropriate level of personal and environmental protection must be extended.

The radiographic process also involves the handling of hazardous materials (see Chapter 19). It is imperative that all personnel involved with the development of radiographs be aware of the chemical hazards inherent to the process. Proper hazardous materials management is based on continuous employee training and active participation to minimize the chances of exposure and possible injury. Employees must know which chemical components are hazardous, the location of the office's hazardous materials list, the labeling system used to identify and describe hazardous chemicals, about the warning signs present, and the location and proper use of material safety data sheets.

Unit, Film, and Patient Preparation

The radiographic process offers the possibility that body fluids will contaminate disposable and reusable items (see Table 15-1). Gloves of some type must be worn when taking radiographs and when handling orally soiled radiographic films. Because taking radiographs is a clinical activity, the protective gowns and masks worn for restorative procedures must also be considered. Protective eyewear is used as a barrier against contact with patient fluids but also to prevent exposure to hazardous chemicals.

Many of the items used to take radiographs are used once and thrown away. Few reusable items touch unintact skin or mucous membranes or enter normally sterile body tissues. These, however, still require sterilization. After cleaning, such materials are sterilized by heat and reused. Since most of these reusable items can withstand sterilization temperatures, it is best to process them in a steam autoclave or an unsaturated chemical vapor sterilizer. Heat-sensitive materials (e.g., some types of plastic) can be treated by immersion in a full-strength glutaraldehyde solution (see Chapters 11 and 12).

Environmental infection control employs surface disinfection and the use of covers. In private practice situations, disinfection is preferred because of cost and efficiency concerns. However, the placement of plastic drapes, bags, or tubing over the x-ray unit (tube head, arm, and cone), chair head rest, and control panel probably is better than disinfection because of the numerous and large surfaces touched during the process (Figures 15-4 and 15-5).

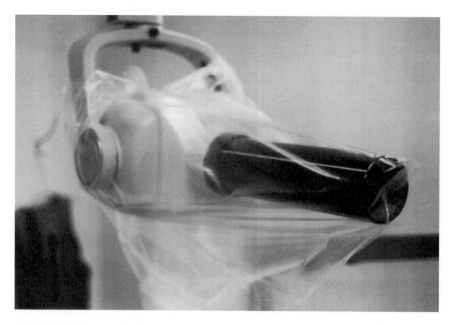

FIGURE 15-4   Use of plastic covers to protect commonly touched surfaces from contamination.

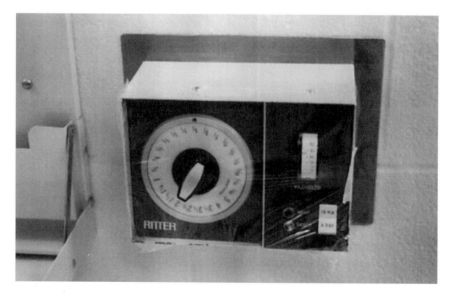

FIGURE 15-5   Protection of x-ray control knobs/buttons with plastic covers.

Taking Radiographs

Using clean gloves (just about any type will work), arrange unexposed films on a paper towel. Exposed films have to be oriented so that exposed films can be easily differentiated from unused ones. A possible solution is to place exposed films into a disposable plastic cup or onto a labeled paper towel. This helps to minimize contamination and also facilitates transport.

Environmental surfaces can be protected from contamination (see Figures 15-4 and 15-5). This can be accomplished by the use of covers, disinfection, or a combination. Contaminated surfaces not covered must be disinfected. See Chapter12 for proper disinfection agents, personal protective barriers, and procedures. Items such as control panel knobs and buttons, because of their shape and design, are best covered. Spraying disinfectant into such areas may cause electrical shorts. Because of time constraints, many offices elect to cover the majority of the involved surfaces, such as x-ray cones, rather than to disinfect.

Darkroom Activities

Exposed films should be transferred to the darkroom in a plastic cup or within a folded paper towel but never in the pocket of a clinic gown or jacket. Avoid touching any surfaces, such as doors, tabletops, or film processing equipment with soiled gloves during transport.

First, all films should be disinfected using an agent known to kill tuberculosis bacterium within ten minutes (see Chapter 12). Use the three-step method of "spray-wipe-spray." A new pair of gloves is then used to open the films onto a new paper towel or sheet. If care is used when opening, further disinfection is not needed. The films are either contained within plastic pouches or they are not. Disinfected pouched films can be carefully opened and the contents expelled. The result is a set of exposed, yet unsoiled, film packets. Disinfected, unopened films are unwrapped using a new pair of gloves. The first step in this process is to open the film packet tab by holding the color-coded end and pulling the tab up and away. The exposed lead foil and black interleaf paper are pulled out. The lead foil is then rotated off the black paper. The black paper is carefully opened and the film is allowed to fall onto a paper towel or into a clean cup.

After all the films have been opened, the gloves, empty packets, and possibly the exterior plastic pouches are discarded into an appropriate container. Hands are then washed and the films developed manually or with the use of an automatic processor. To prevent artifacts, avoid contact between gloves and uncovered film. Note that developer and fixer, even when microbially contaminated, do not sustain bacterial or fungal growth.

For several years, x-ray films have been sold covered with protective plastic pouches. The pouches can also be purchased separately and placed onto x-ray films chairside (Figure 15-6). There are distinct infection control advantages to using radiographic films in pouches. If the pouches are carefully opened in the operatory or the darkroom the result is exposed, but unsoiled, film packets. Testing indicates that when properly placed, the covers do not allow penetration of fluids.

Daylight Loaders

Potential problems can arise with the use of daylight loaders attached to automatic processors or with "portable darkrooms," which contain small beakers or cups of developing so-

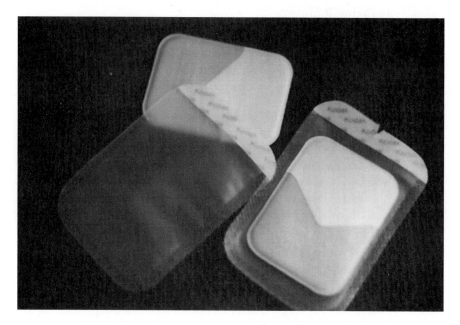

FIGURE 15-6   Protective plastic pouches for radiographic films.

lutions. These units are equipped with portals that allow penetrance of hands and arms with a maximum exclusion of light. This is accomplished with the use of cloth or rubber sleeves, cuffs, or flaps. Because the units have limited operational space, chances of cross-infection are increased. The sleeves are difficult to impossible to disinfect well after soiling.

The only aseptic way to use these units is to insert only disinfected or unsoiled film packets (those formerly in pouches) into the unit. Use powder-free gloves. Film packets can be grouped into plastic cups and placed inside the daylight loader. Unwrapped films can then be placed into another clean cup or onto a paper towel. After all films have been opened, the waste packet wraps can be collected into a cup. Using a bare hand, pick up the films by the edges and feed them into the processor. Manual processing requires gloved hands and clips to dunk the films.

Waste Management

Orally soiled disposable items such as gloves, paper towels, or x-ray film covers are in most locations not considered to be infectious (and thus regulated) medical waste (see Chapter 16). This means that such items do not require special handling, storage, and neutralization procedures before disposal. It is, however, the responsibility of every dental office and clinic to be aware of the current regulations for their location.

SELECTED READINGS

ADA Council on Scientific Affairs and ADA Council on Dental Practice: infection control recommendations for the dental office and the dental laboratory, *Journal of the American Dental Association* 127:672-80, 1996.

Centers for Disease Control: recommended infection-control practices for dentistry, *MMWR* 41(RR-8):1-12, 1993.

Glass BJ, Terezhalmy GT: Infection control in dental radiology. In Cottone JA, Terezhalmy GT, Molinari JA: *Practical infection control in dentistry,* ed 2, Baltimore, 1996, Williams and Wilkins.

Goaz PW, White SC: *Oral radiology - principles and interpretations,* ed 3, St. Louis, 1994, Mosby.

Merchant VA: Infection control in the dental laboratory environment. In Cottone JA, Terezhalmy GT, Molinari JA: *Practical infection control in dentistry,* ed 2, Baltimore, 1996, Williams and Wilkins.

Merchant VA: Infection control in the dental laboratory: concerns for the dentist, *Compendium* 14:382-390, 1993.

Miller CH, Palenik CJ: Infection control in dentistry. In Block S: *Sterilization, disinfection, preservation and sanitation,* ed 4, Philadelphia, 1991, Lea & Febiger.

NADL, Health and Safety Committee. *Infection control compliance manual for dental laboratories,* Alexandria, Virginia, 1992, National Association of Dental Laboratories.

Palenik CJ, Miller CH: Infection control for dental radiology, *Dental Asepsis Review* 17(4):1-2, 1996.

Puttaiah R, Langlais RP, Katz JO, Langland OE: Infection control in dental radiology, *CDA Journal* 23(5):21-28, 1995.

Chapter 16

WASTE MANAGEMENT

COMPREHENSIVE WASTE MANAGEMENT PLAN

Dental offices and clinics are subject to a variety of federal, state, and local regulations concerning infection control, hazardous materials handling, employee safety, and waste management issues. To be in compliance, special efforts must be made by all parties to be aware of an ever-increasing number of governmental mandates.

Because office and clinic personnel must have a working understanding of what is actually required, didactic and in-service training is needed. To meet a perceived need, many organizations and proprietary corporations now offer several consulting services, formal training sessions, and audiovisual materials. Because of the competitive nature of such businesses, the scope and value of some programs tend to be inflated. The question arises, "What kinds of programs do we really need and how can we choose the best ones for us?"

All employees must be knowledgeable of Occupational Safety and Health Administration (OSHA) regulations concerning bloodborne pathogens (Chapter 6), hazardous materials (Chapter 19), and safe use of chemicals in the laboratory (Chapter 19). The Environmental Protection Agency (EPA) has standards, many of which are applicable to dentistry, for workplace exposure levels to chemicals, heat, and radiation, and for discharge and final treatment of waste materials. Employees also must be aware of their state (and possibly local) requirements concerning sterilization, disinfection, and medical waste management. The Centers for Disease Control and Prevention (CDC) and The American Dental Association (ADA) guidelines/recommendations contain important and valuable information (see related topics in Chapters 8, 11, 14, and 17).

Most offices elect to use external sources (including this book) to become more knowledgeable about the involved rules and regulations. After the rules are understood, the process of compliance is far less imposing. OSHA and the ADA indicate that personnel who are knowledgeable about the general rules and the specific discipline(s) of the audience must provide the training. OSHA also requires that training include open opportunities for questions. Even though many audiovisual kits contain elements of programmed learning and sets of review questions, such training aids do not involve the presence of a knowledgeable "live" facilitator.

A bare minimum for personnel training should be attendance at some type of annual program. Unless all required topics are covered, participation in several (more narrow-cast) conferences are required. There currently is a trend in many states to reinstate or increase the number of continuing education hours required to obtain or renew a dental license. It appears that some of the required continuing education time should be devoted to infection control and employee safety issues. The State of California's increased requirement concerning HIV/AIDS and infection control is a recent example.

Table 16-1 Definitions of Waste*

TERM	DEFINITION
Contaminated waste	Items that have had contact with blood or other body secretions
Hazardous waste	Waste posing a risk or peril to humans or the environment
Infectious waste	Waste capable of causing an infectious disease
Medical waste	Any solid waste† that is generated in the diagnosis, treatment, or immunization of human beings or animals in research pertaining thereto, or the production or testing of biologicals. The term does not include hazardous waste or household waste. Only a small percent of medical waste is infectious and needs to be regulated
Regulated waste	Infectious medical waste that requires special handling, neutralization, and disposal.
Toxic waste	Waste capable of having a poisonous effect.

---

*Adapted from EPA (40 CFR Parts 22 and 259. Standard for the tracking and management of medical waste, Federal Register 54:326-395, 1989) and several other sources.
†Solid waste includes discarded solid, liquid, semiliquid, or contained gaseous materials.

TYPES OF WASTE

Many people mistakenly consider the terms *"hospital waste," "medical waste,"* and *"infectious waste"* as being synonymous. "Hospital waste," like "dental office waste" or "household waste," refers to the total discarded solid waste generated by all sources within a given location (Table 16-1). In a hospital, this includes biologic waste materials, such as medical, food services, or animal facility waste, in addition to nonbiologic refuse such as clerical paper and plastic items. "Medical waste" includes materials generated during patient diagnosis, treatment, or immunization. "Infectious waste" is a small subset (estimated at 3% of the total) of "medical waste" that has shown a capability of transmitting an infectious disease. It should be noted that factors such as the number and virulence of the microorganisms present, host resistance, and the presence and availability of portals of entry have important roles in whether an infection occurs.

INFECTIOUS WASTE MANAGEMENT

Over the last five years, differences among federal agencies concerning the definition of Infectious Medical Waste has narrowed. This may be superseded (additional soiled items included) by some states and local jurisdictions. However, no state or local agency can mandate a regulation that does not first encompass all federal rules.

The prevailing view is there is no epidemiologic evidence to suggest that most medical waste is any more infective than residential waste. Also, there is no epidemiologic evidence that current medical/dental waste handling and disposal procedures have caused disease in the community. Therefore identifying wastes for which special precautions are necessary is largely a matter of judgement concerning the relative risk of disease transmission.

It is now commonly agreed that only a limited number/type of medical waste needs to be regulated (requiring special handling, storage, and disposal methods). For dentistry, these include bulk blood or blood products, pathology waste, and sharps. Often, the blood and blood products group is expanded to include liquid or semiliquid blood (and any other potentially infectious materials, OPIM), contaminated items that release liquid or semiliquid blood or OPIM when compressed, items caked with dried blood or OPIM that could be released during handling, and pathologic or microbiologic wastes that contain blood or OPIM. Usually other body fluids are exempt. However, saliva because it often is tainted with blood during treatment is considered by the CDC as infectious waste. Fortunately for dentistry, the generation of infectious waste items is very modest.

BLOOD IN A LIQUID OR SEMILIQUID FORM

All federal agencies consider free-flowing/bulk blood to be infectious medical waste that needs to be regulated. In the overwhelming number of areas, blood (even mixed with other fluids, such as saliva) can be poured or evacuated into the office/clinic waste water system. Sink traps and evacuation lines should be thoroughly rinsed at least daily. It would be helpful if a disinfectant solution (e.g., an iodophor that is going to be disposed of at the end of the day) was drawn through the lines. Final rinsing with water is required, especially if a bleach solution is used.

Although generally allowed, there are several locales that are attempting to restrict the volume of blood entering their sanitary sewers. These areas have had traditional waste disposal problems of all types, especially with EPA water quality requirements. Personnel should always be aware of the regulations in their area and to become actively involved in attempts to change the current situation.

PATHOGENIC WASTE (teeth and other tissues)

Teeth and other waste tissues are considered potentially infectious, and thus their disposal should be regulated. Many areas allow in-house neutralization of such items. The easiest and most effective procedure is sterilization by heat. Steam autoclaving is the method of choice. However, there is published information indicating the effectiveness of an unsaturated chemical vapor sterilizer in the neutralization of pathologic waste. Because the operation parameters (time, pressure, and temperature) of the unsaturated chemical vapor sterilizer are similar to those of the steam autoclave, it seems logical that it would also be capable of pathologic waste sterilization. Dry heat ovens should never be used.

Many areas allow in-house treatment of pathologic waste. The operation of the sterilizer used must be routinely monitored (see Chapter 11). This includes physical examination, chemical indicators, and biologic (spore test) monitors. Pathologic waste should be wrapped for treatment. Any autoclavable plastic/plastic-paper bag or pouch can be used. The bag and its contents are then ready for disposal. Offices and clinics should be discreet about the final disposal of treated infectious medical waste. There have been repeated reports of waste haulers refusing to empty dumpsters boxes or garbage cans if blood and blood soiled items are visible. It is probably best to place treated items into some type of sealed container, such as a cardboard box, before disposal.

One common problem involves the treatment of teeth containing amalgam restorations. The heat of sterilization could create dangerous mercury vapors. Amalgam-restored teeth can be disinfected before disposal. Ideally, a sterilizing chemical (e.g., full-strength glutaraldehyde) should be used. A tooth could be added to a small volume of fresh glutaraldehyde held within a sealed container. Exposure should be for at least 30 minutes. Treated teeth should then be rinsed well.

One stimulus for the return of teeth involves younger children and the "tooth fairy." Jurisdictions vary on the validity of such requests and on the procedures to be followed to satisfy such an inquiry.

Disposal of treated teeth and other tissues must be done according to local regulations. Many areas allow these treated items to be added to the nonregulated waste stream. It would be best that pathologic waste be somehow hidden from the view of the public. Final disposal should be in a secured receptacle.

Treated regulated medical waste is waste treated (usually by the application of heat or by incineration) to substantially reduce or eliminate its pathogenicity. This does not necessarily mean that the waste is destroyed or the volume is significantly reduced. For example, autoclaving does not appreciably affect the volume of treated waste materials.

SHARPS

Another form of medical waste known to be capable of transmitting disease is contaminated sharps. All federal agencies consider sharps to be infectious waste. Sharps are items that can penetrate intact skin. Dental examples include injection needles, scalpel blades, sutures, instruments, and broken glass. OSHA regulations indicate that immediately after use, disposable sharps are to be placed in closeable, leakproof, puncture-resistant containers ("sharps boxes"; Figure 16-1). These containers must be labeled with a biohazard symbol and color-coded for easy identification. The CDC recommend that sharps containers be located as close as is practical to the work area. This means that each operatory should have a minimum of at least one sharps container.

Proper handling of sharps is essential because common personal protective barriers such as gloves will not prevent needlestick accidents. To minimize the potential for accidents, needles should not be recapped, bent, broken, or manipulated by unprotected hands. The use of some type of protective cap-holding device or replacement of the capping sheath by "the scoop technique" (Figure 16-2) with the syringe held in one hand is required.

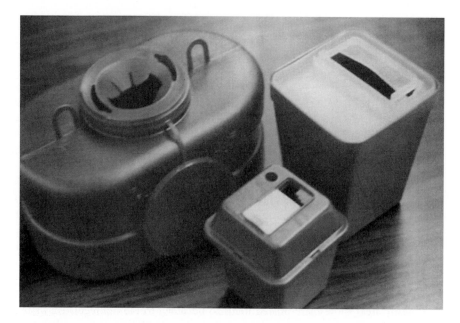

FIGURE 16-1   Acceptable sharps containers are available in several sizes and shapes.

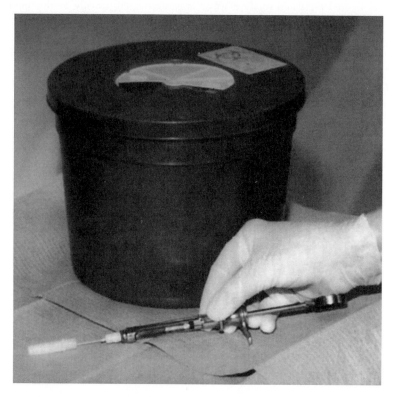

FIGURE 16-2   Recapping a needle using the one-handed "scoop technique."

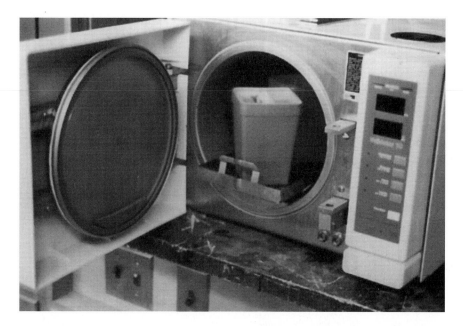

FIGURE 16-3   Filled sharps containers being loaded into a steam autoclave for processing.

Because waste haulers charge a premium price for the removal of medical waste, where legally permissible, dental offices should consider treating their sharps containers in-house. Recent studies have evaluated the effectiveness steam autoclaving had on bacterial endospores placed within a number of different sharps containers. Several container physical orientations (up or on-side, vents open or closed, empty versus three fourths filled) within the autoclave were evaluated (Figure 16-3). Spores were present on commercial spore strips or placed onto capped and uncapped dental needles. All strips and needles in empty or filled containers could be sterilized within 20 minutes when small containers were placed on their sides and their vents left open. Larger containers placed on their sides required more than 20 minutes to achieve sterilization. The contents of all containers processed in an upward position required between 40 and 60 minutes of autoclaving before being sterilized. Offices and clinics prefer to place their sharps containers into the autoclave or unsaturated chemical vapor sterilizer in an upright position. This minimizes the chances of sharps escaping from the container. However, passage of steam or vapor is not as efficient as for containers processed on their sides. The size and shape of the containers can also influence overall efficiency of sterilization.

Specific recommendations for the in-house treatment of sharps containers can be found in Box 16-1. Recent reports indicate that a steam autoclave or an unsaturated chemical vapor sterilizer may be used for treatment. Additional exposure time (e.g., two to three successive cycles) is usually required, however. For example, the State of Indiana requires a 60-minute exposure when treating regulated medical waste in-house.

Box 16-1   Recommended Procedures for Sterilization of Sharps Containers in Moist Heat Sterilizers

---

1. Use only containers specified and labeled by their manufacturers for the collection of sharps (which must be autoclavable)
2. Regularly biologically spore-test the sterilizer (steam or unsaturated chemical vapor) used
3. Consider the following procedural recommendations
   a. Fill containers no more than three-quarters full
   b. Leave container vents open
   c. Place containers in an upright position within the sterilizer chamber (containers placed on their sides are more readily sterilized but this increases the chances of needlestick accidents)
   d. Process the containers for 40 to 60 minutes (usually two cycles unless a longer single cycle can be used) to cover differences in container size, type and fill level, and model and operational status of the sterilizer used
   e. Remove containers after processing and allow them to cool, then carefully close the vents
   f. Label and dispose of containers according to local governmental regulations

---

RECORD KEEPING

In some areas, regulated medical waste must be removed, neutralized, and disposed of by an approved waste hauler. In some cases, facilities, even though not required to do so, elect to contract for such disposal. These services are often expensive, especially if the office or clinic is not in the same building with other practices.

Remember that although another party is physically removing and disposing the medical waste, it is the responsibility of the generating facility to ensure that acceptable and correct methods are used. If the waste were to be illegally dumped, the office or clinic from which the materials derived would be held responsible. Therefore the credentials of any waste hauler should be established. Speaking to other clients and to local health authorities is essential. The EPA usually approves haulers. They are awarded a unique identifying contractor number, which should appear on all your paperwork. A receipt of shipment should be given on removal of the waste. Several weeks later a manifest should come through the mail indicating the exact manner in which the waste was treated and its final site of disposal.

Currently there are a few companies offering disposal by mail. It is imperative to examine the licenses and credentials of such companies. Contact the local post office to ensure that the company involved has the legal right to receive such shipments. Again, a manifest must be received as the deposition of the materials sent. It is also important to note that the legal responsibility for any waste ultimately rests with the generating facility.

SELECTED READINGS

American Dental Association. *Q&A Infectious waste disposal in the dental office,* Chicago, 1989, American Dental Association.

ADA Council on Scientific Affairs and ADA Council on Dental Practice: Infection control recommendations for the dental office and the dental laboratory, *Journal of the American Dental Association* 127:672-80, 1996.

APIC: Position paper: medical waste (revised), *Am J Infect Cont* 20:73-74, 1992.

Centers for Disease Control: Recommended infection-control practices for dentistry, *MMWR* 41 (RR-8):1-12, 1993.

Gooch BF, Cardo DM, McKibben PS *et al.:* Percutaneous exposures to HIV-infected blood among dental workers enrolled in the CDC Needlestick Study, *Journal of the American Dental Association* 126:1237-1242, 1995.

Karpiak J, Pugliese G: Medical waste: declining options in the 90s, *Am J Infect Control* 19:8-15, 1991.

Miller CH, Palenik CJ: Infection control in dentistry. In Block S: *Sterilization, disinfection, preservation and sanitation,* ed 4, Philadelphia, 1991, Lea & Febiger.

Palenik CJ, Miller CH: Be sharp - handle sharps carefully, *Dent Asepsis Rev* 16(3):1-2, 1995.

US Department of Labor, OSHA. 29 CFR Part 1910.1030: *Occupational exposure to blood-borne pathogens; final rule,* Fed Register 56:64004-64182, 1991.

US Environmental Protection Agency: *EPA guide for infectious waste management* (EPA/530-5W-86-014), Washington, DC, 1986, US Environmental Protection Agency.

US Environmental Protection Agency. (1997 - October 15) *Search the U.S. EPA internet site* (WWW document), URL *http://www.epa.gov/epahome/search.html.*

Chapter 17

A CLINICAL ASEPSIS PROTOCOL

Other parts of this book describe a variety of separate infection control procedures. The information here is intended to organize these procedures into a usable protocol based on the sequence of patient treatment activities. Some steps in the protocol may change from one practice to the next. The procedures are grouped into five sets of activities that are conducted:

- Before seating the patient
- After the patient is seated
- During patient treatment
- After patient treatment
- When taking radiographs

BEFORE SEATING PATIENT

1. Put on protective clothing, eyewear, mask, and gloves and clean and then disinfect those surfaces that may be touched during patient treatment and will not be protected by surface covers. These surfaces may be:
   a. Cuspidor rim and control knob
   b. Countertops
   c. Drawer pulls and top edges of drawers that may be used
   d. Sink faucet handles
   e. Handpiece connectors
2. Also, clean and disinfect items brought into the area to be used during patient procedures (e.g., articulators, casts, dies, custom impression trays, record bases, fixed and removable prostheses, facebows).
   a. Disinfection procedure:
      - Spray the surface with the surface disinfectant that has been properly prepared
      - Clean the surface by vigorously wiping with paper towels or 4 × 4 gauze pads
      - Disinfect the precleaned surface by respraying it and let air dry or wipe dry if still wet after 10 minutes
3. Remove and discard mask and gloves and wash your hands
   a. Procedure for removing gloves:
      - Pinch one glove in the wrist area on one hand with the thumb and forefinger of the other hand
      - Stretch the glove out away from the the wrist, slide it off toward the fingertips—but only half-way

- Repeat this on the other hand except slide that glove completely off and drop it directly into the waste receptacle
- Move back to the first hand and place your ungloved thumb under the edge of the glove, which now has the noncontaminated surface inside of the glove turned out. Stretch the glove out away from the hand, slide it completely off toward the fingertips and drop it directly into the waste receptacle

4. Obtain surface covers, supplies, and sterile instruments and other equipment from the supply area
5. Cover the following surfaces with the appropriate cover:
   a. Headrest
   b. Control buttons on side of chair
   c. Light handles
   d. Unit light switch and view box switch
   e. Air/water syringe buttons/handle
   f. High-volume evacuator control
   g. Unit control switches and handpiece, air/water syringe, and HVE holders
   h. Saliva ejector, handpiece and air/water syringe hoses
   i. Bracket table
   j. Stool backs
6. Remove all items not used during patient treatment from countertops (e.g., datebooks, articulator boxes, cardboard and plastic boxes, tackle boxes)

AFTER PATIENT IS SEATED

1. Adjust chair and headrest
2. Place patient napkin
3. Take or update medical history, discuss treatment, do necessary paperwork
4. Remove chart from the countertop
5. Have patient rinse thoroughly with an antimicrobial mouthrinse
6. Open instrument packages and/or tray without touching the instruments
7. Put on mask and eyeglasses
8. Wash hands (preferably in view of patient)
   a. Handwashing procedure:
      - Remove jewelry and gently clean your fingernails
      - Lather for 10 seconds with the liquid detergent
      - Rinse under cool tap water
      - Lather again for 10 seconds
      - Rinse again and towel dry
   b. Perform surgical scrub for procedures so indicated
9. Put on gloves (preferably in view of patient). Use sterile gloves for procedures so indicated; otherwise, use nonsterile examination gloves
10. Rinse nonsterile examination gloves with plain, cool water (no soap) to remove excess powder and towel dry before making impressions and bite registrations. If desired, excess powder may be removed by rinsing with water and drying before other types of procedures. Explain to the patient that these are new gloves being rinsed to remove the powder

11. Flush water/air lines for 20–30 seconds
12. Connect sterile handpieces, air/water syringe tip, HVE tip, saliva ejector tip

DURING PATIENT CARE

1. Restrict spread of microorganisms from patient's mouth
   a. Use rubber dam
   b. Use high volume evacuation (HVE)
   c. Touch as few surfaces as possible with saliva-coated fingers
   d. Keep your gloved hands out of your hair and do not rub your eyes or bare skin or adjust mask or glasses
   e. If you must leave chairside during treatment, remove and discard your gloves. Wash your hands and reglove with fresh gloves when you return. Protective clothing must not be worn in lunchrooms, or outside the building, and must be changed if obviously soiled
   f. Remove gloves and wash hands before handling cameras for intraoral photos
2. Items dropped on the floor or on other nonsterile surfaces are not to be used. Obtain sterile replacements. Remove and replace gloves, preferably in view of patient
3. If gloves are torn during treatment, remove, discard, wash hands, and reglove with fresh gloves
4. Do not recap needles by hand. Insert the needle into the cap using the one-handed "scoop" technique or a cap holder that will not permit contact of the needle with any part of the body. Do not pass syringes with uncapped needles to someone else
5. Look first before reaching for a sharp instrument
6. When placing sharp instruments back on the instrument tray, make sure sharp tips are not pointed up and make sure they are placed in a stable position
7. If equipment is brought to chairside (e.g., light curing apparatus), make sure it is protected with a surface cover or has been disinfected before use
8. Obtain supplies (e.g., amalgam, varnish, cavity liner) from a central storage area. Do not take a container to the unit unless it is covered with plastic wrap or is cleaned and disinfected after use
9. Disinfect contaminated items before they are taken to the dental lab
10. Do not handle charts with contaminated gloves. Use an overglove or remove gloves and wash hands
11. If you are exposed to a patient's blood or saliva, immediately contact the appropriate person to institute a postexposure medical evaluation. An exposure is any eye, mouth, other mucous membrane, nonintact skin, or sharps injury involving blood or saliva

AFTER PATIENT TREATMENT

Anyone who will be cleaning contaminated instruments must wear heavy utility gloves, protective clothing, a mask, and a face shield or protective eyewear. If instruments are hand-scrubbed, they should be submerged in detergent while scrubbing to prevent splattering

1. Remove gloves, then the mask by touching only the ties or elastic band and discard in plastic-lined waste container at the unit and then wash your hands
2. Send the patient to the front desk for dismissal or reappointment
3. Put on fresh gloves and mask
4. Place all instruments back in the tray
5. Place all disposable sharps, including capped or uncapped needles directly into the sharps container at the unit. **Do not place needles or other sharps into the regular trash receptacle.** This would be a serious violation of procedures. Sharps include needles, scalpel blades, carpules, broken instruments and files, burs, orthodontic wire, and other disposable items that could penetrate the skin
6. Place nonsharp disposable items in the plastic-lined waste container at the unit
7. Flush the air/water syringe, highspeed handpiece and ultrasonic scaler into the sink, cuspidor, or container for 30 seconds and disconnect from hoses
8. Remove all surface covers (without touching the underlying surface) and discard in plastic-lined waste container at the unit
9. Clean and then disinfect patient-care-related surfaces that were not covered and were contaminated during treatment. There is no need to clean and disinfect surfaces that were covered unless they become contaminated during removal of the covers (see disinfecting procedures listed above)
10. Take instruments and handpieces to the decontamination/sterilizing area
11. Remove and wash your contaminated eyeglasses, rinse and dry. Avoid contaminating your hair
12. Remove and dispose of the disposable gown (if used) in the plastic-lined waste container at the unit. Untie the gown and pull it off over your gloved hands, and do not touch underlying clothing or skin
13. Remove your gloves and discard in the plastic-lined waste container
14. Wash, rinse and dry your hands

RADIOGRAPHIC ASEPSIS

Unit/Patient Preparation

1. Before seating the patient, prepare the unit by covering or disinfecting all surfaces that will be touched or exposed to potentially infectious fluids
2. Review or update the medical history of the patient
3. After washing hands, gowning, and gloving, determine the appropriate number and type of films to be taken
4. Obtain the films from a central distribution area or film dispenser while wearing clean gloves
5. Reglove and expose the films in the recommended manner
6. Place exposed films on a paper towel or in a cup. If film packs precovered with plastic protectors are used, carefully remove the contaminated covers after exposure and drop the film packs onto a clean surface. Do not touch the film packs with contaminated gloves
7. Remove surface covers from the unit or disinfect contaminated surfaces
8. Remove gloves and wash hands

Darkroom Processing

1. Place new gloves on hands
2. Carry the films to the darkroom using caution not to touch doors, walls, work areas, or processors with contaminated gloves
3. With gloved hands, carefully open the film packets and drop the films onto a clean paper towel. Place contaminated film wrappers into the designated refuse containers
4. Remove contaminated gloves and place the films in the processor
5. After processing, place the films into the appropriate mounts using care not to contaminate the films, mounts, or charts with instruments that were used in the operatory

Daylight Loader Processing

1. Because of the limited operating space inside the loader and because the hand insertion sleeves cannot be disinfected, only films that are **not** contaminated should be placed in the loader. This can be accomplished in two ways
   a. Film disinfection: After the films have been exposed, they can be rinsed with water, soaked in an appropriate bleach or iodophor solution for 10 minutes, and, while wearing clean gloves, rinsed with water and dried with a clean paper towel. The films should be placed into the loader through the top. (Only plastic film packets may be disinfected.)
   b. Pre-exposure wrapping: The film can be wrapped in plastic before being placed in the patient's mouth. Film packs already protected with a removable plastic cover are available. After exposure, the outer wrapping is carefully opened or the cover is removed and the film packet is dropped onto a clean surface. Caution should be used so that the clean packets do not touch the contaminated gloves or wrapping. The films can then be placed in the loader through the top, and the hands, wearing new gloves, passed through the insertion sleeves

III
PART

OFFICE SAFETY

Chapter 18

MANAGING THE OFFICE SAFETY PROGRAM

Practicing infection control procedures, managing hazardous materials and regulated medical waste, and ensuring safety against fire and storms are collectively referred to as *office safety*. The office safety aspects of dentistry are expanding rapidly, with new and revised regulations and recommendations appearing frequently. New asepsis or other safety products and equipment continually appear on the market, and advances in research are bringing new concepts and approaches to controlling the spread of disease agents.

Maintaining and implementing infection control procedures, as well as management of hazardous materials, for protection of the patients and the entire dental team indeed present major challenges to ensuring compliance, maintaining personnel efficiency, and controlling costs.

SAFETY COORDINATOR

Management of the multifaceted office safety program is facilitated if the employer identifies one person in the office to organize and supervise office safety. Such a *safety coordinator* works under the guidance of the employer and could be a hygienist or an assistant.

The safety coordinator must have a basic understanding of microbiology and the modes of disease spread in the office, infection control and other safety procedures, and products and equipment used with these procedures, and also must know the related state and federal regulations. Extra training may be necessary at the time of initial assignment to the position, and continuing education is very important to keep up with changes. The safety coordinator also should possess good written and verbal communication skills, good organizational skills, and must be given time to perform the duties related to office safety.

MANAGEMENT DUTIES

Box 18-1 lists duties involved in managing the office safety program. Although the employer is responsible for all of these duties, most, if not all, can be delegated to the safety coordinator. Chapter 8 provides a review of steps for compliance with the OSHA bloodborne pathogens standard.

Develop Step-By-Step Procedures

Assuring compliance and understanding of office safety procedures to be practiced are greatly facilitated by establishing written step-by-step procedures much like those pre-

---

Box 18-1   Office Safety Management Duties

Continually review infection control, hazardous materials, and other office safety regulations

Prepare, review, and update the office exposure control plan, infection control procedures manual, hazard communication program, and other safety procedures for the office

Develop protocols that provide step-by-step procedures to be followed in practicing office safety

- Provide new and continuing team members with initial and updated training on all office safety policies and procedures
- Assure that the janitorial staff receives proper training related to personal protection during office cleaning procedures

Monitor compliance with office safety procedures and related regulations

Organize and manage procedures for hepatitis B vaccination of new team members and procedures for postexposure medical evaluation and follow-up

Review circumstances surrounding exposure incidents

Evaluate, select, and maintain the stock of products and equipment needed to accomplish office safety

- Assure proper maintenance, availability, cleaning, and disposal of personal protective equipment and all other items needed for office safety

Perform spore-testing of office sterilizers

- Manage disposal of regulated medical waste

Check equipment for decontamination and label contamination portions before shipping for repair

Organize and maintain material safety data sheets, proper labeling, the inventory list, and proper storage for all hazardous chemicals in the office

- Maintain smoke alarms and fire extinguishers and monitor electrical cords and connections
- Keep exit doors and evacuation routes clear and assure other compliance with local fire safety codes

Maintain certification of radiographic equipment

- Maintain appropriate documents and records

Assure that all members of the dental team have constant opportunity to voice concerns about and suggest improvements in office safety

Communicate with patients regarding safety procedures practices in the office

---

sented in some chapters of this book. Writing down the steps allows proper organization of the procedures in a logical fashion, documents their existence, and enhances learning by providing material that may be periodically reviewed.

An example of an overall clinical asepsis protocol that describes step-by-step procedures to be performed before seating the patient, during patient care, and after patient care is given in Chapter 17. The protocol presented may not apply to all practices and should be changed to specifically relate to each office.

Review Regulations and Advances

After all of the current regulations from local, state, and federal agencies have been reviewed, it is necessary to maintain continuing education in this and related areas. Establish contacts with or review educational material from organizations such as the American Dental Association (ADA), Office Safety and Asepsis Procedures Research Foundation (OSAP), Centers for Disease Control and Prevention (CDC), American Dental Hygienists Association (ADHA), American Dental Assistants Association (ADAA), state dental associations, and a local school of dentistry (see Appendix A).

Federal laws are published in the *Federal Register;* state laws are published in state registers. These are available in law schools and some public libraries, or copies of regulations may be obtained by contacting the respective federal or state agency (see Appendix A).

Communication
Among the Dental Team

Office policies and procedures and details of regulations and compliance must be periodically communicated to members of the dental team during the required bloodborne pathogens and management of hazardous materials training sessions. Also, a key aspect of employee satisfaction is open communication among all members of the dental team. The entire team should participate in developing the total office safety program, and lines of communication should be established for constructive criticism and suggestions for improvement. It is best to have an internal mechanism to resolve employee complaints.

With Patients

Communication with patients regarding their safety while in the office is also very important in establishing trust and ensuring return visits. Patients have varying degrees of knowledge about infection control and routes of disease spread. Today, patients are asking more and more questions about their safety in the office because of the news media coverage of issues in dentistry, such as the safety of amalgam fillings, the incident in Florida in which a dentist apparently infected six of his patients with human immunodeficiency virus (HIV) in the late 1980s, and the concern about disease transmission through dental handpieces in the early 1990s. These and other issues erode public confidence in dentistry. Patients must be made aware of office procedures designed for their protection, many of which are conducted "behind the scenes." Box 18-2 lists suggestions for instilling trust in patients regarding the care taken in the office for patient protection.

Maintain Office Safety Documents

Documents and records must be prepared, maintained in proper form, and made readily available to dental team members (Box 18-3).

Develop Responses to Emergencies

Develop mechanisms for rapid responses to body fluid exposures, hazardous material exposures, medical emergencies, fire, and storms. In relation to body fluid exposure, the procedure must involve a medical evaluation and follow-up as described in Chapter 8. Medical emergency kits, smoke alarms, and fire extinguishers should be maintained, an

---

Box 18-2   Developing Patient Trust Regarding Infection Control Procedures in the Office

---

Establish all infection control procedures

Let patients observe you washing your hands at the beginning of their care and especially when you return after being away from chairside

Let patients observe gloving and especially the use of fresh gloves when you return after being away from chairside

Let patients see you unwrap the sterile instruments that will be used so they will know that those instruments have been carefully prepared and protected

Know the facts about infection control procedures and encourage questions

Provide patients with brief written information about the infection control procedures used

Offer tours of the office and the sterilizing room to new or returning patients

Maintain general cleanliness in the office, particularly dust on horizontal surfaces in the operating and waiting room

---

Adapted from Miller CH: Make a lasting positive impression with infection control procedures, *RDH* 13:36, 1993.

evacuation route should be identified in case of fire, and procedures for protection should be identified in case of tornadoes, hurricanes, or earthquakes.

Procure and Manage Safety Products and Equipment

Purchase, maintain, clean, and dispose of all products and equipment needed for infection control, management of hazardous materials, and other office safety procedures (Box 18-4). The costs of providing office safety can be difficult to recover; therefore, managing the supplies inventory, preventive maintenance of equipment, and avoiding infection control overkill can be very important.

Evaluate Products and Equipment

Although adequate supplies need to be maintained, overstocking is a problem. It prolongs changing to another supply item of better quality or lower cost until current supplies have been used. Evaluate products carefully and request samples before ordering. Let the entire dental team assist in the evaluation to ensure proper use when the item is purchased. Make sure an item purchased will be appropriate for the desired use, and do not purchase unproven substitutes or otherwise compromise appropriate quality for low cost. Make sure written and especially verbal claims about products have been appropriately documented with testing or peer-reviewed, published, scientific evaluation.

Use and Maintain Products and Equipment Correctly

Make sure dental team members read, understand, and follow all labels and operating manuals for products and equipment. Misuse of products and equipment can lead to compromises in disease prevention or personal safety, damage to the equipment or surface related to product use, or damage to the equipment itself. It is particularly important to maintain equipment such as sterilizers, ultrasonic cleaners, vacuum traps, radiographic machines, smoke alarms, and fire extinguishers so they will work properly and have maximum use-life.

Box 18-3   Examples of Office Safety Documents and Records

Regulatory Documents

OSHA bloodborne pathogens standard

OSHA hazard communication standard

State, local, or other regulatory documents that may apply (e.g., instrument sterilization, sterilization monitoring, and waste disposal)

Policy Document

OSHA written exposure control plan for the office

OSHA written hazard communication program for the office

Management of fire and other emergencies[*]

Policies not covered by OSHA standards (e.g., state regulations on instrument sterilization, sterilization monitoring, and waste disposal)

OSHA poster (form 2203) on "Job Safety and Health Protection"

Records

OSHA bloodborne pathogens and hazard communication training records

OSHA written schedule for cleaning and disinfecting areas in the office

OSHA form 101 (or equivalent) for individual occupational injury or illness[*]

OSHA form 200 (or equivalent) for annual summary of injury and illness reports[*]

OSHA employee medical records[†]

- Hepatitis B vaccination refusal forms
- Written opinion from physician on vaccination of employees
- Exposure incident reports
- Written opinion from physician on post-exposure medical evaluation and follow-up

Sterilizer spore-testing results

Radiographic equipment certification

Fire extinguisher certification

Manifests from regulated medical waste haulers

Verification of on-site treatment of regulated medical waste

Material safety data sheets

Inventory of hazardous chemicals

---

[*]Written emergency action plan and fire prevention plan and completed 101 and 200 forms are required if there are
eleven or more employees

[†]Confidential

Box 18-4 Examples of Supplies and Equipment For Office Safety

Patient care gloves	Disposable items
Utility gloves	Handpiece cleaner/lubricant
Masks	Sharps containers
Face shields	Biohazard bags
Protective eyeware	Antimicrobial handwash
Protective clothing	Surface covers
Rubber dam	Liquid sterilant
Preprocedure mouthrinse	Surface disinfectant
High-volume evacuation	Eyewash stations
CPR ventilation devices	Fire extinguishers
Ultrasonic cleaner and basket	Smoke alarms
Cleaning solution	Exit signs
Sterilization packaging	Safety signs
Instrument cassettes	Medical emergency kit
Heat sterilizers	Mercury management kit
Biologic indicators	Oxygen
Chemical indicators	Radiation badges
Biohazard labels and signs	Chemical safety cabinets

Periodically check and replace protective equipment such as utility gloves, eyewear, face shields, and reusable protective clothing when necessary. Inventory all incoming chemicals to assure the availability of material safety data sheets (MSDS) and presence of proper labels. Ensure that disinfectants, sterilants, or other items with a specific shelf-life or use-life are replaced when indicated. Make sure sharps containers are located where needed and that they are replaced before they are allowed to overflow.

Infection Control Overkill

Examples of infection control overkill that can be time-consuming and costly are: routinely hand scrubbing and ultrasonically cleaning instruments, routinely cleaning and disinfecting surfaces after removal of surface covers, using more than one layer of sterilization wrap during packaging, routinely disinfecting instruments before sterilization, using thick rather than thin plastic as surface covers, using sterile gloves for routine procedures, and using special disposal mechanisms for items that are not considered as regulated medical waste.

Monitor Procedures

Monitor compliance with office safety procedures by direct observation. This will ensure that the dental team understands how to properly perform procedures and use equipment. Problems with compliance may indicate that further training is needed. Checklists used by the person performing a procedure may be used when direct observation is not possible.

Monitoring the use and functioning of sterilizers is one of the few quality assessment procedures that can be performed in the area of infection control. This involves selecting an appropriate mail-in monitoring service that supplies all materials, analyses, and records of results, or for in-office testing of steam sterilizers, purchasing the appropriate biologic indicators and incubator and performing the testing, analyses, and recordkeeping in the office. Be sure to always use a control biologic indicator (not processed through the sterilizer) with each test. This will ensure the reliability of the test.

CHECKLIST FOR THE INFECTION CONTROL PROGRAM

This checklist can be used in organizing, reviewing, and/or updating an infection control program for the office.

Exposure Control Plan

1. A written exposure control plan (as required by OSHA) for the office is available and contains:
   a. The exposure determination
   b. The schedule and method of implementation of the methods of compliance, the hepatitis B vaccination, the postexposure medical evaluation and follow-up, the communication of biohazards, and the recordkeeping related to the OSHA Bloodborne Pathogens Standard
   c. The procedures for evaluating the circumstances surrounding an exposure incident
2. The Exposure Control Plan is updated at least annually and whenever changes occur in the laws, in modes of exposure, or in procedures, equipment, or supplies used to prevent the spread of disease agents
3. A copy of the Exposure Control Plan is made available to all involved employees

Training the Office Staff

1. The OSHA-required training of appropriate office staff is provided on *ititial* employment at no cost to the staff at a reasonable time and place by a person knowledgeable about the subjects and about the dental office environment, and includes:
   a. A description of the cause, symptoms, epidemiology, spread, and prevention of bloodborne diseases
   b. Details of the office's Exposure Control Plan
   c. The selection, use, limitations, and management of equipment or supplies used to prevent spread of disease agents in the office
   d. The description, safety, efficacy, administration, and benefits of hepatitis B vaccination and immunity
   e. What to do if an exposure to blood or saliva occurs
   f. An explanation of biohazard/color code communication used in the office
   g. The availability of a copy and an explanation of the OSHA Bloodborne Pathogens Standard and other infection control laws that apply
   h. An opportunity for the trained employees to have questions immediately answered

2. Update training of all involved office staff is given at least annually and whenever changes occur in the laws, in modes of exposure, or in procedures, equipment, or supplies used to prevent the spread of disease agents

Hepatitis B Vaccination

1. The hepatitis B vaccination series is offered free of charge at a reasonable time and place by a licensed physician or nurse practitioner within 10 days of employment of a new person who has received proper training (see above) about the vaccine
2. The physician's office involved has a copy of the OSHA Bloodborne Pathogens Standard
3. Prescreening for immunity to hepatitis B is not a condition of employment
4. Employees not accepting the vaccination offer must read and sign the specific vaccination refusal statement given at the end of the OSHA Bloodborne Pathogens Standard
5. Written confirmations are received from the physician indicating that each involved employee has been evaluated/vaccinated

Postexposure Medical Evaluation and Follow-up

1. A medical evaluation and follow-up is offered free of charge at a reasonable time and place by a licensed physician or nurse practitioner to all employees who experience an occupational exposure to blood or saliva
2. Identifiable patients involved in such exposures are requested to be evaluated for their hepatitis B and HIV disease status
3. The physician's office involved has a copy of the OSHA Bloodborne Pathogens Standard.
4. Written confirmations are received from the physician indicating that each involved employee has been informed of the results of the evaluations and of any medical conditions resulting from the exposure that require further evaluation or treatment

General Methods and Aseptic Techniques

1. Universal precautions are practiced
2. Handwashing facilities and handwashing agents are available to staff
3. Hands are washed after removal of gloves or other protective barriers and whenever contaminated with blood, saliva, or other body fluid
4. Eating, drinking, smoking, applying cosmetics, contacts, or lip balm are not done in areas where blood or saliva may be spread from patients
5. Spattering or spraying of blood or saliva during patient treatment is minimized
6. Preprocedure mouthrinsing is used
7. Dental unit water is not used to irrigate surgical sites
8. Unit dosing is used, and/or an aseptic retrieval system (e.g., sterile forceps) is used with every patient if a supply type item must be obtained from a bulk container
9. Disposable items (e.g., plastic air/water syringe tips, evacuation tips, ejector tips, prophy cups, prophy angles) are not cleaned and reused on other patients
10. A one-way CPR airway or oxygen with bagging is available for staff qualified to use such devices

Protective Barriers

1. Appropriate gloves, mask, protective eyewear, and protective clothing are made available and are properly used when there is a potential for exposure to blood or saliva
2. Gloves, mask, protective eyewear, and protective clothing are removed before leaving the work area and are not worn in lunch areas or out of the office
3. Gloves, mask, protective eyewear, and protective clothing are properly cleaned, laundered, maintained, and/or discarded
4. Contaminated, reusable, protective clothing is properly containerized and laundered in the office or by a laundry service and is not taken home by employees for laundering
5. Proper containers/bags are used for handling contaminated laundry
6. Contaminated laundry is properly identified by a biohazard symbol/color coding that is recognizable by the office staff

Management of Regulated Waste

1. Proper barriers, procedures, and containers are used to safely handle sharps, nonsharp waste, liquid waste, and human tissue, including teeth
2. Regulated waste is properly identified by a biohazard symbol/color coding and, where required, name and address labels
3. Recapping of needles is accomplished by a safe technique
4. Sharps containers are located where sharps are used or may be found
5. Sharps containers are not overfilled and are closed when being transported
6. Tongs are available for picking up broken glass, needles, scalpel blades, and other sharps
7. Everyone is instructed to never reach blindly to pick-up or move a sharp item
8. Specimens of human tissue, blood, saliva, or other body fluids are placed in proper containers and properly identified by a biohazard symbol/color coding during collecting, handling, processing, storing, or transporting
9. Regulated waste is properly treated and discarded or transported for final disposal

Decontamination

1. Equipment and instruments are properly decontaminated before servicing or shipping, and if they contain sites that are incompletely contaminated, these sites are identified before servicing or shipping
2. Operatory or other surfaces involved in patient treatment are covered with protective barriers that are changed for every patient, or contaminated surfaces involved in patient treatment are cleaned and then disinfected between patients
3. A written schedule of decontamination of the various work areas is maintained
4. Reusable containers contaminated with body fluids are cleaned and disinfected after use

Instrument Processing

1. Containers of contaminated reusable sharps (e.g., sharp instruments) are properly labeled with a biohazard symbol/color coding, closed on transport, and do not require one to reach inside without being able to see the sharps
2. Contaminated instruments are routinely mechanically cleaned (rather than hand-scrubbed) before rinsing and packaging for sterilization

3. Cleaned and rinsed instruments are dried and packaged before sterilization
4. Packaging materials designed for use in sterilizers and the proper procedures for sealing packages are used
5. Cleaned and packaged reusable instruments, handpieces, handpiece attachments, and other items are sterilized between use on patients
6. Equipment identified by its manufacturer as a sterilizer is used for sterilization
7. Cleaned reusable items that melt in heat sterilizers are sterilized by a low temperature procedure (e.g., glutaraldehyde) between use on patients
8. The use and functioning of each sterilizer is spore-tested at least weekly and a chemical indicator is used with each package
9. Sterilized packages are handled and stored properly

Laboratory Asepsis

1. Items contaminated with oral fluids are sterilized when possible but at least rinsed and disinfected before taken into the in-office laboratory or sent to a commercial laboratory
2. Items from in-office or commercial laboratories are:
   a. Disinfected and rinsed
   b. Confirmed to have been disinfected
   c. Known to be uncontaminated before placed into patients' mouths

Radiographic Asepsis

1. X-ray films are protected with plastic surface covers before being placed into the patient's mouth or are rinsed and disinfected or handled aseptically after removal from the patient's mouth
2. The sleeves of daylight loaders do not come in contact with contaminated gloves or films

Recordkeeping

1. Medical records (name, social security number, written confirmation about hepatitis B evaluation for vaccination, any vaccination refusal statement, written confirmation about postexposure medical evaluation and follow-up) for each employee who may have the potential to be occupationally exposed to body fluids are maintained (to comply with OSHA and some other state requirements) in confidentiality for the duration of employment plus 30 years
2. Records of staff training (names and job classifications of trainees, date and contents of training, name and qualifications of the trainer) are maintained (to comply with OSHA and some other state requirements) for at least three years
3. Records of spore-testing results (identification of the specific sterilizer tested, dates of the testing, results, identification of who performed the tests) are maintained according to state and local requirements
4. Records for the treatment and/or transport and final disposal of regulated waste are maintained

SELECTED READINGS

Miller CH: Make a lasting positive impression with infection control procedures, *RDH* 13:36, 1993.

Miller CH: Implementing an office infection control program, *Dent Assist* 59:11-15, 1990.

Miller CH: Assigning duties to one person reduces infection control errors, *Dent Office* 7:14-15, 1989.

Miller CH: Safety coordinator's duties go beyond casual organization of safety plans, *RDH* 17:52 and 68, 1997.

Runnells RR, Powell L: Managing infection control, hazards communication, and infectious waste disposal, *Dent Clin North Am* 35:299-308, 1991.

Chapter 19

MANAGING CHEMICALS SAFELY IN THE OFFICE

HAZARD COMMUNICATION STANDARD

If you were to ask most dental practitioners about their personal risk of experiencing an occupationally related injury, their responses would most likely include incidents such as needlestick accidents, allergies, burns, abrasions, or muscle strains. Being injured on the job while using or handling a hazardous material, such as a skin exposure to an acid solution, would not often be mentioned. Most health-care workers consider topics such as safer use of chemicals in the workplace to be problems primarily associated with large manufacturing facilities, such as oil refineries, chemical manufacturers, steel mills, coal mines, and metal fabricating shops. Unfortunately, significant numbers of workers in dental environments are exposed and injured each year by hazardous materials while performing normal clinical and laboratory duties.

STATEMENT OF THE PROBLEM

About 32 million workers in the United States are occupationally at risk for exposure to one or more *hazardous chemicals* (Table 19-1). Almost 600,000 chemicals can be purchased in the U.S. and literally thousands of new chemicals are introduced each year. The risk of exposure is continually increasing and the workplace use of toxic chemicals has become commonplace.

Adverse exposure to chemicals can have serious health consequences. Heart, kidney, liver, and lung tissues could be damaged. The result could be a variety of diseases that range from short-term discomfort (e.g., burns or rashes) to life threatening (e.g., cancer, sterility, or organ failure). Preventing exposure to hazardous chemicals is the ultimate goal. Also extremely important is the proper response when an exposure does occur.

OSHA

The U.S. Department of Labor Occupational Safety and Health Administration (OSHA) has for almost 30 years monitored and helped to improve safety conditions in the workplace. The greatest initial need (numbers of employees and severity of injuries), as one would expect, was (and remains) based in large and naturally dangerous worksites. Through a process of improving *engineering controls* and changing *work practices* (see Table 19-1) the number of injuries have begun to decrease.

Table 19-1   Important Definitions for a Hazard Communication Program*

TERM	DEFINITION
Chemical	Any element, chemical compound or mixture of elements and/or compounds
Chemical distributors	A business, other than a chemical manufacturer or importer, that supplies hazardous chemicals to other distributors or to employer
Chemical manufacturers and importers	An employer with a workplace where chemical(s) are produced for use or distribution
Employee	A worker who may be exposed to hazardous chemicals under normal operating conditions or in foreseeable emergencies; some workers, such as office workers or bank tellers, encounter hazardous chemicals only in nonroutine, isolated instances and are not covered by the HazCom Standard
Employer	A person engaged in a business where chemicals are used, distributed, or are produced for use or distribution, including a contractor or subcontractor
Engineering controls	Procedures and materials that help prevent employee exposure to hazardous chemicals. Examples include changing a chemical to a less problematic form or subcontracting of a process to another location or facility
Exposure ("exposed")	An employee subjected to a hazardous chemical in the course of their employment through any route of entry (inhalation, ingestion, skin contact, absorption, etc.), includes potential (e.g., accidental or possible) exposure
Hazardous chemicals	A chemical for which there is statistically significant evidence based on a scientifically designed and conducted study, that describes the acute, and/or chronic health effects that may occur to exposed employee; many chemicals used within dental offices/clinics are considered hazardous
Hazard warning	Words, pictures, symbols, or combinations thereof appearing on a label or other appropriate form of warning that convey the specific physical or health hazard(s), including target organ effects, of the chemical(s) present in a container
HazCom compliance officer	An employee responsible for a clinic/office compliance with the HazCom Standard; they are responsible for the listing of all hazardous chemicals, collection of matching MSDS preparation of labels and warning signs, and the transfer of necessary safety information and training employees

*Adapted from OSHA 29 CFR Part 1910.1030 - Hazard Communication; Final Rule and US Department of Labor, Occupational Safety and Health Administration, *Chemical Hazard Communication* (OSHA 3084). 1995, U.S. Printing Office, Washington, DC.

Table 19-1   Important Definitions for a Hazard Communication Program—cont'd

TERM	DEFINITION
(Written) HazCom program WHCP	A compliance process for the Hazard Communication Standard that includes a written clinic/office program manual, container labeling, and other forms of information transfer and warnings and employee training; best if administered by a HazCom compliance officer
HazCom Standard	The Hazard Communication Standard (aka "Employee Right to Know") has the goal of preventing employee exposures to hazardous chemicals; information from manufacturers of hazardous chemicals must be conveyed by employers to employees; facilities are responsible to assure that the information is received and understood; facilities enhance safety through their HazCom Program
Health hazard	Words, pictures, symbols, or combinations thereof appearing on a label or other appropriate form of warning that conveys the specific physical or health hazard(s), including target organ effects, of the chemical(s) present in a container
Label	Any written, printed or graphic material displayed on or affixed to containers of hazardous chemicals that provides necessary information
MSDS	MSDS (Material Safety Data Sheet) which are written or printed material concerning a hazardous chemical; an MSDS for each hazardous chemical listed within a facility must be obtained
Performance standard	Employers can use a combination of procedures and materials (work practices, engineering controls, PPE and training) to comply with an OSHA standard; OSHA does not usually dictate what process is to be followed, rather it describes the outcome of some behavior, for example, keeping exposures within some limit; how well this is done can be called proper performance or proper achievement (level of compliance)
Personal protective equipment (PPE) and devices	Specialized clothing or equipment worn by an employee for protection against a hazard; general work clothes are not usually designed or intended to prevent exposure to hazardous chemicals
Physical hazard	A chemical for which there is scientifically valid evidence that it is a combustible liquid, a compressed gas, explosive, flammable, an organic peroxide and oxidizer, pyrophoric, unstable (reactive), or water-reactive
Work practice controls	Means that reduce the likelihood of exposure by altering the manner in which a task is performed; for example, the use of a fume hood or vacuum evacuation

In time, OSHA issued comprehensive standards that held the weight of law. Noncompliance even in the absence of injury could result in citation, fines, and even temporary closure for the employer. OSHA also began to describe the required *performance standards* (see Table 19-1) expected from various pieces of work equipment (e.g., ladders, pipes, and electrical service). Then, OSHA applied Environmental Protection Agency (EPA) standards for maximum workplace exposure to chemicals, such as gases and volatile chemicals, radioactivity, and even heat and sound.

Finally, OSHA generated standards for the development, use, and review of *personal protective equipment and devices* (PPE, see Table 19-1). Examples include gloves, masks, respirators, glasses, and uniforms for employees.

The overall goal was to minimize the chances of occupationally related injuries through several mechanisms. Success of such efforts is based on a number of interrelated factors. Of course, issuance of reasonable and reliable standards by OSHA is the guiding force. However, employers must make themselves knowledgeable of what is required and to create within their environments as safe a workplace as possible. Employees must also be aware of the required standards and be active participants in the process. While employers must provide proper safe working environments, employees must be compliant in implementation and performance of the processes.

Over the last few years, dental workers have become very aware of OSHA activities. For example, without the emergence of HIV/AIDS in the U.S. and the involvement of OSHA in health care settings, this book probably would not have been written. Before 1986, there was an overall modest interest in infection control, hazardous materials handling, and waste management. This lack of concern negatively affected employee safety. However, with the growing AIDS epidemic, the interests of health care professionals and the general population grew. A heightened awareness of an increased need for patient and practitioner safety quickly developed.

OSHA's main directive is the protection of employees. Its response to current needs involves development of new standards and broadening the scopes of others. Most dental workers are acutely aware of OSHA *Occupational Exposure to Bloodborne Pathogens; Final Rule* (issued on December 6, 1991). In fact, the majority of interest, effort, and resources with dental environments involves infection control. Conversely, relatively little attention is paid to other OSHA standards. One particularly deficient area is OSHA *Hazard Communication Standard,* CFR 29.1910.1200 (HazCom or HazMat Program; see Table 19-1).

OSHA in an attempt to improve safer use of hazardous materials, on September 23, 1987, began to require chemical manufacturers, importers, and distributors to provide *material safety data sheets* (MSDSs, see Table 19-1) with their shipments of all hazardous chemicals.

Initially, the center of activity involved manufacturing locations. However, with continued evidence of employee injuries, OSHA on May 23, 1988, began to require that employers from the nonmanufacturing sector (including health care facilities) comply with all provisions of the HazCom Standard. Even though the Standard has been in effect for almost ten years, compliance by dental clinics/offices is less than universal. Such deficiencies could be related to heightened concern (and overemphasis) for infection control issues and/or lack of interest or awareness of the HazCom Standard. In any case, dental clinics and offices must comply with all tenets of the Standard. A significant proportion of OSHA inspections involves complaints associated with injuries or the potential for injury involving the handling, use, storage, and disposal of hazardous materials.

PURPOSE OF THE STANDARD

The purpose of the HazCom Standard is to ensure that hazards of all chemicals produced or imported be evaluated and that the information concerning such hazards be transmitted directly to employees by their employers. Information is conveyed through a comprehensive *hazard communication program* (see Table 19-1). The program includes a written clinic/office program manual, container labeling, and other forms of warning, MSDSs, and employee training.

Users of hazardous materials are not in a position to easily evaluate the potential hazards associated with their chemicals. Logically, this responsibility falls to the *manufacturer/importer* (see Table 19-1) and eventually to the *chemical distributors* (see Table 19-1). The responsibility of *employers* (see Table 19-1) is to inform and train their *employees* (see Table 19-1) of all safety materials provided, including all warnings, required personal protective devices, and safer handling and disposal methods.

OSHA has a variety of materials and publications to help employers and employees develop and implement effective hazard communication programs. Brochures on related topics can be obtained by contacting The Department of Labor, OSHA/OSHA Publications, P.O. Box 37535, Washington, DC 20013-7535 (Box 19-1). Single copies can be obtained at no charge by sending a self-addressed mailing label with your request. More extensive information kits can be obtained for a fee from the U.S. Printing Office at Su-

---

Box 19-1   OSHA Related Publications

Available at No Charge From OSHA
All about OSHA - OSHA 2056
Consultation Services for the Employer - OSHA 3047
Employee Workplace Rights - OSHA 3021
How to Prepare for Workplace Emergencies - OSHA 3088
OSHA Inspections – OSHA 2098
Personal Protective Equipment - OSHA 3077
Respiratory Protection - OSHA 3079
Hazard Communication: Final Rule in Federal Register - 59(27):6126-6184, February 9, 1994.

Available For a Fee From the U.S. Printing Office
Hazard Communication - A Compliance Kit - OSHA 3104
   Order No. 029-016-00147-6 - $18.00
Hazard Communication Guidelines for Compliance - OSHA 3111
   Order No. 029-016-00127-1 - $1.00
Job Hazard Analysis - OSHA 3071
   Order No. 029-016-00142-5 - $1.00
Training Requirements in OSHA Standards and Training Guidelines - *OSHA* - OSHA 2254
   Order No. 029-016-00137-9 - $1.00

---

*Adapted from U.S. Department of Labor, Occupational Safety and Health Administration: *Chemical Hazard Communication* (OSHA 3084), 1995, U.S. Printing Office, Washington, DC.

perintendent of Documents, U.S. Printing Office, Washington, DC 20402 or by calling 202.512.1800 (see Box 19-1).

SCOPE AND APPLICATION

As previously stated, chemical manufacturers and importers are charged to assess the hazards associated with the use of their products. Distributors also must inform their clients of the hazards. In turn, employers must inform their employees. The HazCom Standard covers any workplace that employs workers (even one).

Hazardous chemicals involved in the Standard are limited to those present in the workplace to which employees may be exposed under normal working conditions *and* in the case of a foreseeable emergency (e.g., an employee may not directly use a chemical but must be informed and trained about the proper procedures to follow if another employee were to drop and break open a jar of the chemical).

Technically, OSHA considers most health care facilities, including dental clinics/office to be "laboratories." Employers must assure that employees are informed and trained considering the types and amounts of hazardous materials present, the labeling system and warning signs employed, the location and use of MSDSs, and procedures to be followed in case of emergencies.

Some chemicals are exempt from the Standard. These include tobacco and tobacco products, wood and wood products, food, drugs, cosmetics, or alcoholic beverages packaged and sold for consumer use. Foods, drugs, or cosmetics intended for personal consumption by employees while at work are also exempt. Consumer type products (e.g., glass cleaner) used in a manner similar to those used by people at home (applications, amounts used, and duration and frequency of use) are generally considered as not being hazardous. Finally, any chemical defined as a "drug" by the Federal Food, Drug and Cosmetic Act when present in its solid, final form, ready for direct administration to patients (e.g., aspirin) is exempt.

Before reviewing the details of the various parts of the HazCom Standard, a brief review of its design may be helpful. This Standard is different from other OSHA standards in that it covers all hazardous chemicals (not just those associated with a certain type of workplace). The rule incorporates a "downstream flow of information." Producers must inform distributors, who then tell employers, who must transmit information to their employees. The process is described in Table 19-2.

HAZARD DETERMINATION

The quality of a hazard communication program depends on the adequacy and accuracy of the hazard assessment. A hazardous chemical is any *chemical* that is a *physical hazard* or a *health hazard* (see Table 19-1). The EPA specifically designates which chemicals are hazardous. The EPA considers a chemical as hazardous if it can catch fire, if it can react or explode when mixed with other substances, if it is corrosive, or if it is toxic. Included are chemicals that are flammable, spontaneously ignitable, explosive, oxidizers, corrosive, toxic, or radioactive.

The EPA estimates that the average American house with a garage holds about 30 gallons of materials that can be considered hazardous. Consumers readily use many of these

Table 19-2   Responsibilities in a Compliance Scheme that uses "Downstream Flow of Information" Methodology[*]

GROUP	REQUIRED ACTION
Chemical manufacturers/importers	Determine the hazards of each product
Chemical manufacturers/ importers/distributors	Communicate hazard information and associated protective measurers downstream to customers through labels and MSDS
Employers	Identify and list hazardous chemicals in the workplace
	Obtain MSDS and prepare labels for each hazardous chemical
	Develop and implement a written hazard communication program, include list of all hazardous chemicals, chemical labels, MSDS (for each chemical or chemical kit) and employee training
	Communicate hazard information to employees through labels, MSDS, and formal training programs (can include examinations)
Employees	Actively participate in facility training and information sharing
	Know tenets of their facility's hazard communication program, including labels, warning signs, protective equipment and postexposure procedures
	Be able to locate and if necessary complete exposure-related records and reports (e.g., MSDS, accident reports, and postexposure medical treatments)

[*]Adapted from U.S. Department of Labor, Occupational Safety and Health Administration: *Chemical Hazard Communication*. (OSHA 3084). U.S. Printing Office, Washington, DC.

items, including gasoline, fertilizers, pesticides, strong acids or bases, lubricants, paints and varnishes, drain cleaners, and engine coolants. Many chemicals can be considered hazardous for more than one reason (e.g., gasoline is flammable, explosive, toxic, and can at times spontaneously ignite). Although the volume of hazardous materials in a dental clinic/office may not exceed that of many households, the number and forms of potentially harmful chemicals is usually far greater. Of course, the Standard regulates safety in the workplace, not necessary within residences.

The identification, evaluation, and notification of any chemical as being hazardous is the initial responsibility of its manufacturer or importer. They may generate their own scientific data or when appropriate they may cite previously published information. Distributors are required to pass along this information to their clients. Hazardous means any chemical that has shown capability of causing a physical or a health hazard. Toxicity and carcinogenicity are of significant importance. Although many chemicals have been tested, literally thousands of new compounds are produced each year. Many chemicals in common use have not been totally evaluated. Even if considered to be toxic or carcinogenic, debate on a chemical's status can continue for an extended period. The stories associated

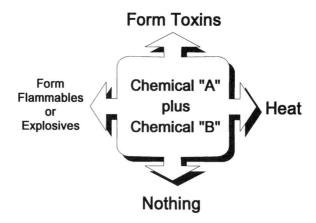

FIGURE 19-1   Potential outcomes of mixing chemicals.

with the investigation of dioxin, asbestos, chlorine, formaldehyde and even the sweetener saccharin have proved legendary. When in doubt, federal chemical registries (e.g., *The Registry of Toxic Effects of Chemical Substances* produced by the National Institute for Occupational Safety and Health) can be consulted. Some hazardous materials are listed in the HazCom Standard itself.

It is uncommon in dental environments that a single pure chemical, like ethanol, is used. A more frequent event is the mixing of chemicals. Kits containing various chemicals are mixed to achieve the desired end product. Trituration of amalgam is a common example of chemical mixing in a dental clinic/office. The manufacturer or importer (and eventually the employer) of a chemical kit must identify the hazards associated with mixing. The combination of chemicals may initially involve more than one hazardous chemical. The result of such combinations can vary (Figure 19-1). Chemicals that are benign when separate can after being mixed produce an end product of significant danger. Warning information as to the type of hazard generated and procedures to safely handle, use, and store the mixture must be provided. Warnings must include specific comments concerning the types of personal protective equipment that need to be worn and the procedures to be used for exposure or for disposal.

WRITTEN HAZARD COMMUNICATION PROGRAM

The HazCom Standard is commonly referred to as the "Employee Right to Know Rule." Another way to look at the Standard is as the "No Surprises Rule." The goal is that by training and the sharing of information, employee injuries involving hazardous chemicals can be kept to a minimum. Employers must develop, implement, and maintain at the workplace a written, comprehensive hazard communication program that includes provisions for container labeling, collection and availability of MSDSs, and an employee-training program.

A central activity to meet this goal is the production of a *written hazard communication program,* WHCP (see Table 19-1). Although such efforts are usually modest (6–8 pages), they cannot be mere reiterations of the HazCom Standard. They are designed to be manuals that reflect the type and size of the dental practice. An outline of a generic WHCP is presented in Table 19-3. Task identification and proper responses follow.

Employers are required to develop, implement, and maintain (monitor) a WHCP for their workplaces. Minimal contents include a list of all known hazardous materials present, the labeling and warning sign system used, the location and use of MSDSs, emergency procedures, and the nature and frequency of employee information and training. The WHCP helps explain how the clinic/office complies with the various criteria of the Standard.

The overall purpose of a WHCP is to provide for the implementation of the Standard's requirements in the workplace and to serve as a reference for employers/employees questions about official clinic/office policies. Because there is great differences even among clinics/offices in the same general locale, the WHCP must be "personalized" to reflect what actually is being performed.

Writing the WHCP involves nine stages or steps. These steps are:

1. **Provide Copies of the HazCom Standard to Each Employee.**   Familiarity with the Standard will increase compliance. Employers may devise a modest examination to assure that employees have read and understood the basic tenets of the Standard.

2. **Determine Who is Responsible for Implementing the WHCP.**   The most effective way for a clinic/office to comply with the Standard is to identify, train, empower, and reward the *HazCom Compliance Officer* (see Table 19-1). Many if not all the various activities associated with HazCom Standard compliance can be completed by a single individual. This is especially important when considering the listing of the hazardous chemicals and the collection of the required MSDSs. The process is improved if all transactions are performed by a single individual. This person's name and title must be formally listed. A back-up officer (e.g., the dentist) should be identified also.

3. **List all Chemicals Used or Produced in the Workplace.**   Specific guidelines on the development of the required list will appear later. The list must be reviewed often because new chemicals are brought into the clinic/office on a regular basis. The goal is to generate and maintain a complete list and location of all hazardous chemicals.

4. **Describe the Methods to be Used to Inform Employees of the Hazards of Nonroutine Tasks.**   Cleaning or repair of some pieces of equipment is an example of nonroutine tasks. Sometimes chemical hazards are released during such process. In other cases, hazardous chemicals are used during the cleaning or repair. Also, some office or clinic employees perform work that does not normally place them at risk for exposure to hazardous chemicals. Such individuals require less information and training.

5. **Describe Methods Used to Inform Contract Employees of the Hazardous Chemicals to Which They Could be Exposed.**   Part-time employees or persons hired to clean or repair must be extended the same level of protection as permanent, full-time employees. Contract employees that bring hazardous materials as part of their work into the clinic/office environment must provide appropriate MSDSs.

Table 19-3 Generic Written Hazardous Chemical Program

STEP	REQUIRED ACTION
Provide copies of the HazCom Standard to each employee	☑ Indicate that their WHCP includes the Standard, introductory comments, a written manual that describes the procedures to be used in the facility, and some definitions
	☑ Provide individual copies of the HazCom Standard
	☑ Discuss in general the materials shared
	☑ Use examinations to ensure employee review of the Standard
Determine who is responsible for implementing the WHCP	☑ Indicate the WHCP date of preparation/review
	☑ Indicate that the subject of the WHCP is to comply with the Hazard Communication Program for General Industry (OSHA 29 CFR 1910.1200)
	☑ Prepare a rationale for workplace compliance (a paragraph or two, describing that workplace injuries and infections can occur—can be gleaned from the Standard)
	☑ Acknowledge the facility's responsibility to determine the hazards associated with all chemicals present and that hazard information and appropriate use of protective measures will be transmitted to employees
	☑ Identify the facility's HazCom Compliance Officer by name and title; establish a trained back-up officer
	☑ Assure that the Compliance Officer will maintain and review at least annually the WHCP, including a written manual, chemical inventory, information dissemination (including MSDS, labels, and warnings) and employee training
List all chemical used or produced in the workplace	☑ Identify, list, and provide the locations of all hazardous chemicals present in the workplace as part of the WHCP (best done by one individual)
	☑ Use a listing scheme (alphabetical, alphanumeric, or numeric) that all employees understand and can readily use
	☑ Inform employees of the locations of the hazardous chemicals list
	☑ Obtain MSDS for each listed chemical and use the MSDS and the list to prepare labels and when necessary warning signs for each hazardous chemical
Describe methods to be used to inform employees of the hazards of nonroutine tasks	☑ Assure that employees are not asked to perform nonroutine tasks for which they are may not be fully trained
	☑ Discuss all nonroutine tasks before initiation (includes training)
	☑ Record the processes used and place within the WHCP

Adapted from U.S. Department of Labor, Occupational Safety and Health Administration: *Chemical Hazard Communication* (OSHA 3084), 1995. U.S. Printing Office, Washington, DC and from U.S. Department of Labor, Occupational Health and Safety Administration: Hazard Communication; Final Rule - 29 CFR 1910.1030. *Fed Register* 59:6126-6184, 1994.

Table 19-3 Generic Written Hazardous Chemical Program—cont'd

STEP	REQUIRED ACTION
Describe methods used to inform contract employees of the hazardous chemicals to which they could be exposed	☑ Assign task to the facility's Compliance Officer ☑ Assure that part-time or contract employees are aware of the chemical hazards associated within their specific work areas ☑ Assure that if such workers bring hazardous chemicals into the facility that they are fully trained regarding their use, storage, and disposal and that they bring appropriate information and hazard signs and MSDS
Describe methods used to label containers	☑ Assure that incoming chemicals are properly labeled, placed on the hazardous chemical list, and have an associated MSDS ☑ Complete labeling for improperly or unmarked containers so that the name and title of the person responsible for labeling is present and a description of the labeling system used (must contain the identity of the chemical, the name and address of the chemical's manufacturer or importer and appropriate hazard warnings, including proper PPE) are present ☑ List and train employees concerning the facility's procedures for reviewing and updating labeling and location information ☑ Keep all hazardous chemicals separate from foods or beverages; this may include processes such as two refrigerators
Collection and maintenance of MSDS	☑ Collect an appropriate MSDS for every chemical that is on the facility's list of hazardous chemicals ☑ Maintain two collections—one in office storage and another where employees have easy access ☑ Train employees concerning the location and proper use of MSDS
Describe employee information transmission and training schemes	☑ List the facility's training coordinator (and back-up) by name and title ☑ Describe procedures used to train employees ☑ Describe procedures used to inform employees of the HazCom Standard, operations that use hazardous chemicals, location of the WHCP, list of hazardous chemicals, and location of MSDS ☑ Collect an appropriate MSDS for every chemical that is on the facility's list of hazardous chemicals ☑ Train employees concerning the facility's written emergency and/or postexposure protocols
Using chemicals that involve trade secrets	☑ Identify chemicals containing "secret ingredients" ☑ Design a protocol for postexposure activities for "secret chemicals" in which a medical emergency exists ☑ Design a protocol for postexposure activities for "secret chemicals" in which no immediate health hazard exists

6. **Describe Methods Used to Label Containers.**   This step has three phases.
    a. Name and title of the person responsible for the proper labeling of all containers
    b. Description of the labeling system used (a proper label must contain the identity of the chemical, the name and address of the chemical manufacturer or importer, and appropriate hazard warnings)
    c. Description of the clinic/office procedures for reviewing and updating labeling information

7. **Collection and Maintenance of MSDSs.**   Use of MSDSs will be described later. However, MSDSs are the center element for information concerning hazardous materials. The WHCP must describe who is responsible for collecting the MSDSs for each hazardous material, as well as the method used to maintain the MSDS collection (e.g., in notebooks and their locations). Also to be listed is how employees can access MSDSs and how the list of MSDSs is kept current.

8. **Describe Employee Information Transmission and Training.**   This step has five phases.
    a. Name and title of the person responsible for employee training
    b. Description of the procedures used to train employees
    c. Description of the procedures for informing employees of the HazCom Standard, the operations that use hazardous materials, the location of the WHCP, a list of hazardous chemicals and the location of the MSDSs
    d. Description of the training program, including hazardous materials monitoring, all physical or health hazards present, and measures used to protect employees
    e. Details of the WHCP, including an explanation of the labeling system used and how the employees are trained to use MSDSs

9. **Using Chemicals That Involve Trade Secrets.**   Some chemical manufacturers are reluctant to share information concerning their products because they think that some trade secret could be gleaned. Although the ratios or percents of the component chemicals can be withheld, it is the manufacturer's/importer's responsibility to inform the user of the hazardous chemicals. This includes specific comments as to which protective equipment or processes should be used when handling their product.

After the WHCP is prepared, it is important that it be reviewed on a regular basis. New employees need to review the WHCP as soon as possible.

INVENTORYING AND LISTING HAZARDOUS CHEMICALS

Each facility is required to inventory their holdings for any hazardous chemicals. Inventories of chemicals can be organized in several ways. Some clinics/offices prefer to use an alphabetical listing; others use a numerical listing in which a chemical is given next available number. Another method is to organize the chemicals by hazard category. Such divisions usually include corrosive, flammable, reactive, and toxic. No matter which listing process is used, it must be understood and used properly by employees.

The list can include scientific and common chemical names and even associated hazards. It would be wise to create an additional column for the PPE and other safety processes to be used for each hazardous chemical. Listing where various hazardous chemicals are located throughout the facility is also very useful. Of course, the list's preparation date (and updates) should be prominently noted. The list should be generated and maintained by the clinic/office HazCom Coordinator. If all purchases and disposals are handled by this individual, there will be little chance that a hazardous chemical will be present but not listed.

Completing a chemical inventory provides an excellent opportunity to discard unwanted chemicals. This could include items never used, those past expiration, samples, and those no longer having clinical value. It is always surprising to learn the volume of unwanted chemicals that are present. Always contact your local environmental regulatory agency concerning proper disposal procedures.

Chemical inventory lists are extremely valuable. All listed chemicals must have their own MSDS. Lists are also important in the generation of informative signs and warnings and should be used for employee training. All employees must know the location of the list of hazardous chemicals and be able to interpret the information present.

LABELS AND OTHER FORMS OF WARNING

Chemical manufacturers and importers and their distributors are required by the HazCom Standard to properly label all products considered as being hazardous. The minimal acceptable label must include a) the identity of the hazardous chemical(s), b) appropriate hazard warning (including target organs or systems and common routes of contact and methods that protect against exposure), and c) the name and address of the chemical manufacturer, importer, or responsible party.

Ideally, the sources of the chemical will properly label all their containers of hazardous chemicals. If an employer determines that a container is properly labeled, there is no requirement to add additional information. You may elect to place extra information (e.g., special labels such as the National Fire Protection Association 704 Diamond System; Figure 19-2) on the container. This could improve the uniformity of the clinic/office labeling system.

"0" = No Hazard - "4" = Maximum Hazard

IDENTIFICATION OF HEALTH HAZARD		IDENTIFICATION OF FLAMMABILITY		IDENTIFICATION OF REACTIVITY (STABILITY)	
Hazard Color Code: BLUE		Hazard Color Code: RED		Hazard Color Code: YELLOW	
Signal	Type of Possible Injury	Signal	Susceptibility of Materials to Burning	Signal	Susceptibility to Release of Energy
4	Materials that on very short exposure could cause death or major residual injury even though prompt medical treatment was given	4	Materials that will rapidly or completely vaporize at atmospheric pressure and normal ambient temperature or that are readily dispersed in air and will burn readily	2	Materials that in themselves are normally unstable and readily undergo violent chemical change but do not detonate, materials may react with water

FIGURE 19-2 Example of the National Fire Protection Association 704 system's diamond identification symbol and description of the various numbers presented.

Unfortunately, some chemicals (especially dental materials kits) are not properly labeled by their sources. In such cases, the clinic/office must complete the labeling process. Action must also be taken when a hazardous chemical is removed from properly labeled containers to an improperly (possibly even blank) container. For example, iodophor surface disinfectant is purchased in a concentrated form and then it is diluted to its working concentration and placed within spray bottles. The new containers must be labeled with a) the identity of the hazardous chemical(s), b) appropriate hazard warning (including target organs/tissues and applicable personal protective equipment and procedures), and c) the name and address of the chemical manufacturer, importer, or responsible party.

There is no official labeling system that must be used. Clinics/offices can photocopy the label from the original container and affix it to the new containers. There are several other labeling schemes available. The most important factors are that the system is easy to use and that employees are proper trained to understand and use the system.

Safe use of hazardous chemicals involves other activities in addition to container labels. Employers can use signs, placards, posted operating procedures, and other written or pictorial information (e.g., international pictograms). Such signage must be in English and when necessary in an alternative language. Warning signs are readily available from many commercial sources. They, however, can also be handmade. The goal is not artistic beauty but simplicity, ease of use, and conveyance of the desired information.

MATERIAL SAFETY DATA SHEETS

There are few more valuable safety constructs than MSDSs. These are written reports prepared by manufacturers or importers who describe an individual chemical or a group collection of chemicals. Valuable information includes the chemicals present, the associated hazards, handling and clean-up procedures, and special PPE that need to be in place.

Chemical manufacturers and importers must obtain or develop an MSDS for each product containing hazardous chemicals. This applies to single chemicals and multiple chemical kits. The employer must obtain an MSDS specific for each hazardous chemical present in the workplace. If a clinic/office uses three types of amalgam, three specific (unique) MSDSs are needed. Generic MSDSs are not acceptable. MSDSs contain phone numbers that are answered 24 hours a day, seven days a week. These contacts are trained to offer highly specific and useful information about the product. Photocopies of MSDSs are acceptable.

Unfortunately, some chemical sources are reluctant, unable, or unwilling to distribute MSDSs. This does not diminish the requirement of employers to obtain MSDSs for all their hazardous chemicals. There are several ways clinics/offices can obtain MSDSs other than from the manufacturer or importer. The American Dental Association (ADA) currently offers advice on MSDSs as a service to its members. Clinics/offices are encouraged to call the ADA about their MSDS collection and any compliance-related issue. Again, a photocopy of an MSDS is as good as an original. In fact, many MSDSs sent with products are actually copies. A small degree of networking among local dental practices (e.g., local study club) can result in a "master list" of MSDSs that can be shared by participants.

Another difficulty facing clinics/offices is that MSDSs are sometimes incomplete or inaccurate. That is, not all of the nine sections are filled out. One reason is the reluctance of suppliers to describe all chemicals present in their products. Another reason is that if common domain information is not available about a hazardous chemical, the manufacturer or importer must pay to have the product evaluated by a laboratory. Clinics/offices when presented an incomplete MSDS should write the source for more specific information.

MSDSs must be readily accessible to employees. Ideally, two copies of an MSDS could be kept in notebooks. One set could remain in an office file cabinet; the other could be placed in a general work area, such as the laboratory or instrument recycling room. MSDSs are essential to a successful clinic/office HazCom Program.

Chemical information presented in MSDSs is essential for the generation of proper labeling, and the development of correct warning signs and notices are present in an MSDS. Emergency exposure guidelines suggest personal protective equipment and mixing; use and disposal tenets are presented also. An example of an actual MSDS is presented in Figure 19-3.

MSDSs contain nine sections.

1. **Product Information.**   This section includes the hazardous chemical names, including generic and scientific names. Chemical formulas may also be present. The name, address, and contact phone number(s) are also listed.

2. **Hazardous Ingredients.**   Chemicals known to be hazardous must be listed. Suspected problem chemicals must also be present, and sometimes hazard data such as flammability, reactivity, or LD_{50}. If the concentration of hazardous chemicals is more than 1%, threshold limit values or permissible exposure limits are commonly noted.

3. **Physical Hazard Data.**   Although very technical, this section provides a great amount of useful information. It describes why the chemical is considered hazardous. Solvents such as ethanol or acetone are commonly used in the dental office and their hazardous properties are described in this section. Data in this section apply to single, pure chemicals and to combination mixtures of several chemicals. Important physical parameters include terms such as boiling point, vapor pressure, solubility, appearance and odor, specific gravity, vapor density, percent volatile by volume, and evaporation rate. These values are extremely important when dealing with any volatile chemical and the vapors produced. It is important to note the levels of acceptable occupational exposures.

4. **Fire and Explosion Data.**   Whenever dealing with flammables, solvents, peroxides, explosives, metal dusts, and any other unstable substances the information presented in this section is extremely important. If a chemical does not pose a fire hazard, it should be stated in this section. Important terms presented include flash point, flammable liquids (lower explosive limit and upper explosive limit), extinguishing media, and special or unusual fire/explosion procedures and hazards.

5. **Health Hazard Information.**   The information presented must reflect an estimate of the total product (e.g., post mixing). This can be expressed as a time weighted average concentration, permissible exposure limit, or threshold limit value. Sometimes an LD_{50} value is mentioned. Expected routes of exposure should also be listed. Information about the potential hazard from absorption of the product, the severity of the effect, and the basis of the hazard determination must be listed. The positions may come from animal studies or reports of human exposures. The effects of acute and chronic exposure should be discussed. This may include some information about a chemical's carcinogenic, teratogenic, or mutagenic potential. Specific

Material Safety Data Sheet

May be used to comply with
OSHA's Hazard Communication Standard.
29 CFR 1910.1200 Standard must be
consulted for specific requirements.

U.S. Department of Labor

Occupational Safety and Health Administration
(Non-Mandatory Form)
Form Approved
OMB No. 1218-0072

IDENTITY *(As Used on Label and List)*
Vapo-Steril   (264253 & 260812)

Note: Blank speaces are not permitted. If any item is not applicable, or no information is available, the space must be marked to indicate that.

Section I

Manufacturer's Name BarnsteadlThermolyne	Emergency Telephone Number: 1-800-424-9300 Chemtrec	To be used only in the event of a chemical emergency involving a spill, leak, fire, exposure or accident involving this product.

Address (Number, Street, City, State, and ZIP Code)	Telephone Number for Information (800) 553-0039
2555 Kerper Boulevard	Date Prepared October 30, 1997
Dubuque, IA 52001	Signature of Preparer (optional)

Section II - Hazardous Ingredients/Identity Information

Hazardous Components (Specific Chemical Identity: Common Name (s))	OSHA PEL	ACGIH TLV	Other Limits Recommended	% (optional)
Ethanol	1000	1000	None	72.38
Formaldehyde (By Weight)	.75	0.3	0.5 ppm action level	.23

NFPA HAZARD RATING:

FLAMMABILITY

HEALTH   REACTIVITY

3

3   1

Section III - Physical/Chemical Characteristics

Boiling Point	172°F	Specific Gravity (H₂O) = 1)	0.825
Vapor Pressure (mm Hg)	50.0 mm Hg	Melting Point	N/A
Vapor Density (AIR = 1)	1.59	Evaporation Rate (Butyl Acetate = 1)	2.7

Solubility in Water   100% @ 20°C.

Appearance and Odor   Clear Liquid - pungent odor

Section IV - Fire and Explosion Hazard Data

Flash Point (Method Used) ASTM D93: 72° - 75°F.	Flammable Limits For Ethyl Alcohol	LEL 3.3%	UEL 19%

Extinguishing Media   Class B Chemical Powder

Special Fire Fighting Procedures   None for small quantities.

Unusual Fire and Explosion Hazards   None for small quantities.

(Reproduce locally)
P/N 260068 • 10/97

OSHA 174, Sept. 1985

FIGURE 19-3   Material Safety Data Sheet (Courtesy of Barnstead/Thermolyne).

Section V - Reactivity Data

Stability	Unstable		
	Stable	X	Keep away from sparks, flames, heat or other ignition sources.

Incompatibility *(Materials to Avoid)*	Concentrated Nitric & Sulfuric Acids, strong Oxidizing Agents.

Hazardous Decomposition or Byproducts	Burning can produce Carbon Monoxide and/or Carbon Dioxide.

Hazardous Polymerization	May Occur		
	Will Not Occur	X	

Section VI - Health Hazard Data

Route(s) of Entry:	Inhalation? X	Skin? X	Ingestion? X

Health Hazards *(Acute and Chronic)*	Acute - Causes eye damage and may cause skin irritation.
	Chronic - Formaldehyde is a suspected carcinogen.

Carcinogenicity:	NTP? YES	IAPC Monographs? YES	OSHA Regulated? YES

Signs and Symptoms of Exposure	Irritation to eye and skin.

Medical Conditions Generally Aggravated by Exposure	None Known

Emergency and First Aid Procedures	Eyes: Immediately flush with large amount of water for 15 minutes. See a physician immediately. Skin Contact: Flush under running water for at least 15 minutes. Ingestion: Give large amount of water if person is conscious.

Section VII - Precautions for Safe Handling and Use

Steps To Be Taken in Case Material is Released or Spilled	Extinguish and do not turn on any ignition source. Flush small spills with water. Wear suitable protective equipment. Collect large spills for disposal.

Waste Disposal Method	Ignitable, should be disposed of as required by hazardous waste regulations.

Precautions to Be Taken in Handling and Storing	Keep away from heat or open flames.

Other Precautions	Store in dry area (40°F - 90°F)

Section VIII - Additional Information

California Prop 65 Warning: This product contains formaldehyde, a chemical known to the State of California to cause cancer

Section IX - Control Measures

Respiratory Protection (Specify Type)	Use in a well ventilated area. Avoid inhalation of fumes.**

Ventilation	Local Exhaust	See OSHA Requirement	Special	Not applicable
	Mechanical (General)	Not applicable	Other	Not applicable

Protective Gloves	Neoprene gloves recommended	Eye Protection	Safety glasses or goggles

Other Protective Clothing or Equipment	None

Work/Hygenic Practices	Employee information and training required.	** California State Department of Food and Agriculture has requested the following be included: Attention: Wear face shield when handling this product and when opening the door of the sterilizer after the treatment cycle.

FIGURE 19-3 Cont'd

signs and symptoms of exposure should be listed. Emergency and first aid procedures to be used by trained response personnel are also presented. Often specific notes to physicians are included. If inhalation is the route of exposure, some further comments can be found in Section 3. Section 8 contains information on the proper respiratory equipment (e.g., gloves, eye, and skin protection). This section also discusses the use of protective glasses.

6. **Reactivity Data.**   The information in this section will assist in determining safe handling and storage procedures for hazardous, unstable substances. Adverse reaction (incompatibility) of chemicals with commonly encountered media (e.g., heat, water, direct sunlight, metal piping, and acids/bases) is usually listed. Stability data are also listed in Sections 2, 4, and 9. After contamination, aging, or burning, a chemical can decompose into hazardous products. These outcomes are also usually listed. Polymerization of some chemicals can release toxic vapors or extremely high or uncontrolled release of heat, which should be noted.

7. **Spill or Leak Procedures.**   Detailed procedures and protective clothing and equipment and/or ventilation to be used for cleaning up a spill and safe disposal are reported in this section. Corresponding information can be found in Sections 2 through 8. Specific recommendations for cleanup need to be delineated. Also presented is whether the substance is incompatible with common cleanup procedures or media (e.g., water). Sometimes the cleanup residue creates a disposal problem (appropriate final disposal method/site [e.g., sanitary landfill, incineration or sanitary sewer]). Disposal recommendations can also be found in Sections 2, 4, 6, and 9.

8. **Special Protection Information.**   If required, specific comments about respiratory protection, ventilation, protective gloves, and eye protection are presented. Most of the other sections also contain information about protective methods and materials.

9. **Special Precautions.**   How to properly label a container or warning sign often is listed in this section. Any safety or health information not previously presented is listed. Some chemical sources will use this section to reiterate some very important safety or health issue.

EMPLOYEE INFORMATION AND TRAINING

Employers must provide employees with information and training on all hazardous chemicals present in the workplace. This includes all chemicals, even if an employee does not use some of them in the course of their normal work. Information and training must be provided at the time of an employee's initial assignment (no matter how experienced or trained the employee may be) or whenever a new hazard is introduced into the work area. To maintain proper clinic/office awareness of hazardous chemicals, annual training sessions are expected.

Employees must be informed of a) the requirements of the HazCom Standard, b) any and all operations in the work area where hazardous chemicals are present and/or used, and c) the location and availability of the WHCP, including the required list of hazardous chemicals and collection of MSDSs. As previously stated, to better comply, each employee must provide a copy of the actual Standard as it appeared in the *Federal Register.*

Training is an essential component of a successful HazCom Standard program. Training is required at the time of hiring, when a new hazard is introduced, and annually for all continuing employees. Training has five major components.

1. **How the HazCom Standard is Implemented in the Workplace.**   Employees must be trained in the reading and interpretation of labels and MSDSs and how they can obtain and use the available hazard information.
2. **Physical and Health Hazards Present.**   Employers are to be trained about the physical and health hazards associated with hazardous chemicals. The use of MSDSs, container labels, and other forms of warning signs reinforce this process.
3. **Personal Protective Devices.**   Employees must be informed of and provided with all the personal protective equipment needed to protect themselves while using hazardous chemicals
4. **Site Specific Information.**   Details of the clinic/office WHCP developed by the employer, including an explanation of the labeling system, and the MSDS collection must be conveyed. Employees must be informed as to how they can obtain and use appropriate hazard information. Protection includes physical pieces of equipment and specific posted procedures. These include appropriate engineering controls, work practice changes, and emergency procedures.
5. **Methods and Observations.**   This section involves knowledge of the visual appearance and/or smell of hazardous chemicals by employees; this should limit exposures to chemicals. This section also assumes that the clinic/office has designed and practiced an emergency plan

TRADE SECRETS

Chemical manufacturers and importers may withhold specific chemical information, including the chemical name or other specific data that could help identify a hazardous chemical on its MSDS. The central argument is whether the source's claim that the information withheld is indeed a trade secret. The rationale being that publication of such information negatively affects market share.

The HazCom Standard attempts to strike a balance between the need to protect exposed employees and a manufacturer's need to maintain the confidentiality of a bona fide trade secret. This is achieved by providing, under specified need and confidentiality, limited disclosure to health professionals who are furnishing medical or other occupational health services to exposed employees, employee representatives, or contract workers.

Chemical manufacturers, importers, and, in some cases, employers must immediately disclose the specific chemical identity of a hazardous chemical to a treating physician or nurse when the information is needed for prompt emergency or first aid treatment. Companies can request the treating physician or nurse to prepare a written statement of need and to complete a confidentiality agreement after the emergency has abated.

When the case is a non-emergency the issue can become protracted. A health care professional (e.g., physician, industrial hygienist, toxicologist, epidemiologist, or occupational health nurse) must write the Source Company, describing the circumstances surrounding their petition.

HOW OSHA SOLVES A PROBLEM

It is interesting to examine the thought processes used to solve potentially complex interpersonal problems within the workplace. Successful resolution of questions concerning

OSHA compliance and other employee health and safety issues is no exception. For example, an employee on the job for a few weeks begins to complain about feeling ill at work. They could state: "I don't know. Something smells funny in here and I'm starting to get headaches." As this person's employer, how should this complaint be best handled?

Employers must take all employee complaints seriously. Most employees are reluctant to report problems, especially if they seem to involve only themselves. It is the employer's responsibility to establish an environment in which employee safety is paramount and in which open communication is the rule. Dismissing out of hand an employee complaint is unfair and unwise. Employees who think their reasonable requests are not being addressed properly are far more likely to seek an answer outside of the office or clinic. In other words, the chances of them reporting the case to a regulatory agency are markedly increased.

The first action taken by the employer should be to determine if a request is reasonable. This is probably more difficult than it sounds. Some employees at times make and maintain unreasonable requests. Fortunately, such cases are the exception. However, separation may be the only viable answer in extreme situations. A guiding rule as to whether a request or a policy, procedure, or piece of equipment has validity is to subject it to three challenges: "Is it reasonable?", "Is it necessary?", and "Is it appropriate?"

Employers must do what is required and proper but they are not obligated to provide more than what is necessary. Regular clinic/office meetings at which compliance issues are discussed in an open manner is central to clinic/office morale and compliance. After such discussions a decision should be made quickly. If the answer is "no," the logic behind the position should be presented. Because the employer is responsible for employee safety, the employer makes the final decision. However, employees usually expect and wish to be active participants in the process. Employers must provide a working environment that is safe; it is the employees' responsibility to comply with established clinic/office procedures.

If after careful review an employer decides that an employee complaint has merit, remedial action is required. It does not necessarily mean that just because an odor is present it is causing the employee's headaches or that it is indeed even potentially harmful. The employer has an obligation to investigate the matter further. Of course, the first temptation is to provide personal protective devices, such as masks. When presented with such a scenario, OSHA would consider its resolution to be a four-step process. A process that progresses from more effective actions to those less effective. These steps are:

1. **Determine if there is a problem.**   The presence of an odor may or may not indicate a potential problem. Of course, some very dangerous chemical vapors have little or no odor. Some types of monitoring devices, such as air samplers attached to color change chemicals or spectrophotometric devices, may be required. Other chemicals can be monitored easily with the use of inexpensive badges. Persistent problems may require consultation with an industrial hygienist or the local health or air quality department. Fortunately, in most cases there is no problem, or one that is readily solved. Problems, of course, can involve issues such as air quality, sound, heat, and lighting (e.g., curing lights).

2. **Engineering controls.**   Engineering controls are measures designed to isolate or remove the chemical hazard from a workplace. If there is a problem, OSHA indicates that the most effective and efficient method of resolution is to remove or change the chemical used or to somehow use it differently. A common dental example is a glutaraldehyde solution. All room temperature sterilizing chemicals are quite harsh and

can easily generate irritating fumes, which could cause allergies. Direct contact with unprotected skin or mucous membranes would likely lead to complaints and possible injury. If an employee complains about the use of glutaraldehydes, it is best to change how reusable instruments and equipment are sterilized. This could include a change to a heat treatment process such as autoclaving. If the items are very heat sensitive, there are other glutaraldehyde solutions commercially available. A change in the chemical used could help eliminate the problem.

3. **Work practices.**   Work practice controls are methods that reduce the likelihood of exposure by altering the manner in which a chemical is used. If engineering controls can not be employed because the chemical is absolutely necessary, work practice controls should be investigated. Again using glutaraldehyde as an example, such solutions can usually be safely used when present in relatively small amounts and when held within tightly sealed containers. Ideally, removing or changing the chemical is the most effective process. However, if the chemical must be used, workplace practices may have to be significantly changed. Of course, an increase in ventilation, such as using a fume hood, would always be beneficial.

4. **Personal protective equipment (PPE).**   PPE includes specialized clothing or equipment worn by an employee for protection against a chemical hazard. General work clothes usually are not sufficiently protective. There are several reasons why PPE is considered to be the least effective and efficient method to prevent employee exposures. One major deficiency is the lack of universal application. It can not be expected that employees will always wear the proper equipment whenever the hazard is present. This includes accidents. Obviously, PPE must be in place whenever there is any risk of exposure. Another fault of PPE involves the physical nature of barriers. Eventually all barriers fail. Newer designs and fabrication materials have improved the longevity of some PPE. Also, technologic advances have helped to improve overall barrier performance. Unfortunately, personal protective barriers will never be as effective as removing or changing a hazardous chemical or the use of improved handling methods.

OCCUPATIONAL EXPOSURE TO HAZARDOUS CHEMICALS IN LABORATORIES

OSHA has promulgated a safety standard (29 CFR Part 1450 - Occupational exposure to hazardous chemicals in laboratories) that helps protect employees engaged in the laboratory use of *hazardous chemicals* (Table 19-4).

In many ways, dental offices and clinics function as laboratories. Although carcinogenic, radioactive, or extremely toxic materials are rarely present, dental workplaces contain significant amounts and varying types of hazardous chemicals. Employees routinely prepare, use, store, and dispose of these materials. This is in addition to daily exposures to infectious agents and physical methods of harm (e.g., heat, sound, light, and air quality).

The major objective of the Standard is to limit employee exposures to specific permissible levels when working in laboratories. For some chemicals there are other OSHA and EPA standards, which are stricter. In some cases, absolutely no exposure is permitted. Some chemicals, however, are exempt. These include chemicals that have no potential for employee exposure, for example, 1) procedures that use chemically impregnated test media ("dipsticks") that are placed into liquid specimens and then the amount of color

Table 19-4   Important Definitions for a Chemical Hygiene Plan*

TERM	DEFINITION
Action plan	A concentration designated in 29 CFR part 1910 for a specific substance, calculated on an eight-hour average exposure. Action usually is in response to a complaint or is part of workplace's regular review program. Appropriate responses include exposure monitoring and medical surveillance
Chemical hygiene officer	An employee who is designated by the employer and who is qualified by training or experience to provide technical guidance in the development and implementation of a Chemical Hygiene Plan. For clinical dentistry, the position is similar to the office infection control hazard communication officer
Chemical Hygiene Plan	A written program developed and implemented by the employer that sets forth procedures, equipment, personal protective equipment, and work practices that 1) are capable of protecting employees from health hazards presented by hazardous chemicals used in a particular workplace and 2) involve the application of the tenets of "prudent practice"
Emergency	Any occurrence such as, but not limited to, equipment failure, rupture of containers or failure of control equipment that results in the uncontrolled release of a hazardous chemical into the workplace
Hazardous chemicals	A chemical for which there is statistically significant evidence based on a scientifically designed and conducted study that describes the acute, and/or chronic health effects that may occur to exposed employees. Many of the chemicals used within dental offices/clinics are considered as hazardous
Prudent practices	A plan originally developed in 1981 by the National Research Council. Useful in the preparation of a workplace's Chemical Hygiene Plan. It helps to better organize identified hazards and offers recommendations for each type of hazard. Deals with both safety and chemical hazards; the laboratory standard is concerned primarily with chemical hazards

*Adapted from OSHA (29 CFR Part 1450 - Occupational Exposure to Hazardous Chemicals in Laboratories Standard and Standard Appendices A and B.

changed is observed and 2) commercial kits in which all the reagents needed to conduct a test are contained within the kit (a pregnancy test is an example).

Limits are not known for all individual chemicals or for groups of chemicals mixed to create a new end product. However, complaints about odors, headaches, runny noses and eyes, nausea, or skin hypersensitivities are relatively common. The initial response is to determine if a problem actually exists (see page 266).

COMPLIANCE

Compliance with the Safe Use of Chemicals in the Laboratory Standard involves seven sections or components. These include: 1) general principles, 2) responsibilities, 3) laboratory facility, 4) components of the Chemical Hygiene Plan, 5) general principles of working with chemicals, 6) safety recommendations, and 7) material safety data sheets. This organization of topics corresponds to sections in the Standard and the recommendations made in the Standard's Appendices A and B. Compliance is mandatory for the Standard; however, the materials presented in Appendices A and B do not have to be followed exactly as presented. These appendices offer valuable organizational help and make valid suggestions. Reviewing (and possibly using) these materials may greatly help any clinic/office's compliance program.

GENERAL PRINCIPLES FOR WORKING WITH LABORATORY CHEMICALS

Each workplace must develop an appropriate *Chemical Hygiene Plan* (see Table 19-4). There is no official form or format. However, information given in Appendices A and B of the Laboratory Standard helps make compliance an easier and more effective process.

Many of the recommendations offered follow those provided by the National Research Council (1981). These are often called Prudent Practices for Handling Hazardous Chemicals in Laboratories or simply as *Prudent Practices* (see Table 19-4). This is actually an assessment of risk and a listing of recommendations that have the ultimate goal of limiting workplace exposure to harmful chemicals. Prudent Practices have a broader scope or intent than does the Laboratory Standard. Prudent Practices deals with safety and chemical hazards, whereas the Laboratory Standard is concerned primarily with just chemical hazards.

It is prudent to minimize all exposures to chemicals. General precautions for the use of chemicals should be developed and implemented effectively. Written general precautions are usually more valuable than the generation of specific guidelines for particular chemicals. An analogy is the concept of universal precautions. In this case, the objective is to prevent contact of health-care workers with patient body fluids. The combination of engineering controls, work practices, and personal protective equipment selected should protect against any infectious agent present in blood and other body fluids.

Avoid underestimation of risk. Even for chemicals that seem to have little or no toxicity, exposure should always be kept to a minimum. Of course, chemicals known to cause problems require special handling. Information on use may come from the manufacturer/importer and is present on the chemical's MSDS. Also, OSHA can provide lists of chemicals that indicate their relative toxicity and acceptable levels of employee exposures. This also involves an *action plan* (see Table 19-4) that is a determination of the levels of chemicals present in the workplace over a specific time and then the generation of an appropriate response.

One of the most effective ways to minimize employee exposure is to limit release and to dilute with air any emissions. Adequate ventilation must be provided. This may include fume hoods and other ventilation devices.

A central activity for compliance with the Laboratory Standard is the mandatory preparation of a chemical hygiene plan designed to minimize exposures. This should always be considered "as a work in progress." It should address all salient issues and be in writing.

CHEMICAL HYGIENE RESPONSIBILITIES

Every person working at a location is responsible for chemical hygiene. The chief executive officer is ultimately responsible; however, all employees must understand the Laboratory Standard and comply with its tenets.

One way to deal with the requirements is to appoint a *chemical hygiene officer* (see Table 19-4) who can serve as liaison between employees and management. Responsibilities include: 1) monitoring procurement, use, and disposal of laboratory chemicals; 2) maintaining lists of chemicals present; 3) being aware of current exposure limits for the chemicals present, and 4) working with management to continually improve the chemical hygiene plan.

The chemical hygiene officer in a dental office or clinic may also serve as laboratory supervisor. The responsibilities of this individual include: 1) assurance that workers know and follow chemical hygiene rules; 2) maintaining that proper PPE and other types of protective equipment are present and in working order; 3) performance of necessary inspections; 4) awareness of current legal requirements concerning regulated substances; 5) evaluation and selection of protective apparel and equipment; and 6) ensuring that the facility and the workers are prepared (usually through training) for the use of a new chemical.

Workers are responsible for planning and conducting each operation according to the office or clinic's chemical hygiene procedures. This usually involves a "safety-first" philosophy. Workers must comply with the tenets of the Laboratory Standard as presented in their facility's written plan.

LABORATORY FACILITIES

Laboratories should have an adequate general ventilation system. In some cases, special air exhaust equipment (e.g., ventilation hood) is needed. PPE is more commonly required. Proper air circulation is needed in all areas of the facility. It is best when handling hazardous chemicals that an eye-face wash fountain and a sink be readily available. It may be necessary that more than one fountain or sink be present. Each facility should also have a formal procedure for the disposal of waste chemicals.

To have the facility's ventilation, exposure control, and PPE materials functioning properly, significant attention must be paid to their maintenance, performance, and applicability. It may be necessary to have the equipment and materials checked by an outside sales and service company.

CHEMICAL HYGIENE PLAN

A Chemical Hygiene Plan is the central element for compliance with the Laboratory Standard. The Plan should be in writing and begins with a listing of the basic rules and procedures to be used in a facility (Table 19-5). Specific comments need to be made for chemical procurement, distribution, and storage. Disposal of chemicals must also be discussed.

Regular instrument monitoring is not usually required. However, such tests can help determine if a problem exists and what changes are needed.

Proper housekeeping, regular maintenance, and periodic inspections need to be performed. Clean floors and surfaces enhance safety. Inspections can identify needed maintenance. For example, eye-face wash fountains should be inspected every three months. Other pieces of equipment can also be inspected at regular intervals. Methods of egress and access to emergency equipment and utility controls in the event of an *emergency* (see Table 19-5) must be available. Passageways, stairways, and hallways must not be used as chemical storage areas.

Each office or clinic must be prepared to provide a medical program. This may involve regular surveillance. More commonly present is the need for first aid, which includes in-house and emergency room activities. Protective apparel and equipment needed include PPE that are compatible with the required degree of protection for the substances being handled, an eye-face wash fountain, fire extinguishers, respiratory protection (including dust), fire alarms, emergency phone numbers, and any other items chosen by the chemical hygiene officer.

Certain records need to be kept to be in compliance. A written record of all accidents must be retained. Because federal and state agencies differ on how long such records need to be kept, it is best to consider their storage as permanent. The office or clinic Plan should be regularly reviewed and when necessary changed. Chemical inventory and use records for hazardous chemicals should also be completed.

One of the most effective safety processes is the placement of signs and labels. Such items need to be posted prominently; there are four categories: 1) emergency telephone numbers (in-house and community rescue), 2) labels that show the contents of containers (including waste receptacles) and associated hazards, 3) location signs for eye-face wash fountains and other safety and first aid equipment and areas where food and beverage consumption and storage are permitted (e.g., refrigerators), and 4) warnings at locations where special or unusual hazards are present.

Accidents and spills should be uncommon events. However, planning and practice of the Plan should minimize employee exposure to harmful chemicals. The written Chemical Hygiene Plan must be communicated to each employee and provide procedures for evacuation, medical care, incident reporting, clean-up (spill control), and drill. Some type of alarm system is helpful. The purpose of a training program is to assure that all individuals at risk are adequately informed about working in the laboratory, its risks, and what to do if an accident occurs. This includes first aid and the use of special chemical abatement equipment.

Table 19-5 Components of a Chemical Hygiene Plan*

COMPONENT	REQUIRED ACTION
Basic rules and procedures	Put everything in writing
	List environmental preventive methods and procedures
	List personal protective equipment and uses
	Outline actions when confronting a spill, accident, or emergency
Chemical procurement, distribution, and storage	List procurement procedures
	Follow established processes concerning introduction of chemicals to a facility's collection
	Store chemicals properly
	Distribute chemicals throughout the facility safely
Environmental monitoring	Do not regularly monitor for chemicals
	Do monitor if required by regulatory agency or if a problem appears to exist
Housekeeping, maintenance, and inspections	Assure cleanliness
	Inspect equipment and safety materials on a regular basis
	Maintain safety items as per inspection or need
	Allow for easy egress and access to safety and emergency equipment and utility controls
Medical program	Provide safety and medical surveillance
	Discover potential exposure outcomes with proper authorities
	Provide necessary first aid
Protective apparel and equipment (PPE)	Provide environmental safety equipment such as fire extinguishers, fire alarms, and adequate ventilation
	Assure that PPE such as eye-face wash fountains, respirators and masks, and special clothing are readily available
	Prohibit eating, drinking, smoking, application of cosmetics, and the use of contact lenses in the presence of chemicals
Records	Maintain written records concerning all accidents
	Establish and maintain a list of all hazardous chemical present and their uses
	Keep any required medical records in accordance with federal state regulations
Signs and labels	Post emergency phone numbers
	Label properly all containers holding hazardous chemicals as to content, hazard, and methods/modes of protection
	Show through signage the locations of safety equipment and materials

*Adapted from OSHA (29 CRF Part 1450 - *Occupational Exposure to Hazardous Chemicals in Laboratories Standard* and Standard Appendices A and B).

Table 19-5 Components of a Chemical Hygiene Plan—cont'd

COMPONENT	REQUIRED ACTION
Spills and accidents	Assure that all employees are aware of the written plan and its tenets
	Plan for accidents, establish procedures
	Analyze the causes of all spills or accidents
Information and training programs	Provide information concerning chemical hazards present
	Train employees as to proper preventive measures
	Train employees concerning postexposure or accident procedures
Waste disposal programs	Identify methods that collect, segregate, and transport waste hazardous chemicals
	Follow federal/state mandates for disposal
	Regularly dispose of waste chemicals

A proper waste disposal system helps assure minimal harm to people, other organisms, and the environment from the disposal of waste laboratory chemicals. This includes collection, segregation, and transportation. An office or clinic must follow local regulations when disposing of chemicals. Waste should be regularly removed. Indiscriminate disposals by pouring down a drain or mixing of chemicals with other refuse and placement in landfills is unacceptable.

WORKING WITH CHEMICALS

A chemical hygiene plan requires workers to know and follow safety rules and procedures. Methods designed to avoid chemical contact must be regularly followed. In the event of an exposure, prompt action is necessary. Extended flushing of eyes with water (usually for 10 to 15 minutes) followed by medical attention is an example. Water rinsing and removal of soiled clothing helps minimize skin contact. Obviously, planning for accidents is essential. You must assume that exposures will occur and that an effective and efficient response is essential.

Preventive behaviors are also very helpful. Eating, smoking, drinking, gum chewing, and applying cosmetics in the presence of hazardous laboratory chemicals must be avoided. Segregation of chemicals from foodstuffs is imperative. It may be necessary to have two refrigerators, one for food and the other for chemicals. Some types of contact lenses will adsorb chemical vapors. Avoid the use of contacts unless necessary.

SAFETY RECOMMENDATIONS

Safety is a two-part equation–prevention and proper handling of accidents and emergencies. If precautions fail there will be increased chances of exposures. It is always better to work hard to prevent injuries, rather than manage exposures.

MATERIAL SAFETY DATA SHEETS

There are few more valuable safety constructs than material safety data sheets. These are written reports prepared by manufacturers or importers who describe an individual chemical or a group collection of chemicals. Valuable information concerns the chemicals present, the associated hazards, handling and clean-up procedures, and special PPE that need to be in place. See page 260 for a detailed discussion of MSDSs.

SELECTED READINGS

Indiana Department of Labor, Bureau of Safety Education and Training: *How to read and understand a material safety data sheet,* 1991, Indianapolis, Indiana, State of Indiana.

Indiana Department of Labor, Bureau of Safety Education and Training: *Guidelines for developing a written hazard communication program,* 1992, Indianapolis, Indiana, State of Indiana.

Meyer E.: *Chemistry of Hazardous Materials,* ed 2, 1989, Englewood Cliffs, New Jersey, Prentice Hall.

Miller CH, Palenik CJ: Infection control in dentistry. In Block S.: *Sterilization, Disinfection, Preservation and Sanitation,* ed 4, 1991, Philadelphia, Lea & Febiger.

Office of the Federal Register, National Archives and Records Administration. *CFR 29 Part 1900-1910.99,* Washington, DC, 1996, US Government Printing Office.

Palenik CJ, Miller CH: All about OSHA - Part I, *Dental Asepsis Review* 18(6):1-2, 1997.

U.S. Department of Labor, Occupational Health and Safety Administration: Hazard Communication Rule, 29 CFR 1910.1200, *Federal Standards and Interpretations* 806.15-806.31, 1991.

U.S. Department of Labor, Occupational Health and Safety Administration: Occupational Exposure to Bloodborne Pathogens; Final Rule, 29 CFR 1910.1030, *Fed Register* 56:64175-64182, 1991.

U.S. Department of Labor, Occupational Health and Safety Administration: Hazard Communication; Final Rule - 29 CFR 1910.1030, *Fed Register* 59:6126-6184, 1994.

U.S. Department of Labor, Occupational Health and Safety Administration. *Workplace fire safety* - Fact Sheet (No. OSHA 93-41), Washington, DC, 1993, U.S. Government Printing Office.

U.S. Department of Labor, Occupational Health and Safety Administration. *All about OSHA* (OSHA 2056), Washington, DC, 1995, U.S. Government Printing Office.

U.S. Department of Labor, Occupational Health and Safety Administration, (1997 - November 7), 1910.38:- *Employee emergency plans and fire prevention plans* (WWW document), URL *http://www.osha-slc.gov/OshStd_data/1910_0038.htm.*

U.S. Department of Labor, Occupational Safety and Health Administration. *Chemical Hazard Communication* (OSHA 3084). 1995, U.S. Printing Office, Washington, DC.

Chapter 20

EMPLOYEE FIRE PREVENTION AND EMERGENCY PLANS

Almost 100 million Americans are employed in various workplace environments. Twenty-seven years ago more than 14,000 workers died annually because of work-related accidents, almost 2.5 million workers had been disabled while working, and an estimated 300,000 new cases of occupational diseases and injuries occurred each year.

The effect of worker injuries in terms of lost productivity and wages, medical expenses, and disability compensation was enormous. Also immense was the amount of human suffering.

In response, Congress passed the Occupational Safety and Health Act (OSHA Act) of 1970. Its mission was ". . . to assure so far as possible every working man and woman in the Nation safe and healthful working conditions and to preserve our human resources." Under the Act, the Occupational Safety and Health Administration (OSHA) was created within the Department of Labor.

OSHA PURPOSES

OSHA was formed to serve several purposes, including: 1) encouragement of employers and employees to reduce workplace hazards and to implement new or existing safety programs, 2) provide research in occupational safety and health problems, 3) establish "separate but dependent responsibilities and rights" for employees and employers to help achieve better working conditions, 4) maintain a reporting and recordkeeping system to monitor injuries and illnesses, 5) establish training programs to increase competence of occupational safety and health personnel, 6) develop and enforce mandatory job safety and health standards, and 7) provide for the development, analysis, evaluation, and approval of state occupational safety and health programs.

COVERAGE OF THE ACT

The Act covers almost all employers and employees in the United States. Coverage is applied directly by federal OSHA or through an OSHA-approved state program (in 24 states plus Puerto Rico and the Virgin Islands). The Act does *not* cover self-employed persons, farms worked by family members, and working environments controlled by other federal agencies. In states and territories that have approved local plans for private sector occupational safety and health programs, there must also be a similar program for state and local government employees.

STANDARDS

OSHA performs its duties by promulgating legally enforceable standards. Standards may describe conditions or the use of practices, means, methods, or processes that are reasonably necessary and appropriate to protect employees on the job. Standards often are "performance standards" or "performance achievements." For example, eight-hour occupational exposure limits to many chemicals have been identified. The employer is challenged to assure that exposures are within the stated limits. This is the expected performance. The employer can use a combination of work practices, engineering controls, and personal protective equipment to achieve the goal. OSHA does not require specific equipment or processes, rather it reviews the outcome of the preventive efforts made by the employers and employees.

Employers must be aware of all standards applicable to their work environments, assure that employees are informed, knowledgeable, and participating in health and safety programs, and provide materials that accomplish the desired protection.

OSHA has produced many standards. However, when a specific standard does not exist for a situation, the OSHA General Duty Clause applies. The Clause states that employers ". . . shall furnish . . . a place of employment which is free from recognized hazards that are causing or are likely to cause death or serious physical harm to their employers." State plans must set standards that are at least as demanding as the federal standards.

Copies of standards can be obtained from several sources. The U.S. Government Printing Office in Washington sells print and electronic copies (202.512.1800). All formative stages of standards, as well as amendments, corrections, insertions, or deletions, appear in the *Federal Register*, which is available in larger libraries. Materials published in the *Federal Register* since 1995 can be obtained electronically *(http://www.access.gpo.gov/nara/index.html)*. The Office of the Federal Register annually publishes all current regulations and standards in the *Code for Federal Regulations* (CFR), which can be found in many libraries. OSHA regulations are collected in Title 29 of the CFR, Part 1900-1999. Information concerning OSHA regulations (various booklets and lists) can be ordered from the U.S. Department of Labor OSHA Publications, PO Box 37535, Washington, DC 20013-7535 (voice - 202.219.4667 or fax - 202.219.9266). Many can be downloaded from the OSHA website (state plans must be obtained directly from state agencies).

STANDARDS DEVELOPMENT

OSHA can begin the standard promulgation process on its own or in response to petitions from other parties, including other federal agencies, state and local organizations, industry self-regulating groups, employers, labor representatives, or any interested person.

If OSHA determines that a specific standard is needed, advisory committees are established. Some are ad hoc; others are standing federal committees. All such committees are composed of governmental workers plus members from management, labor, and local agencies. Recommendations may also come from NIOSH (National Institute for Occupational Safety and Health), which conducts research on safety and health issues and provides technical assistance to OSHA.

If OSHA wants to propose, amend, or revoke a standard, it publishes its intention in the

Federal Register as an "Advanced Notice of Proposed Rulemaking" or as a "Notice of Proposed Rulemaking." Advanced notices usually involve solicitation of information that can be used in drafting the proposal. Usually some time period (e.g., 30-60 days) is allowed for public response. Interested parties who submit written arguments and pertinent evidence may request a formal public hearing. If OSHA schedules one or more hearings, the times, dates, and locations are published in the *Federal Register*. A full report on the comment period and the public hearings, if conducted, and a full, final text version of the new (or amended) standard must be reported in the *Federal Register*. Accompanying the text is an explanation of the standard and a rationale for its implementation. Also, the date the standard becomes effective must be reported. OSHA must also publish if the determination resulted in the decision that no standard or amendment was needed.

Under certain conditions, OSHA can authorize an emergency temporary standard. Such standards become effective immediately and remain in effect until a permanent standard is enacted. OSHA must determine that workers are in grave danger and need immediate protection. Emergency standards are published in the *Federal Register* and serve as proposed permanent standards, which undergo the usual review process. Emergency and permanent standards may be challenged in court.

29 CFR PART 1910.38

OSHA has a safety plan that specifically addresses fire prevention and emergencies in general (Department of Labor, OSHA. 29 CFR Part 1910.38 - Employee emergency plans and fire prevention plans). The Standard is designed to support other OSHA standards that require written emergency action plans. The most important standards for dentistry include the Bloodborne Pathogens (Chapter 6), Hazard Communications (Chapter 19), and Safe Use of Chemicals in the Laboratory (Chapter 19) Standards.

The Standard has two major components: a fire prevention plan and emergency action plan. These plans are a combination of preventive actions and courses of action for anticipated emergencies.

FIRE PREVENTION PLANS

Workplace fire safety is very important. National Safety Council data indicate that workplace fires cause an average of $2.2 billion in losses each year. In 1991, 4,200 people in the U.S. perished in fires. Of these deaths, 327 occurred in the workplace. Fires and burns accounted for 3.3% of all occupational fatalities.

When OSHA conducts a workplace inspection, it monitors employee compliance with the Fire Safety Standard. OSHA also checks if the employer has provided adequate methods of egress, fire fighting equipment, and employee training to reduce (even to the point of prevention) deaths and injuries.

The best way to comply with the Fire Safety Standard is the generation and use of a written office/clinic plan. The written fire safety plan must include a minimum seven elements: a list of major workplace fire hazards; proper use, storage and disposal of potential ignition sources; types of fire protection equipment or systems present; names or regular job titles of persons responsible for equipment/systems maintenance; names or regular job titles of persons responsible for control of fuel source hazards; policing of flammable and combustible materials to minimize fire (housekeeping); and employee training.

An employer must review with each employee on initial assignment all parts of the fire safety plan that the employee must know to protect co-workers (and patients) in the event of an emergency. A written plan must be present in the work environment and made available for employee review. For work sites with less than ten employees, the plan may be communicated orally and the employer is not required to maintain a written plan. However, a written plan offers several advantages, including establishment of a formal office/clinic policy, plan implementation to be used in training and training updates, and more effective communication to employees of any changes in the plan.

Clinical dentistry does not pose the same risk for fire as do many other work environments. However, a fire emergency plan and a fire prevention plan must be established.

An emergency evacuation action plan must list the expected activities of each employee during a fire. This includes accounting for all employees to assure their escape. If some employees are physically impaired, special procedures will have to be developed. If employees must remain temporarily behind (e.g., to shut off utilities or close files), their actions must be fully described.

Employee notification of a problem must be part of the fire safety plan. An alarm system may be a voice communication or a sound signal such as bells, whistles, or horns. Employees must know the signal and help patients and co-workers vacate the premises.

Training is essential. Employees must first become knowledgeable about the plan, especially newly assigned employees. All employees are contacted if the plan is altered. Practicing employee responses helps to assure that the correct actions are taken.

Fire exits are essential for efficient vacating of a workplace. Each workplace must have at least two means of escape. The exits should be as distant from each other as possible. If fire doors are present, they must not be blocked or locked when employees are in the work area. Exit routes must be clearly marked and free of obstructions. Office/clinic signs must match those used in the rest of the building.

Each workplace must have a full complement of the proper types of extinguisher for the fire hazards present. Several large ABC-type extinguishers in a dental office/clinic should be adequate. The presence of portable fire extinguishers indicates that some employees will remain to fight small fires. Those expected or anticipated to use fire extinguishers must receive instruction concerning fire fighting and proper use of the equipment.

Only approved fire extinguishers should be used. They must be kept in good working order. It may be best to hire a fire protection company to estimate an office's/clinic's fire prevention needs and then to maintain and inspect the equipment. Fire suppression systems such as sprinklers could also be considered. These choices are the responsibility of the employer.

Employers need to develop a written fire prevention plan to complement the fire evacuation plan so as to minimize the frequency of evacuation. Fire prevention is always preferable to fire fighting. The employees must review such plans.

Fire prevention is assisted by proper housekeeping procedures for storage, use, and cleanup of flammable materials and proper disposal of flammable waste. Any source of heat, especially open flames must be monitored and controlled. This includes correct maintenance of equipment.

All employees must be knowledgeable of their office's/clinic's fire prevention and fire emergency plans. Again, it is the employer's responsibility to develop the plans and to assure that employees are trained.

EMPLOYEE EMERGENCY PLANS

Each office must generate escape procedures and designate escape routes for any emergency. An emergency plan can be incorporated into the written plans of an applicable standard, such as Hazard Communication Standard. Each employee must know and follow assigned duties and escape routes. In an emergency, some employees will be asked to remain to activate safety equipment or to perform critical operations (e.g., shut off utilities and machinery). Which employees will remain, what they will do, and when they must leave is situational and needs to be described well. During an emergency, an accounting of all employees is essential. The written emergency action plan must include a method to assure that all employees are outside the affected work areas. An established meeting place is one way to meet this requirement. In some situations, employees will perform rescue and medical duties . . . which employees and what actions need to be established. Each workplace must establish a method by which emergencies, including fires, are reported to the proper authorities. Also, official contacts must be determined. The names and titles of this cadre of employees are determined. They serve as contact individuals who can answer questions and provide further information.

An appropriate alarm system should be established for each workplace. With activation of the alarm, certain employee duties and evacuation plans are initiated. To properly implement the emergency action plan, employees must receive training about the types of emergencies that could occur and the written protocol of response activities, including emergency evacuations. Additional training is needed if employee responsibilities or designated areas are changed. Practicing emergency activities on a regular basis increases the probability that employees will respond properly if an actual emergency occurs.

An employer must review with each employee on initial assignment all parts of the emergency plan, or with all employees when the plan is changed. A written plan needs to be present in the work environment and made available for employee review. For work sites with less than ten employees, the plan may be communicated orally and the employer is not required to maintain a written plan. A written plan, however, is considered the superior communication method. It offers several advantages, including the establishment of a formal office policy, the ability to be used in training and training updates, and can be modified easily, with changes more effectively communicated to employees.

SELECTED READINGS

Office of the Federal Register, National Archives and Records Administration. *CFR 29 Part 1900-1910.99,* Washington, DC, 1996, US Government Printing Office.

Palenik CJ, Miller CH: All about OSHA – Part I, *Dental Asepsis Review* 18(6):1-2, 1997.

U.S. Department of Labor, Occupational Health and Safety Administration. *Workplace fire safety* - Fact Sheet No. OSHA 93-41, Washington, DC, 1993, U.S. Government Printing Office.

U.S. Department of Labor, Occupational Health and Safety Administration. *All about OSHA* (OSHA 2056), Washington, DC, 1995, U.S. Government Printing Office.

U.S. Department of Labor, Occupational Health and Safety Administration, (1997 – April 15), 1910.38 – *Employee emergency plans and fire prevention plans* (WWW document), URL *http://www.osha-slc.gov/OshStd_data/1910_0038.htm.*

INFECTION CONTROL AND HAZARDOUS MATERIALS MANAGEMENT RESOURCE LIST

DENTAL-RELATED ORGANIZATIONS

American Dental Association (ADA)
211 E. Chicago Avenue Chicago, IL 60611
(800) 621-8091
Recommendations, manuals, videotapes, brochures, ADA-News journal

American Dental Assistants Association (ADAA)
203 N. LaSalle Street, Suite 1320
Chicago, IL 60601
541-1550
Member support services, journal

American Dental Hygienists Association (ADHA)
444 N. Michigan Avenue, Suite 3400
Chicago, IL 60611
440-8900
Member support services, journal

Dental Assisting National Board, Inc. (DANB)
216 E. Ontario Street
Chicago, IL 60611
(312) 642-3368
Infection Control
Examination (ICE)

INFECTION CONTROL ORGANIZATIONS

Office Safety and Asepsis Procedures Research Foundation (OSAP)
P.O. Box 6297
Annapolis, MD
(800) 298-OSAP
Educational conferences, recommendations, books, brochures, documents, audio tapes, newsletter, member support services

Association for the Advancement of Medical Instrumentation (AAMI)
(Sterilization Standards Committee)
3330 Washington Blvd., Suite 400
Arlington, VA 22201
(703) 525-4890
Standards and recommended monitors, packaging material practices for use of sterilizers, decontamination procedures

FEDERAL AGENCIES

Centers for Disease Control and Prevention (CDC)
Atlanta, GA 30333
(404) 488-4450
AIDS information, recommendations, and disease updates.

(Oral Health Program)
4770 Buffered Highway MS F-10
Chamblee, CA
(770) 488-3034
Voice information service on infection control in dentistry: (404) 332-4552

Environmental Protection Agency (EPA)
401 M Street SW
[Waste Hotline: (800) 424-9364]
[Germicides: (800) 858-7370]
Registration of germicides, solid waste management, water quality

Food and Drug Administration (FDA)
5600 Fishers Lane
Rockville, MD 20857
[Devices/Radiological Health: (800) 638-2041]
[Drug Evaluation Research: (301) 295-8000]
Regulates manufacturing and labeling of medical devices and accessories, handwashing agents, mouthrinses, drugs, food

Occupational Safety and Health Administration
(OSHA) U.S. Department of Labor
200 Constitution Avenue Washington, DC 20210
523-8151
Bloodborne pathogens standard and hazard communications standard

Regional OSHA Offices (States Without OSHA-Approved Programs Are Listed)

  I. Boston (617) 565-7164
    Massachusetts, Maine, New Hampshire, Rhode Island
  II. New York (212) 337-2378
    New Jersey, New York, Puerto Rico

III. Philadelphia (215) 596-1201
District of Columbia, Delaware, Pennsylvania, West Virginia
IV. Atlanta (404) 347-3573
Alabama, Florida, Georgia, Mississippi
V. Chicago (312) 353-2220
Illinois, Ohio, Wisconsin
VI. Dallas (214) 767-4731
Arkansas, Louisiana, Oklahoma, Texas
VII. Kansas City (816) 426-5861
Kansas, Missouri, Nebraska
VIII. Denver (303) 844-3061
Colorado, Montana, North Dakota, South Dakota
IX. San Francisco (415) 744-6670
American Samoa, Guam, Trust Territories of the Pacific
X. Seattle (206) 553-5930
Idaho

States with OSHA Approved Programs

Alaska: Juneau (907) 465-2700
Arizona: Phoenix (602) 542-5795
California: San Francisco (415) 703-4590
Connecticut: Wethersfield (203) 566-5123
Hawaii: Honolulu (808) 548-3150
Indiana: Indianapolis (317) 232-2665
Iowa: Des Moines (515) 281-3447
Kentucky: Frankfort (502) 564-3070
Maryland: Baltimore (301) 333-4179
Michigan: Lansing (517) 373-9600
Minnesota: St. Paul (612) 296-2342
Nevada: Carson City (702) 687-3032
New Mexico: Santa Fe (505) 827-2850
New York: Albany (518) 457-2741
North Carolina: Raleigh (919) 733-7166
Oregon: Salem (503) 378-3272
Puerto Rico: Hato Rey (809) 754-2119
South Carolina: Columbia (803) 734-9594
Tennessee: Nashville (615) 741-2582
Utah: Salt Lake City (801) 530-6900
Vermont: Montpelier (802) 828-2765
Virgin Islands: St. Croix (809) 773-1994
Virginia: Richmond (804) 786-2376
Washington: Olympia (206) 753-6307
Wyoming: Cheyenne (307) 777-7786

CDC INFECTION CONTROL GUIDELINES FOR DENTISTRY

The following CDC staff members contributed to this document:

Coordinators

Jennifer L. Cleveland, D.D.S., M.P.H.
Surveillance, Investigations, and Research Branch
Division of Oral Health
National Center for Prevention Services
Walter W. Bond, M.S.
Hospital Infections Program
National Center for Infectious Diseases

Contributors

Barbara F. Gooch, D.M.D., M.P.H.
Dolores M. Malvitz, Dr. P.H.
Donald W. Marianos, D.D.S., M.P.H.
Chester J. Summers, D.D.S., Dr. P.H., M.S.
Division of Oral Health
National Center for Prevention Services
Linda S. Martin, Ph.D.
HIV Activity
Office of the Director
National Institute for Occupational Safety and Health

This document updates previously published CDC recommendations for infection-control practices in dentistry to reflect new data, materials, technology, and equipment. When implemented, these recommendations should reduce the risk of disease transmission in the dental environment, from patient to dental health-care worker (DHCW), from DHCW to patient, and from patient to patient. Based on principles of infection control, the document delineates specific recommendations related to vaccination of DHCWs; protective attire and barrier techniques; handwashing and care of hands; the use and care of sharp instruments and needles; sterilization or disinfection of instruments; cleaning and disinfection of the dental unit and environmental surfaces; disinfection and the dental laboratory; use and care of handpieces, antiretraction valves, and other intraoral dental devices attached to air and water lines of dental units; single-use disposable instruments; the handling of biopsy specimens; use of extracted teeth in dental educational settings; disposal of waste materials; and implementation of recommendations.

Reprinted from: Centers for Disease Control and Prevention. Recommended infection control practices for dentistry, 1993. *Morbidity Mortality Weekly Report (MMWR)* 41 (No. RR-8): 1-12, May 28, 1993.

This document updates previously published CDC recommendations for infection-control practices for dentistry[1-3] and offers guidance for reducing the risks of disease transmission among dental health-care workers (DHCWs) and their patients. Although the principles of infection control remain unchanged, new technologies, materials, equipment, and data require continuous evaluation of current infection control practices. The unique nature of most dental procedures, instrumentation, and patient care settings also may require specific strategies directed to the prevention of transmission of pathogens among DHCWs and their patients. Recommended infection control practices are applicable to all settings in which dental treatment is provided. These recommended practices should be observed in addition to the practices and procedures for worker protection required by the Occupational Safety and Health Administration (OSHA) final rule on Occupational Exposure to Bloodborne Pathogens (29 CFR 1910.1030), which was published in the *Federal Register* on December 6, 1991.[4]

Dental patients and DHCWs may be exposed to a variety of microorganisms via blood or oral or respiratory secretions. These microorganisms may include cytomegalovirus, hep-atitis B virus (HBV), hepatitis C virus (HCV), herpes simplex virus types 1 and 2, human immunodeficiency virus (HIV), *Mycobacterium tuberculosis,* staphylococci, streptococci, and other viruses and bacteria—specifically, those that infect the upper respiratory tract. Infections may be transmitted in the dental operatory through several routes, including direct contact with blood, oral fluids, or other secretions; indirect contact with contaminated instruments, operatory equipment, or environmental surfaces; or contact with airborne contaminants in droplets, spatter, or aerosols of oral and respiratory fluids. Infection via any of these routes requires that all three of the following conditions be present (commonly referred to as "the chain of infection"): a susceptible host, a pathogen with sufficient infectivity and numbers to cause infection, and a portal through which the pathogen may enter the host. Effective infection-control strategies will break one or more of these "links" in the chain, thereby preventing infection.

A set of infection control strategies common to all health-care delivery settings should reduce the risk of transmission of infectious diseases caused by bloodborne pathogens such as HBV and HIV.[2,5-10] Because all infected patients cannot be identified by medical history, physical examination, or laboratory tests, CDC recommends that blood and body fluid precautions be used consistently for all patients.[2,5] This extension of blood and body fluid precautions, referred to as "universal precautions," must be observed routinely in the care of all dental patients.[2] In addition, specific actions are recommended to reduce the risk of tuberculosis transmission in dental and other ambulatory health-care facilities.[11]

CONFIRMED TRANSMISSION OF HBV AND HIV IN DENTISTRY

Although the possibility of transmission of bloodborne infections from DHCWs to patients is considered to be small,[12-15] precise risks have not been quantified in the dental setting by carefully designed epidemiologic studies. Reports published from 1970 through 1987 indicate nine clusters in which patients were infected with HBV associated with treatment by an infected DHCW.[16-25] In addition, transmission of HIV to six patients of a dentist with acquired immunodeficiency syndrome has been reported.[26,27] Transmission of HBV from dentists to patients has not been reported since 1987, possibly reflecting such factors as incomplete ascertainment and reporting, increased adherence to universal precautions—including routine glove use by dentists—and increased levels of immunity due to use of hepatitis B vaccine. However, isolated sporadic cases of infection are more difficult to link with a health-care worker than are outbreaks involving multiple patients. For HBV and HIV, the precise event or events resulting in transmission of infection in the dental setting have not been determined; epidemiologic and laboratory data indicate that these infections probably were transmitted from the DHCWs to patients, rather than from one patient to another.[26,28] Patient-to-patient transmission of bloodborne pathogens has been reported, however, in several medical settings.[29-31]

VACCINES FOR DENTAL HEALTH-CARE WORKERS

Although HBV infection is uncommon among adults in the United States (1%-2%), sero-logic surveys indicate that 10% to 30% of health-care or dental workers show evidence of past or present HBV infection.[6,32] The OSHA bloodborne pathogens final rule requires that employers make hepatitis B vaccinations available without cost to their employees who may be exposed to blood or other infectious materials.[4] In addition, CDC recommends that all workers, including DHCWs, who might be exposed to blood or blood-contaminated substances in an occupational setting be vaccinated for HBV.[6-8] DHCWs also are at risk for exposure to and possible transmission of other vaccine-preventable diseases[33]; accordingly, vaccination against influenza, measles, mumps, rubella, and tetanus may be appropriate for DHCWs.

PROTECTIVE ATTIRE AND BARRIER TECHNIQUES

For protection of personnel and patients in dental care settings, medical gloves (latex or vinyl) always must be worn by DHCWs when there is potential for contacting blood, blood-contaminated saliva, or mucous membranes.[1,2,4-6] Nonsterile gloves are appropriate for examinations and other nonsurgical procedures[5]; sterile gloves should be used for surgical procedures. Before treatment of each patient, DHCWs should wash their hands and put on new gloves; after treatment of each patient or before leaving the dental operatory, DHCWs should remove and discard gloves, then wash their hands. DHCWs always should wash their hands and reglove between patients. Surgical or examination gloves should not be washed before use; nor should they be washed, disinfected, or sterilized for reuse. Washing of gloves may cause "wicking" (penetration of liquids through undetected holes in the gloves) and is not recommended.[5] Deterioration of gloves may be caused by disinfecting agents, oils, certain oil-based lotions, and heat treatments, such as autoclaving.

Chin-length plastic face shields or surgical masks and protective eyewear should be worn when splashing or spattering of blood or other body fluids is likely, as is common in dentistry.[2,5,6,34,35] When a mask is used, it should be changed between patients or during patient treatment if it becomes wet or moist. Face shields or protective eyewear should be washed with an appropriate cleaning agent and, when visibly soiled, disinfected between patients.

Protective clothing such as reusable or disposable gowns, laboratory coats, or uniforms should be worn when clothing is likely to be soiled with blood or other body fluids. Reusable protective clothing should be washed using a normal laundry cycle, according to the instructions of detergent and machine manufacturers. Protective clothing should be changed at least daily or as soon as it becomes visibly soiled. Protective garments and devices (including gloves, masks, and eye and face protection) should be removed before personnel exit areas of the dental office used for laboratory or patient care activities.

Impervious-backed paper, aluminum foil, or plastic covers should be used to protect items and surfaces (e.g., light handles or x-ray unit heads) that may become contaminated by blood or saliva during use and that are difficult or impossible to clean and disinfect. Between patients, the coverings should be removed (while DHCWs are gloved), discarded, and replaced (after ungloving and washing of hands) with clean material.

Appropriate use of rubber dams, high-velocity air evacuation, and proper patient positioning should minimize the formation of droplets, spatter, and aerosols during patient treatment. In addition, splash shields should be used in the dental laboratory.

HANDWASHING AND CARE OF HANDS

DHCWs should wash their hands before and after treating each patient (i.e., before glove placement and after glove removal) and after barehand touching of inanimate objects likely to be contaminated by blood, saliva, or respiratory secretions.[2,5,6,9] Hands should be washed after removal of gloves because gloves may become perforated during use, and DHCW hands may become contaminated through contact with patient material. Soap and water will remove transient microorganisms acquired directly or indirectly from patient contact[9]; therefore for many routine dental procedures such as examinations and nonsurgical techniques, handwashing with plain soap is adequate. For surgical procedures, an antimicrobial surgical handscrub should be used.[10]

When gloves are torn, cut, or punctured, they should be removed as soon as patient safety permits. DHCWs then should wash their hands thoroughly and reglove to complete the dental procedure. DHCWs who have exudative lesions or weeping dermatitis, particularly on the hands, should refrain from all direct patient care and from handling dental patient care equipment until the condition resolves.[12] Guidelines addressing management of occupational exposures to blood and other fluids to which universal precautions apply have been published previously.[6-8,36]

USE AND CARE OF SHARP INSTRUMENTS AND NEEDLES

Sharp items (e.g., needles, scalpel blades, wires) contaminated with patient blood and saliva should be considered potentially infective and handled with care to prevent injuries.[2,5,6]

Used needles should never be recapped or otherwise manipulated using both hands or any other technique that involves directing the point of a needle toward any part of the body.[2,5,6] A one-handed "scoop" technique or a mechanical device designed for holding the needle sheath should be employed. Used disposable syringes and needles, scalpel blades, and other sharp items should be placed in appropriate puncture-resistant containers located as close as is practical to the area in which the items were used.[2,5,6] Bending or breaking of needles before disposal requires unnecessary manipulation and thus is not recommended.

Before attempting to remove needles from nondisposable aspirating syringes, DHCWs should recap them to prevent injuries. Either of the two acceptable techniques may be used. For procedures involving multiple injections with a single needle, the unsheathed needle should be placed in a location where it will not become contaminated or contribute to unintentional needlesticks between injections. If the decision is made to recap a needle between injections, a one-handed "scoop" technique or a mechanical device designed to hold the needle sheath is recommended.

STERILIZATION OR DISINFECTION OF INSTRUMENTS

Indications for Sterilization or Disinfection of Dental Instruments

As with other medical and surgical instruments, dental instruments are classified into three categories—critical, semicritical, or noncritical—depending on their risk of transmitting infection and the need to sterilize them between uses.[9,37-40] Each dental practice should classify all instruments as follows:

1. **Critical.**   Surgical and other instruments used to *penetrate soft tissue or bone* are classified as critical and should be sterilized after each use. These devices include forceps, scalpels, bone chisels, scalers, and burs.
2. **Semicritical.**   Instruments such as mirrors and amalgam condensers that *do not penetrate soft tissues or bone but contact oral tissues* are classified as semicritical. These devices should be sterilized after each use. If, however, sterilization is not feasible because the instrument will be damaged by heat, the instrument should receive, at a minimum, high-level disinfection.
3. **Noncritical.**   Instruments or medical devices such as external components of x-ray heads that *come into contact only with intact skin* are classified as noncritical. Because these noncritical surfaces have a relatively low risk of transmitting infection, they may be reprocessed between patients with intermediate-level or low-level disinfection (see Cleaning and Disinfection of Dental Unit and Environmental Surfaces) or detergent and water washing, depending on the nature of the surface and the degree and nature of the contamination.[9,38]

Methods of Sterilization or Disinfection of Dental Instruments

Before sterilization or high-level disinfection, instruments should be cleaned thoroughly to remove debris. Persons involved in cleaning and reprocessing instruments should wear heavy-duty (reusable utility) gloves to lessen the risk of hand injuries. Placing instruments into a container of water or disinfectant/detergent as soon as possible after use will prevent drying of patient material and make cleaning easier and more efficient. Cleaning may be accomplished by thoroughly scrubbing with soap and water or a detergent solution, or with a mechanical device (e.g., an ultrasonic cleaner). The use of covered ultrasonic cleaners, when possible, is recommended to increase efficiency of cleaning and to reduce handling of sharp instruments.

All critical and semicritical dental instruments that are heat stable should be sterilized routinely between uses by steam under pressure (autoclaving), dry heat, or chemical vapor, following the instructions of the manufacturers of the instruments and the sterilizers. Critical and semicritical instruments that will not be used immediately should be packaged before sterilization.

Proper functioning of sterilization cycles should be verified by the periodic use (at least weekly) of biologic indicators (i.e., spore tests).[3,9] Heat-sensitive chemical indicators (e.g., those that change color after exposure to heat) alone do not ensure adequacy of a sterilization cycle but may be used on the outside of each pack to identify packs that have been processed through the heating cycle. A simple and inexpensive method to confirm heat penetration to all instruments during each cycle is the use of a chemical indicator inside and in the center of either a load of unwrapped instruments or in each multiple instrument pack[41]; this procedure is recommended for use in all dental practices. Instructions provided by the manufacturers of medical/dental instruments and sterilization devices should be followed closely.

In all dental and other health care settings, indications for the use of liquid chemical germicides to sterilize instruments (i.e., "cold sterilization") are limited. For heat sensitive instruments, this procedure may require up to 10 hours of exposure to a liquid chemical agent registered with the U.S. Environmental Protection Agency (EPA) as a "sterilant/ disinfectant." This sterilization process should be followed by aseptic rinsing with sterile water, drying, and, if the instrument is not used immediately, placement in a sterile container.

EPA-registered "sterilant/disinfectant" chemicals are used to attain high-level disinfection of heat-sensitive semicritical medical and dental instruments. The product manufacturers' directions regarding appropriate concentration and exposure time should be followed closely. The EPA classification of the liquid chemical agent (i.e., "sterilant/ disinfectant") will be shown on the chemical label. Liquid chemical agents that are less potent than the "sterilant/disinfectant" category are *not* appropriate for reprocessing critical or semicritical dental instruments.

CLEANING AND DISINFECTION OF DENTAL UNIT AND ENVIRONMENTAL SURFACES

After treatment of each patient and at the completion of daily work activities, countertops and dental unit surfaces that may have become contaminated with patient material should be cleaned with disposable toweling, using an appropriate cleaning agent and water as necessary. Surfaces then should be disinfected with a suitable chemical germicide.

A chemical germicide registered with the EPA as a "hospital disinfectant" and labeled for "tuberculocidal" (i.e., mycobactericidal) activity is recommended for disinfecting surfaces that have been soiled with patient material. These intermediate-level disinfectants include phenolics, iodophors, and chlorine-containing compounds. Because mycobacteria are among the most resistant groups of microorganisms, germicides effective against mycobacteria should be effective against many other bacterial and viral pathogens.[9,38-40,42] A fresh solution of sodium hypochlorite (household bleach) prepared daily is an inexpensive and effective intermediate-level germicide. Concentrations ranging from 500 to 800 ppm of chlorine (a 1:100 dilution of bleach and tap water of **3** cups of bleach to **1** gallon of water) are effective on environmental surfaces that have been cleaned of visible contamination. Caution should be exercised, since chlorine solutions are corrosive to metals, especially aluminum.

Low-level disinfectants—EPA-registered "hospital disinfectants" that are not labeled for "tuberculocidal" activity (e.g., quaternary ammonium compounds)—are appropriate for general housekeeping purposes such as cleaning floors, walls, and other surfaces. Intermediate- and low-level disinfectants are *not* recommended for reprocessing critical or semicritical dental instruments.

DISINFECTION AND THE DENTAL LABORATORY

Laboratory materials and other items that have been used in the mouth (e.g., impressions, bite registrations, fixed and removable prostheses, orthodontic appliances) should be cleaned and disinfected before being manipulated in the laboratory, whether an on-site or remote location.[43] These items also should be cleaned and disinfected after being manipulated in the dental laboratory and before placement in the patient's mouth.[2] Because of the increasing variety of dental materials used intraorally, DHCWs are advised to consult with manufacturers regarding the stability of specific materials relative to disinfection procedures. A chemical germicide having at least an intermediate level of activity (i.e., "tuberculocidal hospital disinfectant") is appropriate for such disinfection. Communication between dental office and dental laboratory personnel regarding the handling and decontamination of supplies and materials is important.

USE AND CARE OF HANDPIECES, ANTIRETRACTION VALVES, AND OTHER INTRAORAL DENTAL DEVICES ATTACHED TO AIR AND WATER LINES OF DENTAL UNITS

Routine between-patient use of a heating process capable of sterilization (i.e., steam under pressure [autoclaving], dry heat, or heat/chemical vapor) is recommended for all high-speed dental handpieces, low-speed handpiece components used intraorally, and reusable prophylaxis angles. Manufacturer instructions for cleaning, lubrication, and sterilization procedures should be followed closely to ensure effectiveness of the sterilization process and longevity of these instruments. According to manufacturers, virtually all high-speed and low-speed handpieces in production today are heat tolerant, and most heat-sensitive models manufactured earlier can be retrofitted with heat-stable components.

Internal surfaces of high-speed handpieces, low-speed handpiece components, and prophylaxis angles may become contaminated with patient material during use. This retained patient material then may be expelled intraorally during subsequent uses.[44-46] Restricted physical access—particularly to internal surfaces of these instruments—limits cleaning and disinfection or sterilization with liquid chemical germicides. Surface disinfection by wiping or soaking in liquid chemical germicides is *not* an acceptable method for reprocessing high-speed handpieces, low-speed handpiece components used intraorally, or reusable prophylaxis angles.

Because retraction valves in dental unit water lines may cause aspiration of patient material back into the handpiece and water lines, antiretraction valves (one-way flow check valves) should be installed to prevent fluid aspiration and to reduce the risk of transfer of potentially infective material.[47] Routine maintenance of antiretraction valves is necessary to ensure effectiveness; the dental unit manufacturer should be consulted to establish an appropriate maintenance routine.

High-speed handpieces should be run to discharge water and air for a minimum of 20 to 30 seconds after use on each patient. This procedure is intended to aid in physically flushing out patient material that may have entered the turbine and air or water lines.[46] Use of an enclosed container or high-velocity evacuation should be considered to minimize the spread of spray, spatter, and aerosols generated during discharge procedures. Additionally, there is evidence that overnight or weekend microbial accumulation in water lines can be reduced substantially by removing the handpiece and allowing water lines to run, and to discharge water for several minutes at the beginning of each clinic day.[48] Sterile saline or sterile water should be used as a coolant/irrigator when surgical procedures involving the cutting of bone are performed.

Other reusable intraoral instruments attached to, but removable from, the dental unit air or water lines such as ultrasonic scaler tips and component parts and air/water syringe tips should be cleaned and sterilized after treatment of each patient in the same manner as handpieces, which was described previously. Manufacturer directions for re-processing should be followed to ensure effectiveness of the process and longevity of the instruments.

Some dental instruments have components that are heat sensitive or are permanently attached to dental unit water lines. Some items may not enter the patient's oral cavity, but are likely to become contaminated with oral fluids during treatment procedures, including, for example, handles or dental unit attachments of saliva ejectors, high-speed air evacuators, and air/water syringes. These components should be covered with impervious barriers that are changed after each use or, if the surface permits, carefully cleaned and then treated with a chemical germicide having at least an intermediate level of activity. As with high-speed dental handpieces, water lines to all instruments should be flushed thoroughly after the treatment of each patient; flushing at the beginning of each clinic day is recommended.

SINGLE-USE DISPOSABLE INSTRUMENTS

Single-use disposable instruments (e.g., prophylaxis angles; prophylaxis cups and brushes; tips for high-speed air evacuators, saliva ejectors, and air/water syringes) should be used for one patient only and discarded appropriately. These items are not designed nor intended to be cleaned, disinfected, or sterilized for reuse.

HANDLING OF BIOPSY SPECIMENS

In general, each biopsy should be put in a sturdy container with a secure lid to prevent leakage during transport. Care should be taken when collecting specimens to avoid contamination of the outside of the container. If the outside of the container is visibly contaminated, it should be cleaned and disinfected or placed in an impervious bag.[49]

USE OF EXTRACTED TEETH IN DENTAL EDUCATION SETTINGS

Extracted teeth used for the education of DHCWs should be considered infective and classified as clinical specimens because they contain blood. All persons who collect, transport, or manipulate extracted teeth should handle them with the same precautions as a specimen for biopsy.[2] Universal precautions should be adhered to whenever extracted teeth are handled; because preclinical educational exercises simulate clinical experiences, students enrolled in dental education programs should adhere to universal precautions in preclinical and clinical settings. In addition, all persons who handle extracted teeth in dental education settings should receive hepatitis B vaccine.[6-8]

Before extracted teeth are manipulated in dental educational exercises, the teeth first should be cleaned of adherent patient material by scrubbing with detergent and water or by using an ultrasonic cleaner. Teeth should then be stored, immersed in a fresh solution of sodium hypochlorite (household bleach diluted 1:10 with tap water) or any liquid chemical germicide suitable for clinical specimen fixation.[50]

Persons handling extracted teeth should wear gloves. Gloves should be disposed of properly and hands washed after completion of work activities. Additional personal protective equipment (e.g., face shield or surgical mask and protective eyewear) should be worn if mucous membrane contact with debris or spatter is anticipated when the specimen is handled, cleaned, or manipulated. Work surfaces and equipment should be cleaned and decontaminated with an appropriate liquid chemical germicide after completion of work activities.[37,38,40,51]

The handling of extracted teeth used in dental education settings differs from giving patients their own extracted teeth. Several states allow patients to keep such teeth, because these teeth are not considered regulated (pathologic) waste[52] or because the removed body part (tooth) becomes the property of the patient and does not enter the waste system.[53]

DISPOSAL OF WASTE MATERIALS

Blood, suctioned fluids, or other liquid waste may be poured carefully into a drain connected to a sanitary sewer system. Disposable needles, scalpels, or other sharp items should be placed intact into puncture resistant containers before disposal. Solid waste contaminated with blood or other body fluids should be placed in sealed, sturdy impervious bags to prevent leakage of the contained items. All contained solid waste should then be disposed of according to requirements established by local, state, or federal environmental regulatory agencies and published recommendations.[9,49]

IMPLEMENTATION OF RECOMMENDED INFECTION CONTROL PRACTICES FOR DENTISTRY

Emphasis should be placed on consistent adherence to recommended infection control strategies, including the use of protective barriers and appropriate methods of sterilizing or disinfecting instruments and environmental surfaces. Each dental facility should develop a written protocol for instrument reprocessing, operatory cleanup, and management of injuries.[3] Training of all DHCWs in proper infection control practices should begin in professional and vocational schools and be updated with continuing education.

ADDITIONAL NEEDS IN DENTISTRY

Additional information is needed for accurate assessment of factors that may increase the risk for transmission of bloodborne pathogens and other infectious agents in a dental setting. Studies should address the nature, frequency, and circumstances of occupational exposures. Such information may lead to the development and evaluation of improved designs for dental instruments, equipment, and personal protective devices. In addition, more efficient reprocessing techniques should be considered in the design of future dental instruments and equipment. Efforts to protect patients and DHCWs should include improved surveillance, risk assessment, evaluation of measures to prevent exposure, and studies of postexposure prophylaxis. Such efforts may lead to development of safer and more effective medical devices, work practices, and personal protective equipment that are acceptable to DHCWs, are practical and economical, and do not adversely affect patient care.[54,55]

REFERENCES

1. CDC. Recommended infection-control practices for dentistry, *MMWR* 35:237–42, 1986.
2. CDC. Recommendations for prevention of HIV in health-care settings, *MMWR* 36:(No. 2S), 1987.

3. U.S. Department of Health and Human Services. Infection control file: practical infection control in the dental office, Atlanta, Georgia/Rockville, Maryland: CDC/FDA, 1989. (Available through the U.S. Government Printing Office, Washington, DC, or the National Technical Information Services, Springfield, Virginia).

4. Department of Labor, Occupational Safety and Health Administration, 29 CFR Part 1910.1030, occupational exposure to bloodborne pathogens; final rule, *Federal Register* 56(235):64004-182, 1991.

5. CDC. Update: universal precautions for prevention of transmission of human immunodeficiency virus, hepatitis B virus, and other bloodborne pathogens in health-care settings, *MMWR* 37:377-82, 387-8, 1988.

6. CDC. Guidelines for prevention of transmission of human immunodeficiency virus and hepatitis B virus to health-care and public-safety workers. *MMWR* 38(suppl. No. S-6):1-37, 1989.

7. CDC. Protection against viral hepatitis: recommendations of the Immunization Practices Advisory Committee (ACIP), *MMWR* 39(No. RR-2), 1990.

8. CDC. Hepatitis B virus: a comprehensive strategy for eliminating transmission in the United States through universal childhood vaccination, *MMWR* 40(No. RR-13), 1991.

9. Garner JS, Favero MS: Guideline for handwashing and hospital environmental control, 1985, Atlanta: CDC, publication no. 99-1117, 1985

10. Garner JS. Guideline for prevention of surgical wound infections, 1985. Atlanta: CDC publication no. 99-2381, 1985.

11. CDC. Guidelines for preventing the transmission of tuberculosis in health-care settings, with special focus on HIV-related issues, *MMWR* 39(No. RR-17), 1990.

12. CDC. Recommendations for preventing transmission of human immunodeficiency virus and hepatitis B virus during exposure-prone invasive procedures, *MMWR* 40(No. RR-8), 1990.

13. CDC. Update: investigations of patients who have been treated by HIV-infected health-care workers, *MMWR* 41:344-6, 1992.

14. Chamberland ME, Bell DM: HIV transmission from health care worker to patient: what is the risk? *Ann Intern Med* 116:871-3, 1992.

15. Siew C, Chang B, Gruninger SE, Verrusio AC, Neidle EA: Self-reported percutaneous injuries in dentists: implications for HBV, HIV transmission risk, *J Am Dent Assoc* 123:37-44, 1992.

16. Ahtone J, Goodman RA: Hepatitis B and dental personnel: transmission to patients and prevention issues, *J Am Dent Assoc* 106:219-22, 1983.

17. Hadler SC, Sorley DL, Acree KH et al.: An outbreak of hepatitis B in a dental practice, *Ann Intern Med* 5:133-8, 1981.

18. CDC. Hepatitis B among dental patients—Indiana, *MMWR* 34:73-5, 1985.

19. Levin ML, Maddrey WC, Wands JR et al.: Hepatitis B transmission by dentists, *JAMA* 228:1139-40, 1974.

20. Rimland D, Parkin WE, Miller GB et al.: Hepatitis B outbreak traced to an oral surgeon, *N Engl J Med* 296:953-8, 1977.

21. Goodwin D, Fannin SL, McCracken BB: An oral surgeon-related hepatitis B outbreak, *Calif Morbid* 14, 1976.

22. Reingold AL, Kane MA, Murphy EL et al.: Transmission of hepatitis B by an oral surgeon, *J Infect Dis* 145:262-8, 1982.

23. Goodman RA, Ahtone JL, Finton RJ: Hepatitis B transmission from dental personnel to patients: unfinished business, *Ann Intern Med* 96:119, 1982.

24. Shaw FE, Barrett CL, Hamm R et al.: Lethal outbreak of hepatitis B in a dental practice, *JAMA* 255:3261-4, 1986.

25. CDC. Outbreak of hepatitis B associated with an oral surgeon, New Hampshire, *MMWR* 36:132-3, 1987.
26. Ciesielski C, Marianos D, Chin-Yih OU et al.: Transmission of human immunodeficiency virus in a dental practice, *Ann Intern Med* 116:798-805, 1992.
27. CDC. Investigations of patients who have been treated by HIV-infected health-care workers—United States, *MMWR* 42:329-31, 337, 1993.
28. Gooch B, Marianos D, Ciesielski C et al.: Lack of evidence for patient-to-patient transmission of HIV in a dental practice, *J Am Dent Assoc* 124:38-44, 1993.
29. Canter J, Mackey K, Good LS et al.: An outbreak of hepatitis B associated with jet injections in a weight reduction clinic, *Arch Intern Med* 150:1923-7, 1990.
30. Kent GP, Brondum J, Keenlyside RA, LaFazia LM, Scott HD: A large outbreak of acupuncture-associated hepatitis B, *Am J Epidemiol* 127:591-8, 1988.
31. Polish LB, Shapiro CN, Bauer F et al.: Nosocomial transmission of hepatitis B virus associated with the use of a spring-loaded finger-stick device, *N Engl J Med* 326:721-5, 1992.
32. Siew C, Gruninger SE, Mitchell EW, Burrell KH: Survey of hepatitis B exposure and vaccination in volunteer dentists, *J Am Dent Assoc* 114:457-9, 1987.
33. CDC. Immunization recommendations for health-care workers, Atlanta, Georgia, CDC, Division of Immunization, Center for Prevention Services, 1989.
34. Petersen NJ, Bond WW, Favero MS: Air sampling for hepatitis B surface antigen in a dental operatory, *J Am Dent Assoc* 99:465-7, 1979.
35. Bond WW, Petersen NJ, Favero MS, Ebert JW, Maynard JE: Transmission of type B viral hepatitis B via eye inoculation of a chimpanzee, *J Clin Microbiol* 15:533-4, 1982.
36. CDC. Public Health Service statement on management of occupational exposure to human immunodeficiency virus, including considerations regarding zidovudine postexposure use, *MMWR* 39(No. RR-1), 1990.
37. Miller CH, Palenik CJ: Sterilization, disinfection, and asepsis in dentistry. In Block SS, editor: *Disinfection, sterilization, and preservation,* ed 4, Philadelphia, 1991, Lea & Febiger.
38. Favero MS, Bond WW: Chemical disinfection of medical and surgical materials. In Block SS, editor: *Disinfection, sterilization, and preservation,* ed 4, Philadelphia, 1991, Lea & Febiger.
39. FDA, Office of Device Evaluation, Division of General and Restorative Devices, Infection Control Devices Branch. Guidance on the content and format of premarket notification [510 (k)] submissions for liquid chemical germicides. Rockville, Maryland, FDA, January 31, 1992.
40. Rutala WA. APIC guideline for selection and use of disinfectants, *Am J Infect Control* 18:99-117, 1990.
41. Proposed American National Standard/American Dental Association Specification No. 59 for portable steam sterilizers for use in dentistry, Chicago: ADA, April 1991.
42. CDC. Recommendations for preventing transmission of infection with human T-lymphotropic virus type III/lymphadenopathy-associated virus in the workplace, *MMWR* 34:682-6, 691-5, 1995.
43. Council on Dental Materials, Instruments, and Equipment; Dental Practice; and Dental Therapeutics. American Dental Association. Infection control recommendations for the dental office and the dental laboratory, *J Am Dent Assoc* 1126:241-8, 1988.
44. Lewis DL, Boe RK: Cross infection risks associated with current procedures for using high-speed dental handpieces, *J Clin Microbiol* 30:401-6, 1992.
45. Crawford JJ, Broderius RK: Control of cross infection risks in the dental operatory: prevention of water retraction by bur cooling spray systems, *J Am Dent Assoc* 116:685-7, 1988.

46. Lewis DL, Arens M, Appleton SS et al.: Cross-contamination potential with dental equipment, *Lancet* 340:1252-4, 1992.
47. Bagga BSR, Murphy RA, Anderson AW, Punwani I: Contamination of dental unit cooling water with oral microorganisms and its prevention, *J Am Dent Assoc* 109:712-6, 1984.
48. Scheid RC, Kim CK, Bright JS, Whitely MS, Rosen S: Reduction of microbes in handpieces by flushing before use, *J Am Dent Assoc* 105:658-60, 1982.
49. Garner JS, Simmons BP: CDC guideline for isolation precautions in hospitals, Atlanta, Georgia, CDC, HHS publication no. (CDC)83-8314. 1983.
50. Tate WH, White RR: Disinfection of human teeth for educational purposes, *J Dent Educ* 55:583-5, 1991.
51. Favero MS, Bond WW: Sterilization, disinfection, and antisepsis in the hospital. In Balows A, Hausler WJ, Hermann KL, Isenberg HD, Shadomy HJ, editors: *Manual of clinical microbiology,* ed 5, Washington, DC, 1991, American Society for Microbiology.
52. The Michigan Medical Waste Regulatory Act of 1990, Act No. 368 of the Public Health Acts of 1978, Part 138, Medical Waste, Section 13807—Definitions.
53. Oregon Health Division. Infectious waste disposal; questions and answers pertaining to the Administrative Rules 333-18-040 through 333-18-070. Portland, Oregon, Oregon Health Division, 1989.
54. Bell DM: Human immunodeficiency virus transmission in health care settings: risk and risk reduction, *Am J Med* 91(suppl. 3B):294-300, 1991.
55. Bell DM, Shapiro CN, Gooch BF: Preventing HIV transmission to patients during invasive procedures: the CDC perspective, *J Public Health Den* (in press).

CDC GUIDELINES FOR PREVENTION OF TUBERCULOSIS IN DENTAL SETTINGS

The CDC published "Guidelines for Preventing the Transmission *of Mycobacterium tuberculosis* in Health-Care Facilities, 1994" in *Morbidity and Mortality Weekly Report (MMWR)* volume 28, No. RR-13, October 28, 1994. All of the details are in that publication but the information related to dental setting (which is section II. M. 2. E. on page 52 of the above-referenced *MMWR*) is presented here. Further information related to tuberculosis (TB) prevention in the dental office can be found in the May, 1995, issue of the *Journal of the American Dental Association.*[*]

In general, the symptoms for which patients seek treatment in a dental care setting are not likely to be caused by infectious TB. Unless a patient requiring dental care coincidentally has TB, it is unlikely that infectious TB will be encountered in the dental setting. Furthermore, generation of droplet nuclei containing *M. tuberculosis* during dental procedures has not been demonstrated.[†] Therefore the risk of transmission of *M. tuberculosis* in most dental settings is probably quite low. Nevertheless, during dental procedures, patients and dental workers share the same air for varying periods of time. Coughing may be stimulated occasionally by oral manipulations, although no specific dental procedures have been classified as "cough-inducing." In some instances, the population served by a dental care facility, or the HCWs (health-care workers) in the facility, may be at relatively high risk for TB. Because the potential exists for transmission of *M. tuberculosis* in dental settings, the following recommendations should be followed.

- A risk assessment (Box C-1) should be done periodically, and TB infection control policies for each dental setting should be based on the risk assessment. The policies should include provisions for detection and referral of patients who may have undiagnosed active TB; management of patients with active TB, relative to provision of urgent dental care; and employer-sponsored HCW education, counseling, and screening (Box C-2).
- While taking patients' initial medical histories and at periodic updates, dental HCWs should routinely ask all patients whether they have a history of TB disease and symptoms suggestive of TB.
- Patients with a medical history or symptoms suggestive of undiagnosed active TB should be referred promptly for medical evaluation of possible infectiousness. Such patients should not remain in the dental care facility any longer than required to arrange a referral. While in the dental care facility, they should wear surgical masks and should be instructed to cover their mouths and noses when coughing or sneezing.

[*]Cleveland JT et al.: *J Amer Dent Assoc* 126:593-600, 1995.
[†]Dueli RC, Madden RN: Droplet nuclei produced during dental treatment of tubercular patients, *Oral Surg* 30:711-716, 1970.

- Elective dental treatment should be deferred until a physician confirms that the patient does not have infectious TB. If the patient is diagnosed as having active TB, elective dental treatment should be deferred until the patient is no longer infectious.
- If urgent dental care must be provided for a patient who has, or is strongly suspected of having, infectious TB, such care should be provided in facilities that can provide TB isolation (see Section II. E. and G. of the original publication for details). Dental HCWs should use respiratory protection while performing procedures on such patients.
- Any dental HCW who has a persistent cough (i.e., a cough lasting ≥3 weeks), especially in the presence of other signs or symptoms compatible with active TB (e.g., weight loss, night sweats, bloody sputum, anorexia, and fever), should be evaluated promptly for TB. The HCW should not return to the workplace until a diagnosis of TB is excluded or until the HCW is on therapy and a determination is made that the HCW is noninfectious.
- In dental care facilities that provide care to populations at high risk for active TB, it may be appropriate to use engineering controls similar to those used in general-use

---

Box C-1   Conducting a Tuberculosis Risk Assessment in a Dental Setting

ASSESSMENTS AND RESULTS	RISK CATEGORY
Review the community TB profile from public health records and determine the number of patients with active TB seen in the office in the last year. If patients with active TB have been in the office, skin test (PPD*) office staff.	
Active TB patients not treated in office and none reported in the community	Minimal risk
Active TB patients not treated in office but some were reported in the community; plan to screen and refer known or suspected TB patients to a collaborating facility for evaluation and management if treatment is required	Very low risk
Provided treatment to fewer than six active TB patients and no evidence of PPD skin test conversions among office staff	Low risk
Provided treatment to six or more active TB patients and no evidence of PPD skin test conversions among office staff	Intermediate risk
Evidence of transmission of TB in the office based on skin testing data	High risk

*PPD, Purified protein derivative from *Mycobacterium* used in skin testing.

Box C-2   Tuberculosis Prevention Program for the Dental Office*

For Offices in *Minimal Risk* Category
- Assign specific person responsibility for the TB infection control program in the office
- Conduct a baseline risk assessment (see Box C-1) for the office and reassess annually
- Develop a written TB infection control plan
- Develop and implement protocols for identifying and referring patients who may have active TB for evaluation, management, or urgent dental treatment
- Educate, train, and counsel the office staff regarding TB
- Develop a protocol for identifying and referring dental workers who may have active TB and/or positive PPD skin tests
- Develop a protocol for investigating unprotected occupational exposure to TB

For Offices in *Low Risk* Category
- Perform all activities in the minimal and very low risk categories above
- Provide TB isolation when treating patients with known or suspected active TB (see details in original *MMWR* publication)
- Perform engineering controls in the general use areas such as the waiting room to include general ventilation, HEPA filtration, or UVGI

For Offices in *Very Low Risk* Category
- Perform all activities in the minimal risk category above
- As an optional activity, develop protocols and implement engineering controls in general use areas of the office such as the waiting room that may include general ventilation, high-efficiency particulate air (HEPA) filtration, or ultraviolet light germicidal irradiation (UVGI)

---

*Only minimal, very low, and low risk categories are considered here, since this will include essentially all private dental offices. Consult the original *MMWR* publication for prevention related to intermediate or high risk categories.

OFFICE SAFETY AND ASEPSIS PROCEDURES (OSAP) RESEARCH FOUNDATION

GENERAL INFORMATION AND MISSION STATEMENT

The OSAP Research Foundation is the premiere dental infection control organization in the world, and anyone with an interest in dental infection control should join this organization. Its members include dental assistants, dental hygienists, dentists, dental laboratory technologists, researchers, university professors, military personnel, writers, consultants, insurance people, inventors, manufacturers and distributors of infection control products and equipment, and others. The mission of the foundation is:

The Office Safety & Asepsis Procedures (OSAP) Research Foundation is dedicated to promoting infection control and related health and safety policies and practices supported by science and research. OSAP supports this commitment to health care workers and the public through quality education and information dissemination.

MEMBERSHIP CATEGORIES

A person in every dental office and every educational institution and others interested in dental infection control should join this organization. This will assure being kept up to date with the latest information about disease spread in the office; occupational exposures to infectious agents; tips on infection control procedures; changes in laws and recommendations; diseases in dentistry, including tuberculosis, hepatitis, and herpes; HIV disease; reactions to latex gloves; and infection control supplies and equipment. Members also have access to a telephone "hotline" to receive quick answers to infection control and other safety related questions. Various infection control texts, guidelines, official documents, brochures, and copies of laws are also available from this organization and there are regional and national meetings and seminars that foster invaluable interactions and provide current information for immediate use. The membership categories in the OSAP Research Foundation are:

1. Healthcare Professionals
   Allied health
   DDS/DMD/PhD
2. School
   Institution
   Student
3. State Board or State Association

4. Associate
   National Associations
   Consultants
   Individual branch locations of dealers who have been accepted as Corporate members
5. Regional Industry
   Distributors with branches in 1 to 4 states
6. Corporate
   Manufacturers and national distributors with an interest in infection control

Further information about membership or any other aspect of the organization can be obtained by calling the foundation headquarters at 1–800–298–OSAP.

OSAP RESEARCH FOUNDATION INFECTION CONTROL IN DENTISTRY GUIDELINES (SEPTEMBER, 1997)

These infection control guidelines include appropriate procedures to protect dental patients and all dental health care workers (DHCW) whether employers or employees from occupational transmission of infectious diseases (including but not limited to bloodborne pathogens) in the dental office.

1. **Universal Precautions**

   Universal precautions as defined by the Centers for Disease Control and Prevention (CDC) must be used in all patient care in dentistry. The term refers to a set of precautions designed to prevent transmission of human immunodeficiency virus (HIV), hepatitis B virus (HBV), and other bloodborne pathogens in health care settings. Under universal precautions, blood and saliva (in dentistry) of all patients are considered potentially infectious for HIV, HBV, and other bloodborne pathogens. Applied universal precautions means that the same infection control procedures for any given dental procedure must be used for all patients. Thus the required infection control policies and procedures to be used for any given dental procedure are determined by the characteristics of the procedure. Therefore universal precautions are procedure specific not patient specific.

2. **Hepatitis B Immunization**

   All DHCWs who have direct or indirect contact with patient's blood and/or saliva should be immunized with hepatitis B vaccine or show serologic evidence (anti-HBs) to hepatitis B virus infection. The U.S. Occupational Safety & Health Administration (OSHA) requires that the hepatitis B vaccine must be offered to employees at no charge within 10 days of employment. Those who receive the vaccine series should be serologically tested six weeks–six months after the third injection to determine if they have developed immunity. (This testing is not required by current OSHA regulations.) Employees who do not develop immunity should be serologically evaluated to determine past exposure to HBV or possible need for additional hepatitis B immunizations. For adults and children with normal immune status, the antibody response to properly administered vaccine is excellent, and protection lasts for at least 10 years. Booster doses of vaccine are not routinely recommended nor is routine serologic testing to assess antibody levels in vaccine recipients necessary during this period unless a person has a documented percutaneous, mucous membrane, or nonintact skin exposure to blood and/or saliva. In these exposure incidents, the latest CDC guidelines should be followed to assess and manage the exposure.

3. **Percutaneous Injuries**

Percutaneous and permucosal exposure to blood and other body fluids of dental patients poses the single greatest risk of transmission of HIV, hepatitis B, C, and D, and other bloodborne diseases from patient to DHCW. Emphasis should be placed on prevention of these incidents by assessing safer devices and work practices. Review of the dental literature is also useful in determining which practices may be associated with dental exposure incidents.

Despite efforts to prevent such injuries, every dental practice safety program should include preparation for response to these incidents. Postexposure management as required by OSHA includes gathering information related to the exposure, offering medical follow-up to the exposed worker, and requesting that the source patient be tested for HIV and hepatitis B and C. It is imperative that the postexposure management program be in place before an incident occurs. Delay in referral to a qualified medical practitioner in assessing the injury may affect the availability of prophylactic medications that can now be offered to exposed health care workers.

4. **Mouth Rinse**

A pre-procedure mouth rinse should be used to reduce the number of microorganisms in the patient's mouth. The mouth rinse should have residual activity to help maintain reduced microbial levels throughout the appointment.

5. **Handwashing and Hand Care**

The skin of DHCW hands harbors resident and transient microorganisms. Most resident microorganisms on superficial layers of the skin are not highly virulent but may be responsibile for some skin infections. DHCW contact with infected patients is a source of transient microorganisms on DHCW hands. Transient microorganisms pose the greatest risk of cross-infection. Adequate handwashing will remove or inhibit transient and resident organisms.

DHCWs should wash hands before donning gloves, after removal of gloves, and after inadvertent barehand touching of contaminated surfaces or objects.

For most routine procedures, washing with plain soap appears adequate. Use antimicrobial soap for more invasive procedures such as surgery. For all handwashing, convenient placement of sinks, towels, and soaps will encourage use by workers. When possible, use alternative sink controls such as foot or sensor activated faucets. Vigorously rubbing lathered hands together under a stream of water for a minimum of ten seconds is adequate for routine handwashing. Thorough rinsing under a stream of water should follow. Dry hands well before donning gloves. DHCWs with open sores or weeping dermatitis must refrain from direct patient contact and handling of patient care equipment until the condition is resolved.

6. **Personal Protective Equipment**

DHCW must wear protective attire such as eye wear or a chin-length shield, disposable gloves, a disposable surgical quality mask, and protective clothing when performing procedures capable of causing splash, spatter, or other contact with body fluids and/or mucous membranes. Protective attire must also be worn when touching items or surfaces that may be contaminated with these fluids and during other activities that pose a risk of exposure to blood, saliva, or tissue.

Gloves are single use items and <u>must not</u> be reused. Single use gloves may not be washed, disinfected, or sterilized. They must be rinsed with water only to remove excess powder. Torn or compromised gloves must be replaced immediately. Latex, vinyl, or other disposable medical quality gloves may be used for patient examinations and procedures. Plastic or foodhandler gloves may be worn over contaminated treatment gloves (overgloving) to prevent contamination of clean objects handled during treatment. These overgloves may never be used alone as a hand barrier or for intraoral patient care procedures. Overgloves must be handled carefully to avoid contamination during handling with contaminated procedure gloves. If overgloves are not used, contaminated procedure gloves should be removed before leaving chairside during patient care and replaced with new gloves after returning to patient care. Hands must be washed after glove removal and before re-gloving.

Surgical masks that have at least 95% filtration efficiency for particles 3 to 5 microns in diameter must be worn whenever splash or spatter is anticipated. Masks should be changed for every patient or more often, particularly if heavy spatter is generated during treatment. Some literature suggests that masks should be worn a maximum of 20 minutes in areas of high humidity and a maximum of 60 minutes in dry climates. Masks should be handled by touching the periphery only; avoid handling the body of the mask. Masks should not contact the mouth while being worn because the moisture generated will decrease mask filtration efficiency. A mask should be selected that conforms well to the shape of the face. A faceshield does not substitute for a surgical mask.

Protective eye wear must have solid side-shields and be decontaminated between patients by immersion in a cleaning agent. A faceshield may substitute for protective eye wear. If protective eye wear or a faceshield is used to protect against damage from solid projectiles, the protective eye wear should meet American National Standards Institute (ANSI) Occupational and Educational Eye and Face Protection Standard (Z87.1-1989) and be clearly marked as such.

Protective clothing must have a high neck and protect the arms if splash and spatter are reasonably anticipated. Cotton or cotton/polyester or disposable clinic jackets or lab coats are usually satisfactory attire for routine dental procedures. The type and characteristics of protective clothing depend on the type of exposure anticipated. Gowns or jackets worn as protective attire should be changed at least daily, or more often if visibly soiled. Protective gowns or covers must be removed before leaving the work area. Protective attire may not be taken home and washed by employees. It may be laundered in the office if equipment is available and universal precautions are followed for handling and laundering contaminated attire. Contaminated linens transported away from the office for laundering should be in appropriate bags to prevent leaking, with a biohazard label or appropriate color-code, unless the laundry facility employees practice universal precautions in the handling of all laundry. Disposable gowns may be used but must be discarded daily or more often if visibly soiled.

Utility gloves that are puncture resistant, a mask, protective clothing, and protective eyewear must be worn when handling and cleaning contaminated instruments, when performing operatory cleanup, and for surface cleaning and disinfecting. Utility gloves must be discarded if their barrier properties become compromised. Utility gloves, protective eye wear or face shields, and masks must be worn when mixing and/or using chemical sterilants or disinfectants. Used utility gloves must be considered contaminated and handled appropriately until properly disinfected or sterilized.

NOTE: Increased use of latex gloves for infection control purposes has increased incidences of latex allergies and other sensitivities. Certain individuals are considered at increased risk of latex sensitivity. These individuals include persons who have had multiple surgeries (especially involving the placement of rubber tubes or drains), spina bifida patients, health care workers, and individuals with other documented allergies. Medical histories should include questions that may alert the DHCW that a patient is latex-sensitive. If a person is sensitive to latex, precautions such as non-latex gloves, non-latex rubber dams, and avoidance of any other latex-containing products should be implemented in the treatment of those patients. Latex-sensitive patients should also be scheduled at the beginning of the day to minimize exposure to latex residue and powder.

DHCWs who experience symptoms consistent with sensitivity, including skin rash, itching, or wheezing, should seek the advice of a qualified medical professional for diagnosis of the symptoms. Because a variety of materials may be responsible for the sensitivity, including resin materials that may permeate the gloves, self-diagnosis is ill-advised and could increase the risk of a serious allergic response.

7. **Instrument Sterilization**

Puncture-resistant utility gloves, a mask, protective eyewear, and a protective gown or apron must be worn throughout instrument processing.

Single use disposable items must be disposed after each use. All reusable items that contact patient's blood, saliva, or mucous membranes must be sterilized in an autoclave, unsaturated chemical vapor sterilizer, dry heat sterilizer (must be FDA-cleared for use as a medical device), or ethylene oxide gas sterilizer before reuse. Ethylene oxide is inappropriate for use with lubricated items such as handpieces due to failure of the gas to penetrate lubricants.

Sterilization by immersion in a chemical sterilant that has been FDA-cleared for use as a sterilizing agent is appropriate only for items that may be damaged by the sterilization method referred to in the paragraph above. Use the concentration, contact time, and temperature stated on the product label to achieve chemical sterilization. During use the solution should be routinely checked with a glutaraldehyde indicator to assure a minimum effective glutaraldehyde concentration. NOTE that glutaraldehyde cannot be biologically monitored to verify sterilization, nor can items be packaged before chemical sterilization.

The procedure for processing reusable instruments begins at chairside. It is important to keep instruments moist to facilitate cleaning. Therefore, if instruments are not immediately processed, they should be placed in a "holding" solution (soapy water or a commercially available surfactant solution) to prevent the drying of blood and debris. All items must be properly cleaned in an ultrasonic cleaning unit or instrument washer. Only cleaners intended for use in an ultrasonic cleaner or instrument washer should be used. Chemical germicides are inappropriate for use with these devices. Hand scrubbing of sharp instruments should be avoided. However, if hand scrubbing is required, use a clean long-handled brush and keep instruments submerged while scrubbing to reduce spatter. Brushes should be disposable or autoclavable. Care must be taken to avoid injuries with hand (brush) scrubbing. Instruments must be dry if ethylene oxide gas, dry heat, or unsaturated chemical vapor sterilizers are used. Instruments must be packaged (using proper pouches, bags or wrapped cassettes, or packs) before steam, chemical vapor, or dry heat or gas sterilization and remain packaged for storage to protect the items from environmental contamination after sterilization. Mark packages with date and sterilizer number for tracking purposes.

NOTE: Do not write with ink directly on the paper (wrap or pouches). Autoclave tape, bar code stickers, or writing on plastic side of pouches is acceptable.

8. **Handpiece Sterilization**

All high-speed handpieces, nose cones, contra-angles, low-speed motors, motor-to-angle adapters and prophylaxis angles (unless disposable prophylaxis angles are used) must be heat sterilized between patients. The cleaning, sterilization, and maintenance procedures described by the handpiece manufacturer must be meticulously followed to ensure proper sterilization and maximum longevity from the handpiece.

After patient treatment flush the water/air lines for 20 to 30 seconds with the high-speed handpiece still attached. Remove the handpieces and thoroughly clean the external/internal surfaces as directed. Package before sterilization and process through the sterilizer according to the sterilizer and handpiece manufacturer instructions. If lubrication is indicated by the handpiece manufacturer before or after sterilization, follow the procedures as outlined by the manufacturer. It is recommended that a separate container of lubricant be reserved for this purpose as a cross-contamination avoidance strategy.

9. **Sterilization Monitoring**

The use and functioning of heat sterilizers should be biologically monitored at least weekly, or more often if the practice demands it, with appropriate spore tests. Place the spore strips or vials inside a pouch, bag, pack, or cassette, and include this package as part of the normal load through a normal sterilizer cycle. Always use a control spore strip or vial (not heat processed but otherwise treated identically to the test strips or vials) with each spore test performed. Additionally, chemical indicators should be used on the inside of each package during every sterilizer load. Accurate records of sterilization monitoring must be maintained. A chemical indicator from inside each pack may be initialed and dated for each day of patient care and kept in a file. The weekly spore test for each heat sterilization unit may be kept in the same file. Biologically monitor 1) whenever there is a change in packaging, 2) after equipment repair, 3) to retest after failure, and 4) when training new employees.

10. **Environmental Surface and Equipment Asepsis**

Current CDC guidelines recommend that all waterlines for syringes and/or handpieces should be turned on and flushed for several minutes with handpieces disconnected at the beginning of the day and 20 to 30 seconds between patients. However, research shows this protocol alone to be temporary and inadequate in controlling water contamination.

Sterile cooling and irrigating solutions must be used as an irrigant during surgical procedures. This water must be delivered from a source separate from the dental unit. Dental unit water that contains fewer than 200 CFU/mL of heterotrophic mesophilic bacteria is acceptable for use as a coolant or irrigant for all nonsurgical dental procedures. Dental water delivery systems that are fitted with antiretraction valves must be checked weekly. Alternatively, systems that provide constant positive pressure may be used. All vacuum lines must be flushed after every patient procedure to prevent drying of blood and debris in the lines.

To develop an effective asepsis protocol, operatory surfaces, including walls, floors, cabinetry, and equipment, should be classified and managed under three categories: touch surfaces, transfer surfaces, and splash/spatter surfaces.

a. *Touch Surfaces* Surfaces that are usually touched and contaminated during dental procedures. Examples include dental light handles, dental unit handle and controls, headrest adjustment mechanism, or dental chair switches. Touch surfaces should be kept at a minimum. If a surface must or might be touched, it should be cleaned and disinfected, or covered with a barrier that is impervious to liquid. Barriers must be single-use and replaced between patients. Offices should develop a standard procedure for installing and removing barriers that will prevent cross-contamination. All office staff responsible for operatory turnover between patients should be trained in this standard procedure. Contaminated barriers must be properly discarded. If a covered touch surface is compromised and becomes visibly contaminated, it should be cleaned and disinfected with a low or intermediate-level disinfectant before applying the barriers for the next patient. Touch surfaces that have been covered with barriers should be cleaned and disinfected at the end of each clinical day. Before the first patient of the next clinical day, new barriers should be installed.

b. *Transfer Surfaces* Surfaces that are not touched but are usually contacted by contaminated instruments. Examples include instrument trays and dental unit handpiece holders. Asepsis for transfer surfaces is the same as for touch surfaces.

c. *Splash/Spatter Surfaces* All surfaces in the operatory other than touch or transfer surfaces. Splash and spatter surfaces need not be disinfected but should be cleaned (at least daily, or more often if possible).

11. **Laboratory Asepsis**

Open communication must exist between the dental office and the dental laboratory concerning infection control protocols and delineation of responsibilities between the office and lab. Materials, impressions, and intraoral appliances must be cleaned and disinfected before being handled, adjusted, or sent to a dental lab. Personal protective equipment, including gown, gloves, mask, and protective eyewear, should be worn.

Before selecting a disinfecting agent, consult manufacturers of specific materials about the stability of their material relative to disinfection agents and procedures. Disinfect for the specified length of time with the appropriate chemical (1:10 sodium hypochlorite solution or an EPA-registered, tuberculocidal disinfectant that also kills hydrophilic and lipophilic [enveloped and nonenveloped] viruses). Finally, rinse thoroughly. Do not transfer to laboratory in container containing disinfectant.

If items are properly disinfected before taking into or sent out to the laboratory, lab equipment and surfaces should not become contaminated. However, a laboratory that provides services to numerous clients may become subject to contamination from other sources. All items returned from a commercial laboratory should be considered clean for handling but should be disinfected before placement in a patient's mouth. If laboratory equipment, surfaces, and attachments become contaminated with blood or saliva, they must be thoroughly cleaned and then sterilized or disinfected before use on another case.

12. **Waste Disposal**

a. *General* All waste must be disposed according to applicable federal, state, and local regulations and recommendations. Generally, blood and/or saliva-tinged items are not regulated waste. Hard and soft tissue and soaked items, that is, items from which blood or saliva can be squeezed out, or items from which blood may flake, are considered regulated medical waste. Always consult the state or local government agency regarding specific exemptions and disposal/treatment requirements.

b *Infectious Disease Hazard (biohazard) Communication* Containers of regulated medical waste (as defined above) are to be labeled and/or identified in compliance with local regulations. These containers include contaminated sharps containers, contaminated reusable sharps containers (i.e., pans used for holding contaminated instruments), bags of contaminated laundry, specimen containers, and storage containers.

c. *Handling and Disposing Sharps* Place needles and other disposable sharps, such as scalpel blades, orthodontic wires, and broken glass into a puncture resistant, leakproof container that is closable and color-coded or labeled with the biohazard symbol. The container must be located as close as possible to the point of use for immediate disposal. Do not cut, bend, break, or remove needles by hand before disposal, and do not remove needles from disposable syringes. To recap a needle on a nondisposable anesthetic syringe, lay the needle cover on a firm surface and guide the needle into the cover using only one hand; **or** use one-handed resheathing with a resheathing device. Alternatively, self-sheathing needles may also be used. If the device is one that is hand-held, it must provide full hand protection for the hand holding the device. When the sharps container is three fourths full, securely close and treat or dispose according to state and local laws.

d. *Non-sharp Disposable Items* Non-sharp disposable items that are considered regulated waste by state or local laws must be disposed of and/or transported according to specific state and/or local regulations. At a minimum, these items must always be placed in labeled, leak-proof bags or containers. Disposable items that may contain the body fluids of patients but are not subject to medical waste regulations, such as gloves and patient bibs, should be placed in a lined trash receptacle. Red bags should not be used for nonregulated waste. Check the specific requirements of the local regulatory agency (usually state or county health departments).

13. **Tuberculosis**

    With the reemergence of *Mycobacterium tuberculosis* (TB) infection and active tuberculosis as demonstrated risk factors for health care workers (HCW), consult the reference CDC: "Guidelines for preventing the transmission of TB in health care facilities, 1994", and Box D-1.

14. **Training**

    All DHCWs involved in the direct supervision of patient care should receive regular training in infection control and safety issues. Training should include coverage of OSHA pertinent regulations such as Bloodborne Pathogens and Hazard Communication standards.

15. **Other**

    a. *A dental dam and high volume evacuation* may be used during dental procedures, when indicated, to minimize the amount of potentially contaminated splash and spatter and to minimize direct contact with patient's oral mucosa.

    b. *Ventilation devices* such as a one-way CPR airway (e.g., a pocket mask with a one-way valve) or oxygen with bagging capability must be available for those qualified to provide such care.

c. *Eating, Drinking, Smoking* Do not eat, drink, smoke, apply cosmetics or lip balm, handle contact lenses, or store food or drink in areas of possible exposure to (or storage of) blood, saliva, tissue, or other potentially infectious materials. This includes the dental operatory, dental laboratory, sterilization area, and darkroom/x-ray processing area.

d. *Decontamination of Equipment for Servicing or Maintenance* Contaminated equipment or instruments that are to be repaired on site or shipped for service are first to be cleaned and sterilized or disinfected. If a portion of the equipment cannot be cleaned and sterilized or disinfected, that portion should be identified with a biohazard label and an explanation to those who may handle the contaminated item. Utility gloves, masks, and protective eyewear must be worn when routine maintenance is performed on equipment such as replacing filters on suction pumps, etc. Infection control policy and procedures should be communicated to the repair personnel.

e. *Radiographic Asepsis* Wear gloves while exposing films in the patient's mouth. Place exposed films in a paper cup. When all films are exposed, remove and discard gloves. Reglove and transport films to the darkroom, carefully open the packs and drop the films on a clean surface. Discard the contaminated wrappers, remove and discard the gloves; process the films.

(1) Daylight loaders

When using an x-ray processor with a daylight loader, extra precautions are required to avoid contamination of the sleeves and external and internal components of the processor. Place films in a paper cup as they are exposed. When all films are taken, remove gloves and place the paper cup containing exposed film packets into the daylight loader. Wearing clean gloves, insert gloves through the sleeves of the daylight loader. Open all film packets, allowing films to drop onto a clean surface. Do not touch films with gloved hands. After all the film packets have been opened, discard empty film wrappers, remove gloves, and process films with bare hands. For disposal, empty film packets and used gloves may be placed in the paper cup that was originally used to transport the films into the daylight loader. If the insides of the insertion sleeves have ever been contaminated, double gloving may be used for protection when removing hands from the daylight loader. One pair of gloves should be removed after opening film packets, leaving a clean pair of gloves for handling films and touching the sleeves of the daylight loader.

(2) Barrier pack films

X-ray films packaged in fluid impervious barriers are available. A slight modification of the recommended x-ray and darkroom protocol is indicated. After exposing the film, pull on the edges of the barrier pack, allowing the film to drop into a clean paper cup without contaminating the inner film packet. When all films are exposed and collected in the cup, remove procedure gloves and take films to the darkroom or daylight loader for processing.

Disclaimer

The Office Safety and Asepsis Procedures (OSAP) Research Foundation Infection Control in Dentistry Guidelines updated September, 1997 are based on the recommendations of the Centers for Disease Control and Prevention and other publications in the dental and medical literature. The guidelines here are intended to offer general guidance on infection control.

OSAP assumes no responsibility for actions taken based on the information herein.

From Centers for Disease Control and Prevention: Guidelines for preventing the transmission of *Mycobacterium tuberculosis* in health care facilities, 1994.

Box D-1   Policy for Treatment of Dental Patients with Active or Suspected Infection with Tuberculosis

---

A. During initial medical history and periodic updates ask patients about a history of TB disease and symptoms suggestive of TB. Symptoms include chronic cough, coughing blood, night sweats, and weight loss. NOTE: positive TB skin test without symptoms does not indicate active infection in most cases.

B. Patients with history and symptoms suggestive of active TB should be promptly referred to a physician for evaluation for possible infectiousness.

C. Elective dental treatment should be postponed until a physician confirms, using recognized diagnostic evaluations, that the patient does not have active TB.

D. If urgent dental care must be provided for a patient who has, or is suspected of having, active TB infection, TB isolation practices must be implemented. Treatment provided should be limited to the minimum necessary to relieve the patient's immediate pain. Generally, referral to a medical center with proper isolation rooms will be required. Respiratory protection (HEPA-filter masks) must be used by the dental care providers when performing procedures on these patients. The respirators must be fit-tested before each use.

E. DHCWs with persistent cough and other symptoms suggestive of active TB should be evaluated promptly for TB. The individual should not return to work until a diagnosis of TB is excluded or until the individual is on therapy and a determination is made that the worker is not infectious.

EXPOSURE INCIDENT REPORT

Name of Exposed Person:_____

Job Classification: _____

Name of Employer: _____

Date of Exposure:_____ Time:_____

Description of the Incident:_____

_____

_____

_____

_____

_____

_____

_____

What barriers were used by exposed person during the incident?_____

_____

_____

Describe corrective measures to minimize possible recurrence:_____

_____

_____

Was source (patient) sent for medical evaluation?   Yes_____ No_____

Patient's name: _____ Comments: _____

_____

Was exposed person sent for medical evaluation?   Yes_____ No_____

Comments: _____

_____

Was the exposed person informed by the evaluating physician of the results of the medical evaluation as required by OSHA?   Yes_____ No_____

Was the employer informed by the evaluating physician that the exposed person was medically evaluated as required by OSHA?   Yes_____ No_____

_____

Signature of exposed person   Date

_____

Signature of employer   Date

CHEMICALS USED FOR INFECTION CONTROL

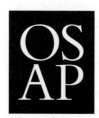

Office **S**afety & **A**sepsis **P**rocedures (OSAP) Research Foundation

P.O. Box 6297 • Annapolis, MD 21401 • www.osap.org • 410-798-5665
Fax:410-798-6797 • Email:osap@clark.net

Chemical Agents for Surface Disinfection Reference Chart

CHEMICAL CLASSIFICATION				PRODUCTS
	ADVANTAGES	DISADVANTAGES	EXAMPLE OF ACTIVE INGREDIENT AND LISTED ON PRODUCT LABEL	NAME
Alcohols	**Do not use for environmental surface disinfection. Rapid evaporation rate. Diminished activity with bioburden.**			
Chlorines	Rapid acting; Broad spectrum Economical (bleach)	Discard diluted solutions daily Diminished activity by organic matter Corrosive	Sodium hypochlorite; Chlorine dioxide	Bleach (5.25%) Clorox Dispatch (0.55%)
Iodophors	Broad spectrum Few reactions Residual biocidal activity	Unstable at high temperatures Dilution and con- tact time critical Discard daily Discoloration of some surfaces Inactived by hard water	Butoxpolypropoxy- polyethoxyethanol iodine complex	IodoFive Biocide Iodophor disinfectant Asepti-IDC
Synthetic Phenolics	Broad spectrum Residual biocidal activity	Discard daily for most diluted solu- tions Degrades certain plastic over time Difficult to rinse Film accumulation	WATER BASED Dual Phenolics Phenylphenol and benzylchlorophenol or tertiary amylphenol	Omni II ProPhene Vital Defense-D ProSpray Birex$_{se}$ Lysol IC disinfec- tant cleaner Lysol IC disinfectant Dual Phenol ger- micidal cleaner

*Temperature: 20° C = 68° F; 25° C = 77° F
†Studies by Klein and DeForest suggest that hydrophilic are more resistant than lipophilic viruses and therefore rep-resent a better gauge of a disinfectant's virucidal efficacy. Hydrophilic viruses include various strains of *Polio, Coxsackie, Rhinovirus* and *Rotavirus.*
‡Demonstrates activity toward *Adeno* virus (resistance level between hydrophilic and lipophilic.)
All products to be used as disinfectants on precleaned surfaces must be EPA-registered. Listing does not imply en-dorsement, recommendation, or warranty. Other products available. Purchasers are legally required to consult the package insert for changes in formulation and recommendation product uses. Check compatibility of material be-fore use on dental/medical equipment.
This chart is a publication of the Office Safety & Asepsis Procedures (OSAP) Research Foundation. OSAP assumes no liability for actions taken based on the information herein.

EPA REG #	DILUTION	TB TIME	TB TEMPERATURE*	HYDROPHILIC VIRUS KILL[†]	TOTAL TIME FOR SURFACE DISINFECTION	FOR MORE INFORMATION CONTACT
N/A	1:100	10 min	20° C	Yes	10 min	Clorox
5813-1	1:100	10 min	20° C	Yes	10 min	Caltech
56392-7	None	2 min	20-25° C	Yes	2 min	
4959-16	1:213	10 min	20° C	Yes	10 min	Cottrell, Ltd
4959-16	1:213	10 min	20° C	Yes	10 min	Biotrol
4959-16	1:213	10 min	20° C	Yes	10 min	Smart Practice
303-63	1:256	10 min	20° C	Yes	10 min	Huntington
46851-1	1:32	10 min	20° C	Yes	10 min	Cottrell
46851-1	1:32	10 min	20° C	Yes	10 min	Cottrell
46851-1	1:32	10 min	20° C	Yes	10 min	Block
46851-5	none	10 min	20° C	Yes	10 min	Cottrell, Ltd
1043-92	1:256	10 min	20° C	No[‡]	10 min	Biotrol
675-46	1:128	10 min	20° C	No[‡]	10 min	Reckitt Colman
675-43	1:200	10 min	20° C	No[‡]	10 min	Reckitt Colman
67813-3	1:256	10 min	20° C	No[‡]	10 min	Smart Practice

Continued

Chemical Agents for Surface Disinfection Reference Chart—Cont'd

	CHEMICAL CLASSIFICATION			PRODUCTS
	ADVANTAGES	DISADVANTAGES	EXAMPLE OF ACTIVE INGREDIENT AND LISTED ON PRODUCT LABEL	NAME
Synthetic Phenolics–cont'd				BiArrest-2
			<u>Tri-Phenolics</u> Phenylphenol Benzylchlorophenol Tertiary amylphenol ALCOHOL-BASED Tertiary amylphenol and/or phenylphenol plus ethyl alcohol or isopropyl alcohol	Tri-cide Dencide Asepti-phene 128 PUMP CoeSpray Asepti-phene RTU AEROSOL Lysol IC disinfectant Asepti-Steryl Discide disinfectant spray Citrace Medicide/ADC Disinfectant deodorant
Dual or Synergized Quaternaries (do not use older generations of quats as surface disinfectants)	Broad spectrum Contains detergent for cleaning Few reactions	Easily inactivated by anionic detergents and organic matter; Deleterious to some materials	Diisobutylphenoxy-ethoxyethyl dimethyl benzyl ammonium chloride Isopropanol	Cavicide DisCide TB Precise QTB GC Spray-Cide SaniTex Plus Asepticare TB
Sodium Bromide and Chlorine	Broad spectrum Reduced storage (tablets)	May not be used for immersion (hard surfaces only); Chlorine smell	Sodium bromide Sodium dichloro-isocyanurate dihydrate	Microstat 2

EPA REG #	DILUTION	TB TIME	TB TEMPERATURE*	HYDROPHILIC VIRUS KILL†	TOTAL TIME FOR SURFACE DISINFECTION	FOR MORE INFORMATION CONTACT
67813-1	1:256	10 min	20° C	No	10 min	Infection Control Technology
11725-1	1:256	10 min	20° C	Yes	10 min	Health-Sonics
63281-4	1:256	10 min	20° C	Yes	10 min	Dentsply
303-223	1:128	10 min	20° C	Yes	10 min	Huntington
334-417	none	10 min	20° C	Yes	10 min	GC America
334-417	none	10 min	20° C	Yes	10 min	Huntington
777-53	none	10 min	20° C	Yes	10 min	Reckitt Colman
706-69	none	10 min	25° C	Yes	10 min	Huntington
706-69	none	10 min	25° C	Yes	10 min	Palmero
56392-2	none	10 min	20-25° C	Yes	10 min	Caltech
334-214	none	10 min	25° C	No	10 min	ADC
46781-6	none	10 min	20° C	Yes	10 min	Kerr
1839-83	none	10 min	20° C	Yes	10 min	Palmero
1839-83	none	10 min	20° C	Yes	10 min	Caltech
1130-15	none	6 min	20° C	Yes	10 min	GC America
1130-15	none	6 min	20° C	Yes	10 min	CrossTex
1130-13	none	10 min	20° C	Yes	10 min	Huntington
70369-1	2 tablets per quart	5 min	20° C	Yes	5 min	Septodont

Office Safety & Asepsis Procedures (OSAP) Research Foundation: Glutaraldehydes for Immersion Sterilization of Instruments

CHEMICAL CLASSIFICATION	PRODUCT	EPA REG #	INTERMEDIATE-LEVEL DISINFECTION			STERILIZATION		FOR MORE INFORMATION
			TB DIRECTIONS		TEST*			
			Temp	Time		Temp	Time	
Alkaline								
3.4%	Cidex Plus	7078-14	25° C	20 min	Quant	25° C	10 hrs	J&J Medical
	Procide Plus	46851-9	20° C	45 min	Quant	20° C	10 hrs	Cottrell, Ltd.
	Banicide Plus	46781-4	25° C	90 min	Quant	25° C	10 hrs	Pascal
	Cida-Steryl Plus	46781-4	25° C	90 min	Quant	25° C	10 hrs	Huntington/Ecolab
	CoeCide XL Plus	46781-4	25° C	90 min	Quant	25° C	10 hrs	GC America
	Security 3.4%	46781-4	25° C	90 min	Quant	25° C	10 hrs	Kerr
2.5%	Cida-Steryl 28	46781-2	25° C	90 min	Quant	25° C	10 hrs	Huntington/Ecolab
	CoeCide XL	46781-2	25° C	90 min	Quant	25° C	10 hrs	GC America
2.4%	ProCide	46851-2	20° C	45 min	Quant	20° C	10 hrs	Cottrell, Ltd.
Acidic								
2.5%	Banicide	15136-1	22° C	45 min	Quant	22° C	10 hrs	Pascal
	Sterall	15136-1	22° C	45 min	Quant	22° C	10 hrs	Colgate

NOTE: Sterilization by immersion in glutaraldehydes is appropriate only for items that may be damaged through steam, dry heat, or chemical vapor sterilization. Glutaraldehydes may **not** be used as surface disinfectants. Please refer to the OSAP Research Foundation resource entitled "Environmental Asepsis Steps" for additional information. All products for immersion must be FDA-cleared.

20° C = 68° F; 22° C = 72° F; 25° C = 77° F.

*Tests for TB label claim: Quant, Quantitative; AOAC, Association of Official Analytical Chemists.

All products are to be used full strength, undiluted on precleaned instruments. Other products are available. Listing does not imply endorsement, recommendation, or warranty. Purchasers are legally required to consult the package insert for changes in formulation and recommended product uses. This chart is a publication of the Office Safety & Asepsis Procedures (OSAP) Research Foundation. OSAP assumes no liability for actions taken based on the information herein.

Updated tables are available from the OSAP Research Foundation 410-798-5665; Fax:410-798-6797

INFECTION CONTROL RECOMMENDATIONS FOR THE DENTAL OFFICE AND THE DENTAL LABORATORY

Dental professionals are exposed to a wide variety of microorganisms in the blood and saliva of patients. These microorganisms may cause infectious diseases such as the common cold, pneumonia, tuberculosis, herpes, hepatitis B, and acquired immune deficiency syndrome. The use of effective infection control procedures and universal precautions in the dental office and dental laboratory will prevent cross-contamination that could extend to dentists, dental office staff, dental technicians, and patients. The American Dental Association has advocated the use of infection control procedures in the dental practice for many years.[1-6] As new information becomes available, the Association disseminates it to the profession and will continue to do so. Currently available Association publications that provide detailed information about infection control and treatment of patients with infectious diseases are Dental Management of the HIV-Infected Patient,[7] Monograph on Safety and Infection Control,[8] Infection Control in the Dental Environment,[9] and now this report. The Association also provides The American Dental Association Regulatory Compliance Manual[10] and a videotape entitled "OSHA: What You Must Know"[11]; both are designed to help dentists comply with OSHA Standards on Occupational Exposure to Bloodborne Pathogens and Hazard Communication.

This report is based on the recommendations of the Centers for Disease Control and Prevention[12-15] and other publications in the medical and dental literature. The recommendations in this document have been accepted by the Council on Scientific Affairs and the Council of Dental Practice. The Councils strongly urge practitioners and dental laboratories to comply with these infection control practices. With the enactment of the OSHA Standard on Occupational Exposure to Bloodborne Pathogens in December 1991,[16] many of these infection control procedures are required by law.

Dentists should recognize an important distinction between OSHA requirements and acceptable infection control practices. OSHA has a Congressional mandate to institute workplace procedures that protect the employee and, by law, is able to write regulations and enter the workplace to conduct inspections and impose financial penalties. The 1991 OSHA Standard on Occupational Exposure to Bloodborne Pathogens is thus written to protect employees. OSHA is not mandated to institute practices that protect the patient or the employer. The OSHA Standard, although providing some patient and employer

Reprinted with permission from: ADA Council on Scientific Affairs and ADA Council on Dental Practice. *J Amer Dent Assoc* 127:672-680, 1996.

protection, does not encompass all the infection control practices recommended by the U.S. Public Health Service (CDC) and the American Dental Association (ADA) to protect patients, employees, and employers from occupational transmission of infectious disease. Conversely, it is also important to note that OSHA has many requirements in the Bloodborne Pathogens Standard that neither the U.S. Public health Service nor the Association include in their infection control recommendations (for example, where contaminated gowns should be laundered, the requirement to retain an employee's medical records for the duration of employment plus 30 years, the requirement that the employer pay for hepatitis B vaccination, and for medical follow-up after an exposure incident).

Therefore although dentists have a legal requirement to comply with the OSHA Standard, the Association believes that they should be aware of and practice proper infection control procedures designed for the safety of everyone. These infection control procedures are detailed in this report, and also in various publications from the CDC and ADA referenced at the end of this report. Since this document is not intended to cover every aspect of infection control compliance, the dentist, his or her staff and that of dental laboratories should refer to the referenced publications.[2,6,15,16]

PREVENTION OF TRANSMISSION OF INFECTIOUS DISEASES

It is generally accepted that the dental health team is far more at risk from hepatitis B virus, or HBV, than from the human immunodeficiency virus that causes AIDS. However, because of increasing acceptance of the HVB vaccine among practicing dentists in recent years—86 percent (American Dental Association Health Screening Program. October 1995. Unpublished data.)—the risk of HBV infection is generally limited to those who have not been vaccinated.[17] Patients with hepatitis B or who are HBV carriers can be treated safety or with minimal risk of transmission of disease in the dental office when infection control procedures are used. HIV appears to be much more difficult to transmit than HBV but there is confidence that the same procedures will prevent transmission of HIV in the dental office.[17-18]

Vaccination Against Hepatitis B

Dental health care workers are at a greater risk than the general population of acquiring hepatitis B through contact with patients. It is the policy of the ADA that all dentists and their staffs having patient contact should be vaccinated against hepatitis B.[19] The OSHA Standard now requires that employers make the hepatitis B vaccine available to occupationally exposed employees, at the employer's expense, within 10 working days of assignment of tasks that may result in exposure.[16]

INFECTION CONTROL PRACTICES FOR THE DENTAL OFFICE: UNIVERSAL PRECAUTIONS

A thorough medical history should be obtained for all patients at the first visit and updated and reviewed at subsequent visits.

However, since not all patients with infectious diseases can be identified by medical history, physical examination, or readily available laboratory tests, the CDC introduced the concept of universal precautions.[20] This term refers to a method of infection control in which all human blood and certain human body fluids (saliva in dentistry) are treated as if known to be infectious for HIV, HBV, and other bloodborne pathogens. Universal precautions means that the same infection control procedures are used for all patients.

Barrier Techniques
Gloves

Gloves must be worn when skin contact with body fluids or mucous membranes is anticipated, or when touching items or surfaces that may be contaminated with these fluids. After contact with each patient, gloves must be removed and hands must be washed and then regloved before treating another patient. Repeated use of a single pair of gloves by disinfecting them between patients is not acceptable. Exposure to disinfectants or other chemicals often causes defects in gloves, thereby diminishing their value as effective barriers.[21] Latex or vinyl gloves should be used for patient examinations and procedures. Heavy rubber gloves, also called utility gloves, preferably should be used for cleaning instruments and environmental surfaces. Dentists should know that allergic reactions to latex gloves or the cornstarch powder in gloves have been reported in health care workers and patients.[22-23] To reduce the possibility of such reactions, nylon glove liners for use under latex, rubber, or plastic gloves are available. Polyethylene gloves, also known as food-handler gloves may be worn over treatment gloves to prevent contamination of objects such as drawer or light handles or charts.

Protective Clothing

Gowns, aprons, lab coats, clinic jackets, or similar outer garments, either reusable or disposable, must be worn when clothing or skin is likely to be exposed to body fluids. Professional judgment should be used to determine the degree of exposure anticipated in a given procedure. Protective clothing should be changed when visibly soiled or penetrated by fluids. OSHA requires that these garments not be worn outside the work area and that protective clothing be removed and placed in laundry bags or containers that are properly marked after use. Contaminated articles should be laundered using a normal laundry cycle.[13]

Masks

Surgical masks or chin-length face shields must be worn to protect the face, the oral mucosa, and the nasal mucosa when spatter of body fluids is anticipated. Masks should be changed when visibly soiled or wet. Face shields should be cleaned when necessary.

Protective Eyewear

Protective eyewear in combination with a mask must be worn to protect the eyes when spatter and splash of body fluids are anticipated and a face shield is not chosen. The OSHA Standard specifies that protective eyewear be fitted with solid side shields.[16] Eyewear should be cleaned as necessary.

Limiting Contamination

Three principal means of limiting contamination by droplets and spatter are the use of high-volume evacuation, proper patient positioning, and rubber dams. Dental personnel should also limit contamination by avoiding contact with objects such as charts, telephones, and cabinets during patient treatment procedures. A second pair of disposable gloves, such as food-handler gloves, or a sheet of plastic wrap or foil may be used over gloves when it is necessary to prevent contamination of these objects.

Hands

Hand Washing

Hands must always be washed at the start of each day, before gloving, after removal of gloves, and after touching inanimate objects likely to be contaminated by body fluids from patients. For many routine dental procedures, such as examinations and nonsurgical procedures, handwashing with plain soap appears to be adequate, since soap and water will remove transient microorganisms acquired directly or indirectly from patient contact. For surgical procedures, an antimicrobial surgical handscrub should be used.[9] Handwashing facilities should be designed to avoid cross-contamination at the scrub sink from water valve handles and soap dispensers.

Care of Hands

Precautions should be taken to avoid hand injuries during procedures. If an injury such as a needlestick occurs or gloves are torn, cut, or punctured, gloves should be removed as soon as is compatible with the patient's safety. Hands should be washed thoroughly and regloved before completing the dental procedure.

Handling Sharp Instruments and Needles

Needles, scalpel blades, and other sharp instruments should be handled carefully to prevent injuries. Syringe needles may be recapped after they are used. If a patient requires multiple injection over time from a single syringe, the needle should be recapped between each use to avoid the possibility of a needlestick injury. Needles can be safely recapped by placing the cap in a special holder, by using a forceps or other appropriate instrument to grasp the cap, or by simply laying the cap on the instrument tray and then guiding the needle into the cap until the cap can be completely seated. Therefore when recapping, the cap must not be held in the operator's hand, as this poses a great risk of needlestick injury.

Disposable needles should not be bent or broken after use. Needles should not be removed manually from disposable syringes or otherwise handled manually. Forceps or other appropriate instruments may be used to handle sharp items. Disposable syringes, needles, scalpel blades, and other sharps items should be discarded into puncture-resistant biohazard (sharps) containers that are easily accessible.

Sterilization and Disinfection

Sterilization is the process by which all forms of microorganisms, including viruses, bacteria, fungi, and spores, are destroyed. Suitable methods of sterilization include the use of steam under pressure (autoclave), dry heat, chemical vapor, and ethylene oxide gas (only for instruments that can be thoroughly cleaned and dried). Immersion in a cold chemical sterilant solution instead of the use of physical means of sterilization is not recommended for several reasons:

- Sterilization by chemical solutions cannot be monitored biologically
- Instruments sterilized by chemical solutions must be handled aseptically, rinsed in sterile water and dried with sterile towels
- Instruments sterilized by chemical solutions are not wrapped and therefore must be used immediately or stored in a sterile container

Disinfection is generally less lethal to pathogenic organisms than sterilization. The disinfection process leads to a reduction in the level of microbial contamination and covers, depending on the disinfectant used and treatment time: a broad range of activity that may extend from sterility at one extreme to a minimal reduction in microbial contamination at the other.[24] Disinfection may be accomplished by using a chemical disinfectant according to the directions on the product label. When chemical solutions are used for disinfection, manufacturer instructions must be followed carefully. Particular attention should be given to dilution requirements (if any), contact time, temperature requirements, antimicrobial activity spectrum, and reuse life. A chemical agent for disinfection (other than sodium hypochlorite) in the dental setting must be registered by the Environmental Protection Agency (EPA) as a hospital disinfectant and must be tuberculocidal. Virucidal efficacy must include, as a minimum, lipophilic and hydrophilic viruses. Table G–1 summarizes appropriate sterilization and disinfection methods for dental instruments, dental materials, and other commonly used items. Consideration should be given to the effect of sterilization or disinfection on materials and instruments. The use of a rust-inhibitor solution on instruments before autoclaving can be helpful in avoiding corrosion problems. Manufacturers should be consulted on appropriate sterilization or disinfection of specific products.

Instruments and Equipment

Surgical and other instruments that normally penetrate soft tissue or bone (for example, forceps, scalpels, bone chisels, scalers, and surgical burs) must be sterilized after each use or discarded. Instruments that are not intended to penetrate oral soft tissues or bone (such as amalgam condensers and plastic instruments) but that may come into contact with oral tissues should also be sterilized after each use. If, however, sterilization is not feasible because the instrument will be damaged by heat, the instrument should be discarded or immersed for six to 10 hours in an EPA-registered chemical sterilant according to manufacturers' instructions.

If instruments are to be stored after sterilization, they should be wrapped or bagged before sterilization, using a suitable wrap material such as muslin, clear pouches or paper as recommended by the manufacturer of the sterilizer. The wrap or bag should be sealed with appropriate tape. Pins, staples, or paper clips should not be used because these make holes in the wrap that permit entry of microorganisms. After sterilization, the instruments should be stored in the sealed packages until they are used. Process indicators should be used with each load. Biologic monitors should be used routinely to verify the adequacy of sterilization cycles. Weekly verification should be adequate for most dental practices.[6,15,25]

Instruments and equipment that come in contact with intact skin, that may be exposed to spatter or spray of body fluids, or that may have been touched by contaminated hands (such as physical measurement devices and amalgamators) should be disinfected.

Instruments and equipment intended for sterilization or disinfection procedures must first be carefully prepared. Patient debris and body fluids must be removed from the instruments and surfaces before sterilization or disinfection. This can be done by scrubbing the instruments with hot water and soap or detergent or by using a device such as an ultrasonic cleaner with an appropriate cleaning solution. Dental personnel responsible for handling instruments should wear heavy-duty utility gloves to prevent hand injuries. After cleaning, the instruments should be dried before being wrapped or packaged.

Handpieces

Although no documented cases of disease transmission have been associated with high-speed dental handpieces, low-speed handpiece components used intraorally or prophy an-

Table G-1   Sterilization of Dental Instruments, Materials, and Some Commonly Used Items*

	STEAM AUTOCLAVE	DRY HEAT OVEN	CHEMICAL VAPOR	ETHYLENE OXIDE†	OTHER METHODS AND COMMENTS
Angle attachments*	+	+	+	++	
Burs					
Carbon steel	−	++	++	++	Discard
Steel	+	++	++	++	Discard
Tungsten-carbide	+	++	+	++	Discard
Condensers	++	++	++	++	
Dapen dishes	++	+	+	++	
Endodontic instruments (broaches, files, reamers)	++	++	++	++	
Stainless steel handles	+	++	++	++	
Stainless steel w/plastic handles	++	++	−	++	
Fluoride gel trays					
Heat resistant plastic	++	=	−	++	
Nonheat resistant plastic	=	=	−	++	Discard (++)
Glass slabs	++	++	++	++	
Hand instruments					
Carbon steel	−	++	++	++	
	(Steam autoclave with chemical protection [2% sodium nitrite])				
Stainless steel	++	++	++	++	
Handpieces*	(++)*	−	(+)★	++	
Contra-angles	++	−	++	++	
Prophylaxis angles* (disposable preferred)	+	+	+	+	Discard (++)
Impression trays					
Aluminum metal	++	+	++	++	
Chrome-plated	++	++	++	++	
Custom acrylic resin	=	=	=	++	Discard (++)
Plastic	=	=	=	++	Discard (++) preferred
Instruments in packs	++	+ Small packs	++	++ Small packs	

*Since manufacturers use a variety of alloys and materials in these products, confirmation with the equipment manufacturers is recommended, especially for handpieces and their attachments.
†Ethylene oxide should be used only to sterilize instruments that can be thoroughly cleaned and dried.
+Effective and acceptable method.
++Effective and preferred method.
−Effective method, but risk of damage to materials.
=Ineffective method with risk of damage to materials.

Table G-1 Sterilization of Dental Instruments, Materials, and Some Commonly Used Items*—cont'd

	STEAM AUTOCLAVE	DRY HEAT OVEN	CHEMICAL VAPOR	ETHYLENE OXIDE†	OTHER METHODS AND COMMENTS
Instrument tray setups					
Restorative or surgical	+	+	+	++	
	Size limit		Size limit	Size limit	
Mirrors	−	++	++	++	
Needles					
Disposable	=	=	=	=	Discard (++)
					Do not reuse
Nitrous oxide					
Nose piece	(++)*	=	(++)*	++	
Hoses	(++)*	=	(++)*	++	
Orthodontic pliers					
High-quality stainless	++	++	++	++	
Low-quality stainless	−	++	++	++	
w/plastic parts	=	=	=	++	
Pluggers and condensers	++	++	++	++	
Polishing wheels and disks					
Garnet and cuttle	=	−	−	++	
Rag	++	−	+	++	
Rubber	+	−	−	++	
Protheses, removable	−	−	−	+	
Rubber dam equipment					
Carbon steel clamps	−	++	++	++	
Metal frames	++	++	++	++	
Plastic frames	−	−	−	++	
Punches	−	++	++	++	
Stainless steel clamps	++	++	++	++	
Rubber items					
Prophylaxis cups	−	−	−	++	Discard (++)
Saliva evacuators, ejectors (plastic)	−	−	−	−	Discard (++) (single use/ disposable)
Stones					
Diamond	+	++	++	++	
Polishing	++	+	++	++	
Sharpening	++	++	++	−	
Surgical instruments					
Stainless steel	++	++	++	++	
Ultrasonic scaling tips	+	=	=	++	
Water-air syringe tips	++	++	++	++	Discard (++)
X-ray equipment					
Plastic film holders	(++)*	=	(+)*	++	
Collimating devices	−	=	=	++	

gles, sterilization between patients with acceptable methods that ensure internal, as well as external sterility is recommended. Acceptable sterilization methods include steam under pressure (autoclave), dry heat, or chemical vapor. Ethylene oxide sterilization is not recommended for high-speed dental handpieces, low-speed handpiece components used intraorally, or prophy angles. Disposable prophy angles are available and are to be discarded after one-time use.

Manufacturer instructions must be followed for proper sterilization of handpieces and prophy angles and for the use and maintenance of waterlines and check valves. The first step before sterilization is to flush the handpiece with water by running it for 20 to 30 seconds and discharging the water into a sink or container. An ultrasonic cleaner should be used to remove adherent material, but only if recommended by the handpiece manufacturer. Otherwise, the handpiece should be scrubbed thoroughly with a detergent and hot water. Many manufacturers recommend spraying a cleaner/lubricant into the assembled handpiece before and after sterilization. If in doubt as to whether a handpiece can be sterilized, contact the manufacturer. Some manufacturers will replace the handpiece components that cannot be sterilized, making the handpiece sterilizable. This is often automatically done when a handpiece is serviced.

Air/Water Syringes and Ultrasonic Scalers

Units should be flushed as described for handpieces. These attachments should be sterilized in the same manner as handpieces, or in accordance with manufacturer instructions. It is recommended that removable or disposable tips be used for these instruments if used only one time for one patient.

X-ray Equipment and Films

Protective coverings or disinfectants should be used to prevent microbial contamination of position-indicating devices. Intraorally contaminated film packets should be handled in a manner to prevent cross-contamination. Contaminated packets should be handled in a manner to prevent cross-contamination. Contaminated packets should be opened in the darkroom, using disposable gloves. The films should be dropped out of the packets without touching the films. The contaminated packets should be accumulated in a disposable towel. After all packets have been opened, they should be discarded and the gloves removed. The films can then be processed without contaminating darkroom equipment with microorganisms from the patient.[26] Alternatively, film packets can be placed in protective pouches before use. The uncontaminated packets can then be dropped out of the pouches before processing.

Operatory Surfaces

Countertops and dental equipment surfaces such as light handles, X-ray unit heads, amalgamators, cabinet and drawer pulls, tray tables, and chair switches are likely to become contaminated with potentially infectious materials during treatment procedures. These surfaces can be covered or disinfected. Surfaces can be covered with plastic wrap, aluminum foil, or impervious-backed absorbent paper. These protective coverings should be changed between patients and when contaminated.

Alternatively, surfaces can be precleaned to remove extraneous organic matter and then disinfected with an EPA-registered disinfectant that is tuberculocidal following manufacturer instructions. These include certain combination synthetic phenolics and iodophors, phenolic-alcohol combinations, and chlorine compounds. A solution of sodium hypochlorite (household bleach) prepared fresh daily is an effective germicide. Concentrations of sodium hypochlorite ranging from 5,000 to 500 parts per million, achieved by diluting household bleach in a ratio ranging from 1:10 to 1:100, is effective, depending on the amount or organic matter (blood and mucus) present on the surface to be cleaned and disinfected. Sodium hypochlorite should be used with caution because it is corrosive to some metals, especially aluminum. Corrosiveness is less of a problem with some commercial disinfectants. Glutaraldehydes of 2 and 3.2 percent strength are not suitable for this purpose. Surfaces should be disinfected between patients and when they are visibly contaminated by splashes of body fluids.

Housekeeping surfaces including floors, sinks, and related objects are not likely to be associated with the transmission of infection. Therefore extraordinary attempts to disinfect these surfaces are not necessary. However, cleaning and the removal of visible soil should be undertaken on a routine basis. Cleaners with germicidal activity may be used.

Impressions, Prostheses, Casts, Wax Rims, Jaw Relation Records

Items such as impressions, jaw relation records, casts, prosthetic restorations, and devices that have been in the patient's mouth should be properly disinfected before shipment to a dental laboratory (Table G-2). Disinfected impressions that are sent to a dental laboratory should be labeled as such to prevent duplication of the disinfection protocol. Impressions must be rinsed to remove saliva, blood, and debris and then disinfected. Impressions can be disinfected by immersion in any compatible disinfecting product. Since the compatibility of an impression material with a disinfectant varies, manufacturer recommendations for proper disinfection should be followed.[27] The use of disinfectants requiring time of no more than 30 minutes for disinfection is recommended.

Disposal of Waste Materials

Disposable materials such as gloves, masks, wipes, paper drapes, and surface covers that are contaminated with body fluids should be carefully handled with gloves and discarded in sturdy, impervious plastic bags to minimize human contact. Blood, disinfectants, and sterilants may be carefully poured down a drain connected to a sanitary sewer system. Care should be taken to ensure compliance with applicable local regulations. It is recommended

---

Table G-2   Disinfection of Prostheses, Casts, Wax Rims, and Jaw Relation Records

MATERIAL	METHOD
Stone casts	Spray or immerse in hypochlorite or iodophor
Fixed (metal/porcelain)	Immerse in glutaradehyde
Removable dentures (acrylic/porcelain)	Immerse in iodophors or chlorine compound
Removable partials (metal/acrylic)	Immerse in iodophors or chlorine compound
Wax rims/bites	Spray, wipe, spray with iodophors

that drains be flushed or purged each night to reduce bacteria accumulation and growth. Sharp items such as needles and scalpel blades should be placed in puncture-resistant containers marked with the biohazard symbol. Human tissue may be handled in the same manner as sharp items but should not be placed in the same container. Regulated medical waste (sharps and tissues, for example) should be disposed of according to the requirements established by local or state environmental regulatory agencies.

PRACTICES FOR THE DENTAL LABORATORY

Dental laboratories should institute appropriate infection control programs.[28] Such programs should be coordinated with the dental office.

Receiving area. A receiving area should be established separate from the production area. Countertops and work surfaces should be cleaned and then disinfected daily with an appropriate surface disinfectant used according to manufacturer directions.

Incoming cases. Unless the laboratory employee knows that the case has been disinfected by the dental office, all cases should be disinfected as they are received. Containers should be sterilized or disinfected after each use. Packing materials should be discarded to avoid cross-contamination.

Disposal of waste materials. Solid waste that is soaked or saturated with body fluids should be placed in sealed, sturdy impervious bags. The bag should be disposed of following regulations established by local or state environmental agencies.

Production area. Persons working in the production area should wear a clean uniform or laboratory coat, a face mask, protective eyewear, and disposable gloves. Work surfaces and equipment should be kept free of debris and disinfected daily. Any instruments, attachments, and materials to be used with new prostheses or appliances should be maintained separately from those to be used with prostheses or appliances that have already been inserted in the mouth. Ragwheels can be washed and autoclaved after each case. Brushes and other equipment should be disinfected at least daily. A small amount of pumice should be dispensed in small disposable containers for individual use on each case. The excess should be discarded. A liquid disinfectant (1:20 sodium hypochlorite solution) can serve as a mixing medium for pumice.[29] Adding three parts green soap to the disinfectant solution will keep the pumice suspended.

Outgoing cases. Each case should be disinfected before it is returned to the dental office. Dentists should be informed about infection control procedures that are used in the dental laboratory.

SELECTED READINGS

1. Council on Dental Materials and Devices and Council on Dental Therapeutics: Infection control in the dental office, *JADA* 97(4):673-7, 1978.
2. Council of Dental Therapeutics and Council on Prosthetic Services and Dental Laboratory Relations: Guidelines for infection control in the dental office and the commercial dental laboratory, *JADA* 110(6):969-72, 1985.
3. Council on Dental Materials, Instruments and Equipment: *Dentists' desk reference,* Chicago, 1983, American Dental Association.

4. Council on Dental Therapeutics: *Accepted dental therapeutics,* Chicago,1984, American Dental Association.

5. Council on Dental Materials, Instruments and Equipment, Council on Dental Practice, and Council on Dental Therapeutics: Infection control recommendations for the dental office and the dental laboratory, *JADA* 116(2):241-8, 1988.

6. Council on Dental Materials, Instruments and Equipment, Council on Dental Practice, and Council on Dental Therapeutics: Infection control recommendations for the dental office and the dental laboratory, *JADA* 123(8) (supplement), 1992.

7. American Dental Association, American Academy of Oral Medicine: Dental management of the HIV-infected patient, *JADA* 126(12) (supplement), 1995.

8. Council on Dental Therapeutics and Council on Dental Materials, Instruments and equipment: *Monograph on safety and infection control,* ed 1, Chicago, 1990, American Dental Association.

9. Department of Veterans Affairs, American Dental Association, and Department of Human and Health Services: Infection control in the dental environment [video and training manual], Chicago, 1989, American Dental Association.

10. American Dental Association: *The American Dental Association regulatory compliance manual,* Chicago, 1990, American Dental Association.

11. American Dental Association: *OSHA: what you must know* [video], Chicago, 1992, American Dental Association.

12. Centers for Disease Control: Recommended infection control practices for dentistry, *MMWR* 35:237-42, 1986.

13. Centers for Disease Control: Recommendations for prevention of HIV transmission in health care settings, *MMWR* 36(supplement 2S), 1987.

14. Centers for Disease Control: Recommendations for prevention of transmission of human immunodeficiency virus and hepatitis B virus to patients during exposure-prone invasive procedures, *MMWR* 40:1-9, 1991.

15. Centers for Disease Control and Prevention: Recommended infection-control practices for dentistry, 1993, *MMWR* 41(RR-8):1-12, 1993.

16. U.S. Department of Labor, Occupational Safety and Health Administration: 29 CFR Part 1910.1030, Occupational exposure to bloodborne pathogens, final rule, *Federal Register* 56(235):64004-182, 1991.

17. Centers for Disease Control: Protection against viral hepatitis, *MMWR* 39:1-26, 1990.

18. Henderson DK, Fahey BJ, Willy M et al.: Risk for occupational transmission of human immunodeficiency virus type 1 (HIV-1) associated with clinical exposures, *Ann Intern Med* 113:740-46, 1990.

19. American Dental Association: Hepatitis B vaccination and post-vaccination testing for dentists and their staffs, 1987 Transactions, Chicago, 1988, American Dental Association 509.

20. Centers for Disease Control:. Recommendations for preventing transmission of infection with human T-lymphotropic virus type III/lymphadenopathy-associated virus in the workplace, *MMWR* 34:681-95, 1985.

21. Ready MA, Schuster GS, Wilson JT Hanes CM: Effects of dental medicaments on examination glove permeability, *J Prosthet Dent* 61:499-503, 1989.

22. U.S. Food and Drug Administration: Allergic reactions to latex-containing medical devices, *FDA Medical Alert* MDA91-1, March 29, 1991.

23. Stewart J: Professional management of allergic hypersensitivity reactions to gloves, *J Mich Dent Assoc* 72(3)148-9, 1990.

24. Block SS: *Disinfection, sterilization and preservation,* ed 4, Philadelphia, 1991, Lea & Febiger.

25. Council on Dental Materials, Instruments and Equipment, Council of Dental Practice and Council on Dental Therapeutics: Biological indicators for verifying sterilization, *JADA* 117(5):653-4, 1988.
26. Council on Dental Materials, Instruments and Equipment: Recommendations for radiographic darkrooms and darkroom practices, *JADA* 104(6):886-7, 1982.
27. Council on Dental Materials, Instruments and Equipment: Disinfection of impressions, *JADA* 122(3):110, 1991.
28. National Board for Certification of Laboratories: Infection control requirements for certified dental laboratories, Alexandria, Virginia, National Association of Dental Laboratories, 1986.
29. Council of Dental Therapeutics, Council on Prosthetic Services and Dental Laboratory Relations: Guidelines for infection control in the dental office and the commercial dental laboratory, *JADA* 110(6)969-72, 1985.

THE OSHA BLOODBORNE PATHOGENS STANDARD

XI. The Standard

General Industry

Part 1910 of title 29 of the Code of Federal Regulations is amended as follows:

PART 1910—[AMENDED]

Subpart Z—[Amended]

1. The general authority citation for subpart Z of 29 CFR part 1910 continues to read as follows and a new citation for 1910.1030 is added:

Authority: Secs. 6 and 8. Occupational Safety and Health Act. 29 U.S.C. 655, 657, Secretary of Labor's Orders Nos. 12-71 (36 FR 8754). 8-76 (41 FR 25059), or 9-83 (48 FR 35736), as applicable; and 20 CFR part 1911.

★ ★ ★ ★ ★

Section 1910.1030 also issued under 29 U.S.C. 653.

★ ★ ★ ★ ★

2. Section 1910.1030 is added to read as follows:

1910.1030 Bloodborne Pathogens.

(a) *Scope and Application.* This section applies to all occupational exposure to blood or other potentially infectious materials as defined by paragraph (b) of this section.

(b) *Definitions.* For purposes of this section, the following shall apply:

Assistant Secretary means the Assistant Secretary of Labor for Occupational Safety and Health, or designated representative.

Blood means human blood, human blood components, and products made from human blood.

Bloodborne Pathogens means pathogenic microorganisms that are present in human blood and can cause disease in humans. These pathogens include, but are not limited to, hepatitis B virus (HBV) and human immunodeficiency virus (HIV).

Clinical Laboratory means a workplace where diagnostic or other screening procedures are performed on blood or other potentially infectious materials.

Contaminated means the presence or the reasonably anticipated presence of blood or other potentially infectious materials on an item or surface.

Contaminated Laundry means laundry that has been soiled with blood or other potentially infectious materials or may contain sharps.

Reprinted from: Department of Labor, Occupational Safety and Health Administration. 29 CFR Part 1910.1030. Occupational exposure to bloodborne pathogens; Final Rule. Federal Register 56(No. 235):645175-64182, December 6, 1991.

Contaminated Sharps means any contaminated object that can penetrate the skin, including, but not limited to, needles, scalpels, broken glass, broken capillary tubes, and exposed ends of dental wires.

Decontamination means the use of physical or chemical means to remove, inactivate, or destroy bloodborne pathogens on a surface or item to the point where they are no longer capable of transmitting infectious particles and the surface or item is rendered safe for handling, use, or disposal.

Director means the Director of the National Institute for Occupational Safety and Health, U.S. Department of Health and Human Services, or designated representative.

Engineering Controls means controls (e.g., sharps disposal containers, self-sheathing needles) that isolate or remove the bloodborne pathogens hazard from the workplace.

Exposure Incident means a specific eye, mouth, other mucous membrane, non-intact skin, or parenteral contact with blood or other potentially infectious materials that results from the performance of an employee's duties.

Handwashing Facilities means a facility providing an adequate supply of running potable water, soap and single use towels or hot air drying machines.

Licensed Healthcare Professional is a person whose legally permitted scope of practice allows him or her to independently perform the activities required by paragraph (f) Hepatitis B Vaccination and Post-exposure Evaluation and Follow-up.

HBV means hepatitis B virus.

HIV means human immunodeficiency virus.

Occupational Exposure means reasonably anticipated skin, eye, mucous membrane, or parenteral contact with blood or other potentially infectious materials that may result from the performance of an employee's duties.

Other Potentially Infectious Materials means

(1) The following human body fluids: semen, vaginal secretions, cerebrospinal fluid, synovial fluid, pleural fluid, pericardial fluid, peritoneal fluid, amniotic fluid, saliva in dental procedures, any body fluid that is visibly contaminated with blood, and all body fluids in situations where it is difficult or impossible to differentiate between body fluids;

(2) Any unfixed tissue or organ (other than intact skin) from a human (living or dead), and

(3) HIV-containing cell or tissue cultures, organ cultures, and HIV - or HBV-containing culture medium or other solutions; and blood, organs, or other tissues from experimental animals infected with HIV or HBV.

Parenteral means piercing mucous membranes or the skin barrier through such events as needlesticks, human bites, cuts, and abrasions.

Personal Protective Equipment is specialized clothing or equipment worn by an employee for protection against a hazard. General work clothes (e.g., uniforms, pants, shirts or blouses) not intended to function as protection against a hazard are not considered to be personal protective equipment.

Production Facility means a facility engaged in industrial-scale, large-volume or high concentration production of HIV or HBV.

Regulated Waste means liquid or semi-liquid blood or other potentially infectious materials; contaminated items that would release blood or other potentially infectious materials in a liquid or semi-liquid state if compressed; items that are caked with dried blood or other potentially infectious materials and are capable of releasing these materials during handling; contaminated sharps; and pathological and microbiological wastes containing blood or other potentially infectious materials.

Research Laboratory means a laboratory producing or using research-laboratory-scale amounts of HIV or HBV. Research laboratories may produce high concentrations of HIV or HBV but not in the volume found in production facilities.

Source Individual means any individual, living or dead, whose blood or other potentially infectious materials may be a source of occupational exposure to the employee. Examples include, but are not limited to, hospital and clinic patients; clients in institutions for the developmentally disabled; trauma victims; clients of drug and alcohol treatment facilities; residents of hospices and nursing homes; human remains; and individuals who donate or sell blood or blood components.

Sterilize means the use of a physical or chemical procedure to destroy all microbial life, including highly resistant bacterial endospores.

Universal Precautions is an approach to infection control. According to the concept of Universal Precautions, all human blood and certain human body fluids are treated as if known to be infectious for HIV, HBV, and other bloodborne pathogens.

Work Practice Controls means controls that reduce the likelihood of exposure by altering the manner in which a task is performed (e.g., prohibiting recapping of needles by a two-handed technique).

(c) *Exposure control—(1) Exposure Control Plan.* (i) Each employer having an employee(s) with occupational exposure as defined by paragraph (b) of this section shall establish a written Exposure Control Plan designed to eliminate or minimize employee exposure.

(ii) The Exposure Control Plan shall contain at least the following elements:

(A) The exposure determination required by paragraph (c)(2).

(B) The schedule and method of implementation for paragraphs (d) Methods of Compliance, (e) HIV and HBV Research Laboratories and Production Facilities, (f) Hepatitis B Vaccination and Post-Exposure Evaluation and Follow-up, (g) Communication of Hazards to Employees, and (h) Recordkeeping, of this standard, and

(C) The procedure for the evaluation of circumstances surrounding exposure incidents as required by paragraph (f)(3)(i) of this standard.

(iii) Each employer shall ensure that a copy of the Exposure Control Plan is accessible to employees in accordance with 29 CFR 1910.20(e).

(iv) The Exposure Control Plan shall be reviewed and updated at least annually and whenever necessary to reflect new or modified tasks and procedures that affect occupational exposure and to reflect new or revised employee positions with occupational exposure.

(v) The Exposure Control Plan shall be made available to the Assistant Secretary and the Director upon request for examination and copying.

(2) *Exposure determination.* (i) Each employer who has an employee(s) with occupational exposure as defined by paragraph (b) of this section shall prepare an exposure determination. This exposure determination shall contain the following:

(A) A list of all job classifications in which all employees in those job classifications have occupational exposure;

(B) A list of job classifications in which some employees have occupational exposure, and

(C) A list of all tasks and procedures or groups of closely related tasks and procedures in which occupational exposure occurs and that are performed by employees in job classifications listed in accordance with the provisions of paragraph (c)(2)(i)(B) of this standard.

(ii) This exposure determination shall be made without regard to the use of personal protective equipment.

(d) *Methods of compliance*—*(1) General*—Universal precautions shall be observed to prevent contact with blood or other potentially infectious materials. Under circumstances in which differentiation between body fluid types is difficult or impossible, all body fluids shall be considered potentially infectious materials.

(2) *Engineering and work practice controls.* (i) Engineering and work practice controls shall be used to eliminate or minimize employee exposure. Where occupational exposure remains after institution of these controls, personal protective equipment shall also be used.

(ii) Engineering controls shall be examined and maintained or replaced on a regular schedule to ensure their effectiveness.

(iii) Employers shall provide handwashing facilities that are readily accessible to employees.

(iv) When provision of handwashing facilities is not feasible, the employer shall provide either an appropriate antiseptic hand cleanser in conjunction with clean cloth/paper towels or antiseptic towelettes. When antiseptic hand cleansers or towelettes are used, hands shall be washed with soap and running water as soon as feasible.

(v) Employers shall ensure that employees wash their hands immediately or as soon as feasible after removal of gloves or other personal protective equipment.

(vi) Employers shall ensure that employees wash hands and any other skin with soap and water, or flush mucous membranes with water immediately or as soon as feasible following contact of such body areas with blood or other potentially infectious materials.

(vii) Contaminated needles and other contaminated sharps shall not be bent, recapped, or removed except as noted in paragraphs (d)(2)(vii)(A) and (d)(2)(vii)(B) below. Shearing or breaking of contaminated needles is prohibited.

(A) Contaminated needles and other contaminated sharps shall not be recapped or removed unless the employer can demonstrate that no alternative is feasible or that such action is required by a specific medical procedure.

(B) Such recapping or needle removal must be accomplished through the use of a mechanical device or a one-handed technique.

(viii) Immediately or as soon as possible after use, contaminated reusable sharps shall be placed in appropriate containers until properly reprocessed. These containers shall be:

(A) Puncture resistant;

(B) Labeled or color-coded in accordance with this standard;

(C) Leakproof on the sides and bottom; and

(D) In accordance with the requirements set forth in paragraph (d)(4)(ii)(E) for reusable sharps.

(ix) Eating, drinking, smoking, applying cosmetics or lip balm, and handling contact lenses are prohibited in work areas where there is a reasonable likelihood of occupational exposure.

(x) Food and drink shall not be kept in refrigerators, freezers, shelves, cabinets or on countertops or benchtops where blood or other potentially infectious materials are present.

(xi) All procedures involving blood or other potentially infectious materials shall be performed in such a manner as to minimize splashing, spraying, spattering, and generation of droplets of these substances.

(xii) Mouth pipetting/suctioning of blood or other potentially infectious materials is prohibited.

(xiii) Specimens of blood or other potentially infectious materials shall be placed in a container which prevents leakage during collection, handling, processing, storage, transport, or shipping.

(A) The container for storage, transport, or shipping shall be labeled or color-coded according to paragraph (g)(1)(i) and closed prior to being stored, transported, or shipped. When a facility utilizes Universal Precautions in the handling of all specimens, the labeling/color-coding of specimens is not necessary provided containers are recognizable as containing specimens. This exemption only applies while such specimens/containers remain within the facility. Labeling or color-coding in accordance with paragraph (g)(1)(i) is required when such specimens/containers leave the facility.

(B) If outside contamination of the primary container occurs, the primary container shall be placed within a second container that prevents leakage during handling, processing, storage, transport, or shipping and is labeled or color-coded according to the requirements of this standard.

(C) If the specimen could puncture the primary container, the primary container shall be placed within a secondary container that is puncture-resistant in addition to the above characteristics.

(xiv) Equipment that may become contaminated with blood or other potentially infectious materials shall be examined prior to servicing or shipping and shall be decontaminated as necessary, unless the employer can demonstrate that decontamination of such equipment or portions of such equipment is not feasible.

(A) A readily observable label in accordance with paragraph (g)(1)(i)(H) shall be attached to the equipment stating which portions remain contaminated.

(B) The employer shall ensure that this information is conveyed to all affected employees, the servicing representative, and/or the manufacturer, as appropriate, prior to handling, servicing, or shipping so that appropriate precautions will be taken.

(3) Personal protective equipment—(i) Provision. When there is occupational exposure, the employer shall provide, at no cost to the employee, appropriate personal protective equipment such as, but not limited to, gloves, gowns, laboratory coats, face shields or masks and eye protection, and mouthpieces, resuscitation bags, pocket masks, or other ventilation devices. Personal protective equipment will be considered "appropriate" only if it does not permit blood or other potentially infectious materials to pass through to or reach the employee's work clothes, street clothes, undergarments, skin, eyes, mouth, or other mucous membranes under normal conditions of use and for the duration of time which the protective equipment will be used.

(ii) Use. The employer shall ensure that the employee uses appropriate personal protective equipment unless the employer shows that the employee temporarily and briefly declined to use personal protective equipment when, under rare and extraordinary circumstances, it was the employee's professional judgement that in the specific instance its use would have prevented the delivery of health care or public safety services or would have posed an increased hazard to the safety of the worker or co-worker. When the employee makes this judgement, the circumstances shall be investigated and documented in order to determine whether changes can be instituted to prevent such occurences in the future.

(iii) Accessibility. The employer shall ensure that appropriate personal protective equipment in the appropriate sizes is readily accessible at the worksite or is issued to employees. Hypoallergenic gloves, glove liners, powderless gloves, or other similar alternatives shall be readily accessible to those employees who are allergic to the gloves normally provided.

(iv) Cleaning, Laundering, and Disposal. The employer shall clean, launder, and dispose of personal protective equipment required by paragraphs (d) and (e) of this standard, at no cost to the employee.

(v) Repair and Replacement. The employer shall repair or replace personal protective equipment as needed to maintain its effectiveness, at no cost to the employee.

(vi) If a garment(s) is penetrated by blood or other potentially infectious materials, the garment(s) shall be removed immediately or as soon as feasible.

(vii) All personal protective equipment shall be removed prior to leaving the work area.

(viii) When personal protective equipment is removed it shall be placed in an appropriately designated area or container for storage, washing, decontamination or disposal.

(ix) Gloves. Gloves shall be worn when it can be reasonably anticipated that the employee may have hand contact with blood, other potentially infectious materials, mucous membranes, and non-intact skin; when performing vascular access procedures except as specified in paragraph (d)(3)(ix)(D); and when handling or touching contaminated items or surfaces.

(A) Disposable (single use) gloves such as surgical or examination gloves, shall be replaced as soon as practical when contaminated or as soon as feasible if they are torn, punctured, or when their ability to function as a barrier is compromised.

(B) Disposable (single use) gloves shall not be washed or decontaminated for re-use.

(C) Utility gloves may be decontaminated for re-use if the integrity of the glove is not compromised. However, they must be discarded if they are cracked, peeling, torn, punctured, or exhibit other signs of deterioration or when their ability to function as a barrier is compromised.

(D) If an employer in a volunteer blood donation center judges that routine gloving for all phlebotomies is not necessary then the employer shall:

(1) Periodically reevaluate this policy;

(2) Make gloves available to all employees who wish to use them for phlebotomy;

(3) Not discourage the use of gloves for phlebotomy; and

(4) Require that gloves be used for phlebotomy in the following circumstances:

(i) When the employee has cuts, scratches, or other breaks in his or her skin;

(ii) When the employee judges that hand contamination with blood may occur, for example, when performing phlebotomy on an uncooperative source individual; and

(iii) When the employee is receiving training in phlebotomy.

(x) Masks, Eye Protection, and Face Shields. Masks in combination with eye protection devices, such as goggles or glasses with solid side shields, or chin-length face shields, shall be worn whenever splashes, spray, spatter, or droplets of blood or other potentially infectious materials may be generated and eye, nose, or mouth contamination can be reasonably anticipated.

(xi) Gowns, Aprons, and Other Protective Body Clothing. Appropriate protective clothing such as, but not limited to, gowns, aprons, lab coats, clinic jackets, or similar outer garments shall be worn in occupational exposure situations. The type and characteristics will depend upon the task and degree of exposure anticipated.

(xii) Surgical caps or hoods and/or shoe covers or boots shall be worn in instances when gross contamination can reasonably be anticipated (e.g., autopsies, orthopaedic surgery).

(4) *Housekeeping.* (i) General. Employers shall ensure that the worksite is maintained in a clean and sanitary condition. The employer shall determine and implement an appropriate written schedule for cleaning and method of decontamination based upon the location within the facility, type of surface to be cleaned, type of soil present, and tasks or procedures being performed in the area.

(ii) All equipment and environmental and working surfaces shall be cleaned and de-contaminated after contact with blood or other potentially infectious materials.

(A) Contaminated work surfaces shall be decontaminated with an appropriate disinfectant after completion of procedures; immediately or as soon as feasible when surfaces are overtly contaminated or after any spill of blood or other potentially infectious materials; and at the end of the work shift if the surface may have become contaminated since the last cleaning.

(B) Protective coverings, such as plastic wrap, aluminum foil, or imperviously-backed absorbent paper used to cover equipment and environmental surfaces, shall be removed and replaced as soon as feasible when they become overtly contaminated or at the end of the workshift if they may have become contaminated during the shift.

(C) All bins, pails, cans, and similar receptacles intended for reuse which have a reasonable likelihood for becoming contaminated with blood or other potentially infectious materials shall be inspected and decontaminated on a regularly scheduled basis and cleaned and decontaminated immediately or as soon as feasible upon visible contamination.

(D) Broken glassware that may be contaminated shall not be picked up directly with the hands. It shall be cleaned up using mechanical means, such as a brush and dust pan, tongs, or forceps.

(E) Reusable sharps that are contaminated with blood or other potentially infectious materials shall not be stored or processed in a manner that requires employees to reach by hand into the containers where these sharps have been placed.

(iii) Regulated Waste.

(A) Contaminated Sharps Discarding and Containment. (1) Contaminated sharps shall be discarded immediately or as soon as feasible in containers that are:

(i) Closable;

(ii) Puncture resistant;

(iii) Leakproof on sides and bottom; and

(iv) Labeled or color-coded in accordance with paragraph (g)(1)(i) of this standard.

(2) During use, containers for contaminated sharps shall be:

(i) Easily accessible to personnel and located as close as is feasible to the immediate area where sharps are used or can be reasonably anticipated to be found (e.g., laundries);

(ii) Maintained upright throughout use; and

(iii) Replaced routinely and not be allowed to overfill.

(3) When moving containers of contaminated sharps from the area of use, the containers shall be:

(i) Closed immediately prior to removal or replacement to prevent spillage or protrusion of contents during handling, storage, transport, or shipping;

(ii) Placed in a secondary container if leakage is possible. The second container shall be:

(A) Closable;

(B) Constructed to contain all contents and prevent leakage during handling, storage, transport, or shipping; and

(C) Labeled or color-coded according to paragraph (g)(1)(i) of this standard.

(4) Reusable containers shall not be opened, emptied, or cleaned manually or in any other manner which would expose employees to the risk of percutaneous injury.

(B) Other Regulated Waste Containment. *(1)* Regulated waste shall be placed in containers which are:

(i) Closable;

(ii) Constructed to contain all contents and prevent leakage of fluids during handling, storage, transport or shipping;

(iii) Labeled or color-coded in accordance with paragraph (g)(1)(i) of this standard; and

(iv) Closed prior to removal to prevent spillage or protrusion of contents during handling, storage, transport, or shipping.

(2) If outside contamination of the regulated waste container occurs, it shall be placed in a second container. The second container shall be:

(i) Closable;

(ii) Constructed to contain all contents and prevent leakage of fluids during handling, storage, transport or shipping;

(iii) Labeled or color-coded in accordance with paragraph (g)(1)(i) of this standard; and

(iv) Closed prior to removal to prevent spillage or protrusion of contents during handling, storage, transport, or shipping.

(C) Disposal of all regulated waste shall be in accordance with applicable regulations of the United States, States and Territories, and political subdivisions of States and Territories.

(iv) Laundry.

(A) Contaminated laundry shall be handled as little as possible with a minimum of agitation.

(1) Contaminated laundry shall be bagged or containerized at the location where it was used and shall not be sorted or rinsed in the location of use.

(2) Contaminated laundry shall be placed and transported in bags or containers labeled or color-coded in accordance with paragraph (g)(1)(i) of this standard. When a facility utilizes Universal Precautions in the handling of all soiled laundry, alternative labeling or color-coding is sufficient if it permits all employees to recognize the containers as requiring compliance with Universal Precautions.

(3) Whenever contaminated laundry is wet and presents a reasonable likelihood of soak-through or leakage from the bag or container, the laundry shall be placed and transported in bags or containers which prevent soak-through and/or leakage of fluids to the exterior.

(B) The employer shall ensure that employees who have contact with contaminated laundry wear protective gloves and other appropriate personal protective equipment.

(C) When a facility ships contaminated laundry off-site to a second facility which does not utilize Universal Precautions in the handling of all laundry, the facility generating the contaminated laundry must place such laundry in bags or containers which are labeled or color-coded in accordance with paragraph (g)(1)(i).

(e) *HIV and HBV Research Laboratories and Production Facilities.* See original publication for this information.

(f) *Hepatitis B vaccination and post-exposure evaluation and follow-up—(1) General.* (i) The employer shall make available the hepatitis B vaccine and vaccination series to all employees who have occupational exposure, and post-exposure evaluation and follow-up to all employees who have had an exposure incident.

(ii) The employer shall ensure that all medical evaluations and procedures, including the hepatitis B vaccine and vaccination series and post-exposure evaluation and follow-up, including prophylaxis are:

(A) Made available at no cost to the employee;

(B) Made available to the employee at a reasonable time and place;

(C) Performed by or under the supervision of a licensed physician or by or under the supervision of another licensed healthcare professional; and

(D) Provided according to recommendations of the U.S. Public Health Service current at the time these evaluations and procedures take place, except as specified by this paragraph (f).

(iii) The employer shall ensure that all laboratory tests are conducted by an accredited laboratory at no cost to the employee.

(2) *Hepatitis B Vaccination.* (i) Hepatitis B vaccination shall be made available after the employee has received the training required in paragraph (g)(2)(vii)(I) and within 10 working days of initial assignment to all employees who have occupational exposure unless the employee has previously received the complete hepatitis B vaccination series, antibody testing has revealed that the employee is immune, or the vaccine is contraindicated for medical reasons.

(ii) The employer shall not make participation in a prescreening program a prerequisite for receiving hepatitis B vaccination.

(iii) If the employee initially declines hepatitis B vaccination but at a later date while still covered under the standard decides to accept the vaccination, the employer shall make available hepatitis B vaccination at that time.

(iv) The employer shall assure that employees who decline to accept hepatitis B vaccination offered by the employer sign the statement (Form H-1).

(v) If a routine booster dose(s) of hepatitis B vaccine is recommended by the U.S. Public Health Service at a future date, such booster dose(s) shall be made available in accordance with section (f)(1)(ii).

(3) *Post-exposure Evaluation and Follow-up.* Following a report of an exposure incident, the employer shall make immediately available to the exposed employee a confidential medical evaluation and follow-up, including at least the following elements:

(i) Documentation of the route(s) of exposure, and the circumstances under which the exposure incident occurred;

(ii) Identification and documentation of the source individual, unless the employer can establish that identification is infeasible or prohibited by state or local law;

(A) The source individual's blood shall be tested as soon as feasible and after consent is obtained in order to determine HBV and HIV infectivity. If consent is not obtained, the employer shall establish that legally required consent cannot be obtained. When the source individual's consent is not required by law, the source individual's blood, if available, shall be tested and the results documented.

Form H-1   Hepatitis B Vaccine Declination (Mandatory)

I understand that due to my occupational exposure to blood or other potentially infectious materials I may be at risk of acquiring hepatitis B virus (HBV) infection. I have been given the opportunity to be vaccinated with hepatitis B vaccine, at no charge to myself. However, I decline hepatitis B vaccination at this time. I understand that by declining this vaccine, I continue to be at risk of acquiring hepatitis B, a serious disease. If in the future I continue to have occupational exposure to blood or other potentially infectious materials and I want to be vaccinated with hepatitis B vaccine, I can receive the vaccination series at no charge to me.

_____   _____
Name   Date

(B) When the source individual is already known to be infected with HBV or HIV, testing for the source individual's known HBV or HIV status need not be repeated.

(C) Results of the source individual's testing shall be made available to the exposed employee, and the employee shall be informed of applicable laws and regulations concerning disclosure of the identity and infectious status of the source individual.

(iii) Collection and testing of blood for HBV and HIV serological status;

(A) The exposed employee's blood shall be collected as soon as feasible and tested after consent is obtained.

(B) If the employee consents to baseline blood collection, but does not give consent at that time for HIV serologic testing, the sample shall be preserved for at least 90 days. If, within 90 days of the exposure incident, the employee elects to have the baseline sample tested, such testing shall be done as soon as feasible.

(iv) Post-exposure prophylaxis, when medically indicated, as recommended by the U.S. Public Health Service;

(v) Counseling; and

(vi) Evaluation of reported illnesses.

(4) *Information Provided to the Healthcare Professional.* (i) The employer shall ensure that the healthcare professional responsible for the employee's Hepatitis B vaccination is provided a copy of this regulation.

(ii) The employer shall ensure that the healthcare professional evaluating an employee after an exposure incident is provided the following information:

(A) A copy of this regulation;

(B) A description of the exposed employee's duties as they relate to the exposure incident;

(C) Documentation of the route(s) of exposure and circumstances under which exposure occurred;

(D) Results of the source individual's blood testing, if available; and

(E) All medical records relevant to the appropriate treatment of the employee, including vaccination status, which are the employer's responsibility to maintain.

(5) *Healthcare Professional's Written Opinion.* The employer shall obtain and provide the employee with a copy of the evaluating healthcare professional's written opinion within 15 days of the completion of the evaluation.

(i) The healthcare professional's written opinion for Hepatitis B vaccination shall be limited to whether Hepatitis B vaccination is indicated for an employee, and if the employee has received such vaccination.

(ii) The healthcare professional's written opinion for post-exposure evaluation and follow-up shall be limited to the following information:

(A) That the employee has been informed of the results of the evaluation; and

(B) That the employee has been told about any medical conditions resulting from exposure to blood or other potentially infectious materials that require further evaluation or treatment.

(iii) All other findings or diagnoses shall remain confidential and shall not be included in the written report.

(6) *Medical recordkeeping.* Medical records required by this standard shall be maintained in accordance with paragraph (h)(1) of this section.

(g) *Communication of hazards to employees— (1) Labels and signs.* (i) Labels. (A) Warning labels shall be affixed to containers of regulated waste, refrigerators and freezers containing blood or other potentially infectious material; and other containers used to store, transport or ship blood or other potentially infectious materials, except as provided in paragraph (g)(1)(i)(E), (F) and (G).

(B) Labels required by this section shall include the following legend:

BIOHAZARD

(C) These labels shall be fluorescent orange or orange-red or predominantly so, with lettering or symbols in a contrasting color.

(D) Labels required be affixed as close as feasible to the container by string, wire, adhesive, or other method that prevents their loss or unintentional removal.

(E) Red bags or red containers may be substituted for labels.

(F) Containers of blood, blood components, or blood products that are labeled as to their contents and have been released for transfusion or other clinical use are exempted from the labeling requirements of paragraph (g).

(G) Individual containers of blood or other potentially infectious materials that are placed in a labeled container during storage, transport, shipment or disposal are exempted from the labeling requirement.

(H) Labels required for contaminated equipment shall be in accordance with this paragraph and shall also state which portions of the equipment remain contaminated.

(I) Regulated waste that has been decontaminated need not be labeled or color-coded.

(ii) Signs. (A) The employer shall post signs at the entrance to work areas specified in paragraph (e), HIV and HBV Research Laboratory and Production Facilities, which shall bear the following legend:

BIOHAZARD

(Name of the Infectious Agent)

(Special requirements for entering the area)

(Name, telephone number of the laboratory director or other responsible person.)

(B) These signs shall be fluorescent orange-red or predominantly so, with lettering or symbols in a contrasting color.

(2) *Information and Training.* (i) Employers shall ensure that all employees with occupational exposure participate in a training program that must be provided at no cost to the employee and during working hours.

(ii) Training shall be provided as follows:

(A) At the time of initial assignment to tasks where occupational exposure may take place;

(B) Within 90 days after the effective date of the standard; and

(C) At least annually thereafter.

(iii) For employees who have received training on bloodborne pathogens in the year preceding the effective date of the standard, only training with respect to the provisions of the standard that were not included need be provided.

(iv) Annual training for all employees shall be provided within one year of their previous training.

(v) Employers shall provide additional training when changes such as modification of tasks or procedures or institution of new tasks or procedures affect the employee's occupational exposure. The additional training may be limited to addressing the new exposures created.

(vi) Material appropriate in content and vocabulary to educational level, literacy, and language of employees shall be used.

(vii) The training program shall contain at a minimum the following elements:

(A) An accessible copy of the regulatory text of this standard and an explanation of its contents;

(B) A general explanation of the epidemiology and symptoms of bloodborne diseases;

(C) An explanation of the modes of transmission of bloodborne pathogens;

(D) An explanation of the employer's exposure control plan and the means by which the employee can obtain a copy of the written plan;

(E) An explanation of the appropriate methods for recognizing tasks and other activities that may involve exposure to blood and other potentially infectious materials;

(F) An explanation of the use and limitations of methods that will prevent or reduce exposure, including appropriate engineering controls, work practices, and personal protective equipment;

(G) Information on the types, proper use, location, removal, handling, decontamination and disposal of personal protective equipment;

(H) An explanation of the basis for selection of personal protective equipment;

(I) Information on the hepatitis B vaccine, including information on its efficacy, safety, method of administration, the benefits of being vaccinated, and that the vaccine and vaccination will be offered free of charge;

(J) Information on the appropriate actions to take and persons to contact in an emergency involving blood or other potentially infectious materials;

(K) An explanation of the procedure to follow if an exposure incident occurs, including the method of reporting the incident and the medical follow-up that will be made available;

(L) Information on the post-exposure evaluation and follow-up that the employer is required to provide for the employee following an exposure incident;

(M) An explanation of the signs and labels and/or color coding required by paragraph (g)(1); and

(N) An opportunity for interactive questions and answers with the person conducting the training session.

(viii) The person conducting the training shall be knowledgeable in the subject matter covered by the elements contained in the training program as it relates to the workplace that the training will address.

(ix) Additional Initial Training for Employees in HIV and HBV Laboratories and Production Facilities, Employees in HIV or HBV research laboratories and HIV or HBV production facilities shall receive the following initial training in addition to the above training requirements.

(A) The employer shall assure that employees demonstrate proficiency in standard microbiological practices and techniques and in the practices and operations specific to the facility before being allowed to work with HIV or HBV.

(B) The employer shall assure that employees have prior experience in the handling of human pathogens or tissue cultures before working with HIV or HBV.

(C) The employer shall provide a training program to employees who have no prior experience in handling human pathogens. Initial work activities shall not include the handling of infectious agents. A progression of work activities shall be assigned as techniques are learned and proficiency is developed. The employer shall assure that employees participate in work activities involving infectious agents only after proficiency has been demonstrated.

(h) *Recordkeeping—(1) Medical Records.*

(i) The employer shall establish and maintain an accurate record for each employee with occupational exposure, in accordance with 29 CFR 1910.20.

(ii) This record shall include:

(A) The name and social security number of the employee;

(B) A copy of the employee's hepatitis B vaccination status including the dates of all the hepatitis B vaccinations and any medical records relative to the employee's ability to receive vaccination as required by paragraph (f)(2);

(C) A copy of all results of examinations, medical testing, and follow-up procedures as required by paragraph (f)(3);

(D) The employer's copy of the healthcare professional's written opinion as required by paragraph (f)(5); and

(E) A copy of the information provided to the healthcare professional as required by paragraphs (f)(4)(ii)(B)(C) and (D).

(iii) Confidentiality. The employer shall ensure that employee medical records required by paragraph (h)(1) are:

(A) Kept confidential; and

(B) Are not disclosed or reported without the employee's express written consent to any person within or outside the workplace except as required by this section or as may be required by law.

(iv) The employer shall maintain the records required by paragraph (h) for at least the duration of employment plus 30 years in accordance with 29 CFR 1910.20.

(2) *Training Records.*

(i) Training records shall include the following information:

(A) The dates of the training sessions;

(B) The contents or a summary of the training sessions;

(C) The names and qualifications of persons conducting the training; and

(D) The names and job titles of all persons attending the training sessions.

(ii) Training records shall be maintained for 3 years from the date on which the training occurred.

(3) *Availability.* (i) The employer shall ensure that all records required to be maintained by this section shall be made available upon request to the Assistant Secretary and the Director for examination and copying.

(ii) Employee training records required by this paragraph shall be provided upon request for examination and copying to employees, to employee representatives, to the Director, and to the Assistant Secretary in accordance with 29 CFR 1910.20.

(iii) Employee medical records required by this paragraph shall be provided upon request for examination and copying to the subject employee, to anyone having written consent of the subject employee, to the Director, and to the Assistant Secretary in accordance with 29 CFR 1910.20.

(4) *Transfer of Records.*

(i) The employer shall comply with the requirements involving transfer of records set forth in 29 CFR 1910.20(h).

(ii) If the employer ceases to do business and there is no successor employer to receive and retain the records for the prescribed period, the employer shall notify the Director, at least three months prior to their disposal and transmit them to the Director, if required by the Director to do so, within that three month period.

(i) *Dates—(1) Effective Date.* The standard shall become effective on March 6, 1992.

(2) The Exposure Control Plan required by paragraph (c)(2) of this section shall be completed on or before May 5, 1992.

(3) Paragraph (g)(2) Information and Training and (h) Recordkeeping shall take effect on or before June 4, 1992.

(4) Paragraphs (d)(2) Engineering and Work Practice Controls, (d)(3) Personal Protective Equipment, (d)(4) Housekeeping, (e) HIV and HBV Research Laboratories and Production Facilities, (f) Hepatitis B Vaccination and Post-Exposure Evaluation and Follow-up, and (g)(1) Labels and Signs, shall take effect July 6, 1992.

Appendix A to Section 1910.1030—Hepatitis B Vaccine Declination (Mandatory)

GLOSSARY

AAMI Association for the Advancement of Medical Instrumentation (see Appendix A)

acidic Condition caused by an abundance of hydrogen ions (H^+) resulting in a pH of less than 7.0

acidogenic organism An organism that produces acids during growth

aciduric organism An organism that survives in acidic environments below pH 5.5

acquired immunity In contrast to innate immunity, this immunity is obtained in some manner other than by heredity

Actinomycosis Infection with endogenous oral *Actinomyces* species resulting in nodular lesions that may form abscesses; cervical facial actinomycosis occurs in the neck-jaw area

acute necrotizing ulcerative gingivitis (ANUG) A severe form of periodontal disease, involving predisposing factors and resulting in inflammation of the gingival tissue (also called **trench mouth)**

acute stage In a disease, the period when symptoms are the greatest

ADA American Dental Association (see Appendix A)

ADAA American Dental Assistants Association (see Appendix A)

ADHA American Dental Hygienists Association (see Appendix A)

adherence The attachment of a microorganism to a host cell or other surface

agar A polysaccharide extracted from seaweed and used as the basic component for semisolid bacterial growth media

AIDS Acquired immunodeficiency syndrome

allergen A foreign substance (e.g., pollen) that acts as an antigen but stimulates an allergic response

allergic contact dermatitis A type IV hypersensitivity resulting from contact with a chemical allergen (e.g., poison ivy, certain reactions to patient care gloves); the cell-mediated reaction occurs only where contact with the allergen has been made

allergy Disorder in which the immune system reacts inappropriately, usually by responding to an antigen it normally ignores (also called **hypersensitivity)**

amino acid An organic acid containing an amino group and a carboxyl group; the building blocks of protein

anabolism The synthesis of large molecules from simpler components

anion A negatively charged ion

antibiotic A chemical substance produced by microorganisms that can inhibit the growth of or destroy other microorganisms

antibody A protein produced in response to an antigen that is capable of binding specifically to that antigen

antigen A substance or cell that the body identifies as foreign and toward which it mounts an immune response

antiseptic A chemical agent that can be safely used externally on tissues to destroy microorganisms or to inhibit their growth

AOAC Association for Official Analytical Chemists; this group devises tests used to characterize sterilants and disinfectants

asepsis The absence of infection or infectious materials or agents

asthma Respiratory distress caused by inhaled or ingested allergens or by hypersensitivity to endogenous microorganisms

ASTM American Society of Testing and Materials; this group devises tests to evaluate a variety of products

asymptomatic carrier A person infected with a pathogen but has no symptoms of the infection

autoclave An instrument for sterilization by means of moist heat under pressure

bacillus (plural: **bacilli**) A rodlike bacterium

bacteremia The presence of bacteria in the blood

bacteria All prokaryotic organisms

bacterial endocarditis A life-threatening infection and inflammation of the lining and valves of the heart

bacterial growth An increase in the number of bacterial cells of one type, also called bacterial multiplication

bactericidal agent An agent that kills bacteria

bacteriophage A virus that infects bacteria

bacteriostatic agent An agent that stops the growth of bacteria, but does not necessarily kill the bacteria

binary fission The process by which bacteria multiply; the cell divides into two cells

binomial nomenclature The system of taxonomy in which each organism is assigned a genus and species name

bioburden The microbial or organic material on a surface or object prior to decontamination

biofilm A mass or layer of live microorganisms attached to a surface

biologic indicator (BI) Paper strips or vials containing bacterial endospores used to monitor heat and gas sterilization procedures

bloodborne pathogens Disease-producing microorganisms that are spread by contact with blood or other body fluids from an infected person

bloodborne pathogens standard A law developed by OSHA and passed by Congress directing employers to protect employees from occupational exposure to blood and other potentially infectious material

candidiasis A fungal infection caused by *Candida albicans* that appears as thrush or denture stomatitis in the mouth

capsid The protein coating of a virus, which protects the nucleic acid core from the environment and determines the shape of the virus

capsule A structure outside the bacterial cell wall that is antiphagocytic and protects the cell from drying

carbohydrates Compounds composed of carbon, hydrogen, and oxygen that serve as the main source of energy for most living things

catabolism The chemical breakdown of molecules in which energy is released

catalase An enzyme that converts hydrogen peroxide to water and molecular oxygen

cation A positively charged ion

CDC Centers for Disease Control and Prevention (see Appendix A)

cell-mediated immunity Immune response carried out at the cellular level by T-lymphocytes

cell wall A layer of most bacterial and fungal cells that maintains the shape of the cell and protects against mechanical damage

cellulitis Inflammation of the loose subcutaneous cellular tissue

chemical indicator A material containing a chemical that changes color or form with exposure to heat, steam, or ethylene oxide gas; used to monitor exposure of items to heat- or gas-sterilizing agents

chemical vapor sterilizer An instrument for sterilization by means of hot formaldehyde vapors under pressure

Chlamydia A group of nonmotile, spherical bacteria that are obligate intracellular parasites with a complex life cycle

chlorination The addition of chlorine to water to kill bacteria

ciliary escalator The physical movement created by the action of cilia (hairlike projections) on the surface of respiratory epithelial cells that moves mucus and trapped particles up and out of the lungs

coccus (plural: **cocci**) A spherical bacterium

collagenase An enzyme that degrades body protein collagen in connective tissue

colony A mass of cells that originated from one cell or one colony-forming-unit

colony-forming-units (CFU) The original cells that begin multiplication to form a colony

communicable disease Infectious disease that can be spread from one host to another (also called **contagious disease**)

complement A set of proteins present in blood and when activated form a nonspecific defense mechanism against many different microorganisms (also called **complement system**)

contact dermatitis A type of allergy mediated by special T-lymphocytes that results in a skin reaction after skin contact with an allergen (e.g., poison ivy)

convalescent stage In a disease, that period when the symptoms are subsiding and the person is recovering

cytoplasm The semifluid substance inside the cytoplasmic membrane

cytoplasmic membrane The structural layer of a bacterial cell immediately internal to the cell wall

cytotoxic Toxic to cells

DANB Dental Assisting National Board, Inc. (see Appendix A)

decontamination Removing bioburden from objects or surfaces

delta hepatitis See **hepatitis**

demineralization Removal of minerals from tooth structures; this causes dental caries

dental aerosols Small droplets of oral fluid and water generated during use of handpieces, ultrasonic scalers, and air/water syringes

dental caries An infectious disease resulting in the destruction of the teeth by microbial acids

deoxyribonucleic acid (DNA) Nucleic acid that carries hereditary information from one generation to the next

direct contact transmission Mode of disease transmission requiring person-to-person body contact

disinfection Reducing the number of pathogenic organisms on objects or in materials so that they pose no threat of disease

droplet infection Contact transmission of disease through small liquid droplets

dry heat sterilizer An instrument for sterilizing by means of heated air

endemic disease A disease that is constantly present in a specific population

endogenous infection An infection caused by opportunistic microorganisms already present in the body

endospore A resistant, dormant structure, formed inside some bacteria such as *Bacillus* and *Clostridium,* that can survive adverse conditions

endotoxin A toxic substance in the gram-negative bacterial cell wall that is released when the bacterium dies

enzymes Protein catalysts that control the rate of chemical reactions in cells

EPA Environmental Protection Agency (see Appendix A)

epidemic Occurs when a disease has a very high incidence in a population over a relatively short period of time

epidemiology The study of factors and mechanisms involved in the spread of disease within a population

epidermis The thin outer layer of the skin

exogenous infection An infection caused by microorganisms that enter the body from the environment

exotoxin A soluble toxin secreted by microorganisms into their surroundings, including host tissues

exposure control plan A written plan required by OSHA that describes how exposure to bloodborne disease agents will be controlled in a given worksite

extracellular enzymes Exoenzymes produced by bacteria, which act in the environment around the organism

facultative anaerobes Bacteria that carry on aerobic metabolism when oxygen is present but shift to anaerobic metabolism when oxygen is absent

FDA Food and Drug Administration (see Appendix A)

fimbriae Short, hairlike projections from bacterial cells that function in adherence

flagella Long, thin structures of some bacteria that provide means of locomotion

fungi Nonphotosynthetic, eukaryotic organisms

fungicidal agent An agent that kills fungi

genome The genetic information in an organism

genus The first name of an organism in binomial nomenclature, e.g., *Streptococcus* in *Streptococcus mutans*

gingivitis A periodontal disease characterized by inflammation of the soft tissue (gingiva) around the teeth

glycocalyx Term used to refer to all substances containing polysaccharides found external to the cell wall

gram-negative bacteria Bacteria that stain pink in the differential Gram stain procedure

gram-positive bacteria Bacteria that stain blue in the differential Gram stain procedure

hay fever Irritation of the eyes and upper respiratory tract caused by inhaled allergens

hazard communication standard A law developed by OSHA and passed by Congress directing employers to provide employees with information on the hazards of chemicals used in the workplace (also called HazMat Standard, HazCom Standard, "Employee Right-to-Know Rule")

HEPA High efficiency particulate air filters; they can filter out microorganisms for air

hepatitis An inflammation of the liver, usually caused by viruses but sometimes by other organisms or toxic chemicals; hepatitis A and E viruses are spread by contaminated food and water; hepatitis B, C, D and G viruses are bloodborne disease agents

herpes labialis Fever blisters (cold sores) on lips

herpetic whitlow Infection of the fingers with herpes simplex virus

histolytic enzyme An enzyme that can degrade a component in tissues or cells of the body

HIV-1 Human immunodeficiency virus type 1

HIV-disease A disease that includes HIV-infection and/or AIDS

HIV-infection Infection with HIV-1 before the development of AIDS

hyaluronidase Bacterially-produced enzyme that digests hyaluronic acid, which holds body cells together

hydrophilic viruses Viruses without lipid envelopes such as polioviruses, adenoviruses, coxsackieviruses; these viruses are generally considered to be more difficult to kill by some germicides than are lipophilic viruses

hypersensitivity Disorder in which the immune system reacts inappropriately, usually by responding to an antigen it normally ignores (also called **allergy)**

immunity The ability to defend against the damage that may be caused by a microorganism

immunodeficiency Disorder in which the immune system responds inadequately to an antigen because of inborn or acquired defects in B- or T-lymphocytes

incidence The number of new cases of a particular disease seen in a specific period of time

incubation stage In a disease, the time between infection and the appearance of signs and symptoms

indirect contact transmission Spread of disease agents through fomites (objects or surfaces)

infection Growth and survival of a microorganism on or in the body

infection control Controlling the spread of disease agents by performing specific procedures

infectious disease Disease caused by a microorganism

innate body defenses Naturally occurring body defense mechanisms against infectious disease agents

interferon A small protein released from virus-infected cells that causes adjacent cells to produce a protein that interferes with viral replication

intermediate viruses Viruses without envelopes; not quite as resistant to chemical killing as the hydrophilic non-enveloped viruses but more resistant to chemical killing than the lipophilic enveloped viruses (see Table 12-3)

irritant contact dermatitis A nonimmunologic irritation of the skin by chemicals

jaundice Yellow skin color due to excessive bilirubin in the blood from the breakdown of erythrocytes; caused by impaired liver function and common in hepatitis

kPa A metric unit for measuring pressure in kilopascals

latex A milky white fluid extracted from the rubber tree *Hevea brasiliensis* that contains the rubber material cis-1,4 polyisoprene

latex allergy A type I hypersensitivity (mediated by IgE antibody) resulting from contact with a chemical allergen in latex materials (e.g., latex gloves) or in materials associated with latex products (e.g., airborne powder from latex gloves)

LD$_{50}$ Lethal Dose 50%, a measure of toxicity; the dose of a substance that kills 50% of the test animals

lipids A diverse group of water-insoluble compounds

lipophilic viruses Viruses with an outer lipid envelope such as influenza viruses, herpes simplex viruses, HIV-1; these viruses are generally considered to be more easily killed by some germicides than are hydrophilic and intermediate viruses (see Table 12-3)

lipopolysaccharide Part of the outer layer of the cell wall in gram-negative bacteria (also called **endotoxin)**

lymphocytes Leukocytes (white blood cells) found in large numbers in lymphoid tissues that contribute to immunity

lymphokines   Chemicals secreted by lymphocytes that help mediate the immune response

lysis   The disruption of a cell

lysozyme   An enzyme in saliva and some other body fluids that acts on peptidoglycan to weaken the bacterial cell walls

lytic cycle   The sequence of events in which a virus infects a cell, replicates, and eventually causes rupture of the cell

macrophages   Phagocytic leukocytes found in tissues

malaise   A symptom of disease in which the person "feels bad" and is usually tired and weak

mesophiles   Organisms that grow best at 37° C

mesosome   A membraneous structure of bacterial cells that contain extracellular enzymes used in nutrition

metabolism   The sum of all chemical reactions that occur in living organisms

microaerophiles   Bacteria that grow best in the presence of a small amount of free oxygen

microbial growth   Increase in the number of cells, due to cell division

microbiology   The study of microorganisms

micrometer (μm)   Unit of measure equal to 0.000001 meters (m) or 10^{-6} m

minimum bactericidal concentration (MBC)   The lowest concentration of an antimicrobial agent that kills microorganisms

minimum inhibitory concentration (MIC)   The lowest concentration of an antimicrobial agent that prevents growth of microorganisms

MSDS   Material safety data sheet; describes composition, properties, and hazards of a chemical

mutans streptococci   A group of *Streptococcus* sp. with properties similar to *S. mutans* (*S. mutans, S. sobrinus, S. cricetus, S. rattus, S. ferus, S. macacae*)

non self-cleansing areas   These are the sights around the teeth that are not kept clean by contact with the tongue and cheeks

non-enveloped viruses   Viruses without envelopes and which are hydrophilic or intermediate in their solubility, being more resistant to chemical killing than enveloped viruses (see Table 12-3)

normal microbiota   Microorganisms commonly found in or on the body

nosocomial infection   An infection acquired in a hospital or other medical facility

nucleoid   Nuclear region in bacteria

obligate aerobes   Bacteria that must have free oxygen to grow

obligate anaerobes   Bacteria that are killed by free oxygen

obligate intracellular parasites   Organisms that can live or multiply only inside a living host cell

opportunistic disease   Disease caused by an organism that is usually harmless but can cause disease under certain conditions

OSAP   The Office Sterilization and Asepsis Procedures Research Foundation (see Appendix A and D)

OSHA   Occupational Safety and Health Administration (see Appendix A)

pandemic   An epidemic that has become worldwide

pasteurization   Mild heating to destroy pathogens and other organisms that cause spoilage (e.g., 71.6° C [161° F] for 15 seconds)

pathogen Any microorganism capable of causing disease in its host

pellicle The thin, saliva-based, protein layer that coats the teeth and forms the base over which dental plaque develops

peptide A short chain of amino acids linked together

peptidoglycan A polymer in bacterial cell wall composed of a peptide and a polysaccharide

periapical infection An infection of the tissue around the apex of the root of a tooth

periodontal disease An infectious disease that results in destruction of the soft tissue and/or bone that support the teeth (e.g., gingivitis, periodontitis)

periodontitis An inflammation of the periodontal tissue resulting in destruction of the bone in which the teeth are set

periodontopathogen A microorganism important in causing a periodontal disease

pH A means of expressing the hydrogen-ion concentration (acidity) of a solution

phagocytosis Ingestion of bacteria and other small particles by white blood cells

pili Projections from the bacterial cell used to attach bacteria to surfaces (fimbriae) or for conjugation (sex pili)

planktonic microorganisms Microorganisms that are free-floating (not attached to surfaces) in their fluid environment; this is in contrast to biofilm microorganisms that are attached to surfaces

plaque A bacterial mass that accumulates on the teeth in the absence of oral hygiene

pneumonia An inflammation of lung tissue caused by bacteria, viruses, protozoa, or fungi

polysaccharide A carbohydrate formed when many monosaccharides are linked together

portal of entry A site at which microorganisms can gain access to body tissues

portal of exit A site at which microorganisms can leave the body

preprocedure mouthrinsing Using a mouthrinse before a dental procedure to reduce the number of microorganisms present

prevalence The number of people infected with a particular disease at any one time

prion A small infectious particle thought to consist of protein without any nucleic acid; their existence is challenged by some investigators

prodomal stage In a disease, the short period during which early nonspecific symptoms such as malaise and headache sometimes appear

prokaryotes Microorganisms that lack a nucleus; all bacteria are prokaryotes

protease An enzyme that degrades protein into peptides or amino acids

protein A polymer of amino acids joined by peptide bonds

protozoa Single-celled, microscopic, eukaryotic organisms in the kingdom Protista

psi A unit for measuring pressure in pounds per square inch

psychrophiles Cold-loving bacteria that grow best at a temperature of 7° C

pulpitis Inflammation of the pulp of a tooth

pure culture A culture that contains only a single species of organism

resident flora Species of microorganisms that are always present on or in the body

retrovirus These RNA viruses use the enzyme reverse transcriptase to synthesize DNA from RNA during multiplication of the virus inside of host cells (e.g., HIV-1)

reuse life For germicides this is the period of time a solution should remain effective as it is used and reused (for contrast see **use-life**)

ribonucleic acid (RNA) Nucleic acid that directs or participates in the assembly of proteins

Rickettsia Small, nonmotile, gram-negative bacteria that are obligate intracellular parasites of mammalian and arthropod cells

septicemia An infection caused by rapid multiplication of pathogens in the blood

sharps containers Puncture-resistant containers for disposal of sharp items that could puncture the skin (also called **sharps boxes)**

shelf life The period of time a solution or products may be stored before activation or use and still retain its effectiveness upon activation or use

species The second name of an organism in binomial nomenclature (e.g., *mutans* in *Streptococcus mutans)*

spirillum (pl: **spirilli**)   A corkscrew-shaped bacterium

spirochete A flexible, wavy-shaped bacterium

sporadic disease A disease that is limited to a small number of isolated cases, posing no great threat to a large population

sporicidal agent An agent that kills bacterial endospores and therefore can be called a sterilant

sterilant An agent capable of killing all microorganisms

sterility The state in which there are no living organisms in or on a material

sterilization The killing or removal of all microorganisms in a material or on an object

subclinical infection An infection that does not produce symptoms (also called **asymptomatic infection)**

sucrose A sugar containing one molecule of fructose and one molecule of glucose (also called **table sugar)**

superoxide dismutase An enzyme that converts toxic superoxide to molecular oxygen and hydrogen peroxide

surface asepsis Procedures that prevent the involvement of environmental surfaces in spreading disease agents

systemic infection An infection that involves the entire body

thermophiles Heat-loving bacteria that grow best at a temperature of 56° C

toxin A poisonous substance

toxoid An inactivated toxin that is immunogenic but not toxin

transient flora Microorganisms that may be present in or on the body under certain conditions and for certain lengths of time

tuberculocidal agent An agent that can kill *Mycobacterium tuberculosis*

universal precautions Consideration of all patients as being infected with pathogens and therefore applying infection control procedures to the care of all patients

universal sterilization The sterilization of all reusable instruments between use on patients

upper respiratory tract The nasal cavity, pharynx, larynx, trachea, bronchi, and larger bronchioles

use-life For germicidal agents this is the period of time a solution is effective after it has been activated or prepared for use (for contrast see **reuse-life**)

vaccine A substance that contains an antigen to which the immune system responds

virucidal agent An agent that kills viruses

viruses Submicroscopic, acellular, obligate intracellular parasites composed of a nucleic acid core inside a protein coat

Whitlow A herpetic lesion on a finger that can result from exposure to oral, ocular, and (probably) genital herpes

INDEX

A

AAMI; *see* Association for the Advancement of
    Medical Instrumentation
Acid-fast bacillus (AFB), 5
Acquired Immunodeficiency syndrome (AIDS); *see*
    also HIV-disease
    as part of HIV disease, 62
    characteristics of, 63
    opportunistic infections in, 63,64
    oral manifestations of, 63
    prevention of, 68
    transmission of, 63-67
Actinobacillus sp., 44
Actinobacillus actinomycetemcomitans
    pathogenic properties and, 29
    periodontitis and, 50
Actinomyces sp., 44,50,51,192
Actinomyces israelii, 51
Actinomyces naeslundii
    pathogenic properties of, 47
    root caries and, 47
Actinomycosis, 51
Action plan, 268
Acute dental infection, 51
Acute stage of disease, 25
ADA; *see* American Dental Association
ADAA; *see* American Dental Assistants Association
ADHA; *see* American Dental Hygienists Associa-
    tion
Adenosine triphosphate, 17
Adenovirus, 71
Adult periodontitis; *see* Chronic periodontitis
Aerobe, 14
Aerosol
    masks and, 127-128
    high volume evacuation and, 205
    OSHA and, 101
    protective eyewear and, 129
    rubber dam and, 206-207
Agar, 6, 15
AIDS; *see* Acquired immunodeficiency syndrome
Alcohol
    as a disinfectant, 186-187
    hepatitis B and, 55
    precleaning and, 182

Alcohol—cont'd
    quaternary ammonium compounds and, 188
Alcohol-phenolics, 186,188
Alginate impression material, 201
Allergen, 34
Allergic contact dermatitis, 120-121
Allergy, 23, 33-34, 121-124
American Dental Assistants Association (ADAA),
    280
American Dental Association (ADA), 90, 280
    dental unit water and, 200
    infection control recommendations and, 317-
        328
    instrument sterilization and, 105
    MSDS and, 260
    resources and, 280
    safety coordinator and, 238
    sterilizer testing and, 158
American Dental Hygienists Association (ADHA),
    238, 280
American National Standards Institute (ANSI), 129
Amino acid, 7, 16
Anabolism, 16
ANSI; *see* American National Standards Institute
Antibiotic, 10, 18
Antibody
    allergies and, 44, 122
    antigen and, 32
    bacterial differentiation and, 6
    formation of, 32-33
    hepatitis B and, 57
    HIV-infection and, 63
    latex allergy and, 122
Antigen
    antibody and, 32
    examples of, 32, 33, 34
    hepatitis B and, 57, 110, 111
    in allergies, 34
Antimicrobial chemical,
    antibiotic, 18
    antiseptic, 182
    chlorhexidine, 125
    disinfectant, 183
    handwashing agent, 125

Antimicrobial chemical—cont'd
  in the body, 31
  mouthrinse, 207
Antimicrobial chemical
  para-chloro-meta-xylenol (PCMX), 125
  sterilant, 173, 183
  povidone iodine, 125
  triclosan, 125
Antiseptic, 182
Appliance disinfection, 110-213
Arachnia sp., 44
Aseptic meningitis, 64
Aseptic retrieval, 188
Aseptic technique
  at chairside, 205-209, 232
  in laboratory, 196-204
  in radiology, 204-209
Association for the Advancement of Medical In-
     strumentation (AAMI), 91, 281
Asthma, 23, 34, 122
Asymptomatic carrier, 24, 58, 61, 72
Athlete's foot, 21
Autoclave; *see* Sterilizer, steam

B

Bacillus sp., 11, 192
Bacillus stearothermophilus
  biologic indicator and, 156
  heat resistance of, 11, 13
  proper incubation of, 158
  spore formation and, 11
  testing sterilizers with, 148, 156-161
Bacillus subtilis
  biologic indicator and, 156
  cell morphology, 8, 10
  dental unit water and, 192
  proper incubation of, 158
  testing sterilizers with, 148, 156-161
  spore formation and, 11
Bacteremia, 51
Bacteria
  acid production and, 113-14, 45, 47
  attachment of, 11, 45-46, 195-196
  control of, 18-19
  culturing of, 15-16
  differentiation of, 5
  growth of, 11-19
  pathogenic properties of, 28-30
  shape of, 7
  staining of, 5
  structure of, 7-11
Bateriology, 2
Bacteriophage, 3
Bacteriostatic agent, 18
Bacteroides sp., 44, 192
Bacteroides forsythus, 50

Bagging, 143
Barrier technique *see also* Personal protective equip-
     ment
  for dental team, 115-134
  for laboratory, 210
  for operatory surfaces, 175-181
  for radiology, 217
Bartonella henselae, 36
Bead "sterilizer," 173
Bifidobacterium sp., 44
Binary fission, 111-13
Biofilm, 195-197
  dental plaque, 45-46
  dental unit waterline, 195-197
Biohazard symbol, 96
Biological indicator, 156-160, 162, 164
Biological monitoring, 156-160
Bleach; *see* Sodium hypochlorite
Bloodborne pathogen; *see* Hepatitis and HIV dis-
     ease
Bloodborne pathogens standard from OSHA, 92-
     105, 329-342
  hepatitis vaccination and, 60, 97-98, 109-113
  office records and, 100
Bloodborne disease, 54-69; *see also* Hepatitis B, C,
     and D and HIV disease
  occupational spread, 59, 66, 67
  viruses and, 19
  regulations and, 92-105
  transmission of, 55-59, 63-66
B-lymphocyte; *see* Lymphocyte
Borrelia burgdorferi, 36
Broth culture, 15

C

Capsid, 19,20
Campylobacter sp., 44
Candida albicans,
  AIDS and, 63, 64
  normal oral flora and, 43
  oral diseases from, 71,73
Candidiasis, 21
  AIDS and, 63, 64
  in the mouth, 71,73
Capnocytophaga sp., 44
Capnocytophaga ochracea, 50
Capsule, bacterial, 10
Cardiobacterium sp., 44
Caries-conducive bacteria, 46-48
Carriers
  hepatitis B and, 58, 59
  hepatitis C and, 61
  HIV-infection and, 63
  of different microbes, 72
  types of, 24

Case, laboratory, 216
Cassette, instrument
    cleaning of, 140-141
    loading in a sterilizer, 152
    wrapping of, 144, 146
Catabolism, 16
CD$_4$-lymphocyte; *see* Lymphocyte
CDC; *see* Centers for Disease Control and Prevention
Cell-mediated immunity, 32
Cellulitis, 51
Cell wall, 8, 9-10
Centers for Disease Control and Prevention
        (CDC)
    Advisory Committee on Immunization Practices and, 108
    Infection control recommendations and, 283-294
    instrument sterilization and, 105
    sterilizer testing and, 158, 287
    resources and, 281
    safety coordinator and, 238
    waste management and, 222, 225
Centipeda sp., 44
Cervicofacial actinomycosis, 51
Chlamydia, 16
Checklist, 242
Chemical disinfectants, 182-188, 311-315
Chemical, hazardous, 247-274
Chemical hygiene officer, 268, 27
Chemical hygiene plan, 268, 271-273
Chemical indicator, 161-163
Chemical monitoring, 161-163
Chemical sterilant, 171-172, 173, 316
Chemical vapor sterilizer; *see* Sterilizer, chemical vapor
Chemiclave; *see* Sterilizer, chemical vapor
Chickenpox, 2, 71, 72, 74
Chlorhexidine digluconate, 9, 125
Chlorine, 185, 312
Chlorine dioxide, 312
p-Chloro-*m*-xylenol (PCMX), 125
Cholera, 36, 37, 38, 107
Chronic active hepatitis, 58
Chronic periodontitis, 50
Chronic persistant hepatitis, 58
Cirrhosis, liver, 58
Ciliary escalator, 30
Cleaning, 136, 139-142, 182
Clinical asepsis protocol, 230-234
Clostridium sp., 30
Clostridium botulinum, 29
Clostridium difficile, 64
Clostridium sporogenes, 11
Clostridium tetani, 29, 107
Clothing, protective, 129, 132

Coccidioidomycosis, 69
Code for Federal Regulations (CFR), 276
Collagenase, 29, 33
Colony-forming-units (CFU), 15
Color-coded bags/containers, 96, 104-105
Complement, 31
Compliance officer, 248
Compound impression material, 214
Contact dermatitis, 434, 121-122
Containers
    for laundry, 104-105
    for non-sharps, 104
    for sharps, 104, 225-226, 332
    for specimens, 101, 102
Contaminated waste, 223
Contra angle, sterilization, 171
Convalescent stage of disease, 25
Corrosion control, 142, 170
Corynebacterium sp., 44
Corynebacterium diphtheriae, 72
Coxsackievirus, 36, 71
Creutzfeldt-Jacob disease, 136
Cross-contamination, 83-89
Cryptococcosis, 21, 64
Cryptosporidiosis, 64
Cryptosporidium parvum, 36, 40-41
Cytomegalovirus, 64, 72
Cytoplasm, 7-9, 16
Cytoplasmic membrane, 8, 9, 16

D

Darkroom asepsis, 219
Delta hepatitis, 54, 55, 56, 57, 60-61; *see also* Hepatitis D
Demineralization, 44, 45
Dental caries
    demineralization and, 44, and 45
    endogenous disease and, 23
    formation of, 44-48
    lactic acid and, 17, 45, 48
Dental plaque
    caries and, 45-46
    composition of, 46
    pathogenic properties of, 46
    periodontal disease and, 48-49
Denture disinfection, 212
Desquamation, 31
Diphtheria
    asymptomatic carrier and, 72
    bacterial attachment and, 11
    immunization for, 41, 107
    spread by oral fluids, 71
    vaccine (DPT), 107
Direct contact, 26
Disease transmission, 26-27

Disinfectant
  activity
    bacteriocidal, 183, 311-315
    fungicidal, 183, 311-315
    tuberculocidal, 183, 185, 311-315
    virucidal, 183, 187, 311-315
  as a cleaner, 182
  damage to surfaces, 185
  hospital type, 183
  single use of, 213
  types of, 186
Disinfection
  at chairside, 230, 233
  in laboratory, 210-215
  in radiology, 219
  of appliances, 212
  of impressions, 214
  precleaning and, 182
  procedures for, 182
  sterilization versus, 136-137
Disposable items, 207-208
DNA
  composition of, 7
  in conjugation, 11
  in nucleoid, 8
  in plasmid, 9
  in spores, 11
  in viruses, 19-20
  function of, 9
DPT, 107
Droplet infection, 26-27
Dry heat sterilizer; *see* Sterilizer, dry heat

E

Ear infection,71, 78
Ebola virus, 36, 41-42
Ehrlichia chaffeenis, 36
Ehrlichiosis, 36
Eikenella sp., 44
Eikenella corrodens, 50
Emerging diseases, 35-42
Emergency, 268, 277, 279
Employee right-to-know (OSHA), 254
Employees and OSHA, 92, 248
Employers and OSHA, 92, 248
Endocarditis, 51
Endospores, bacterial, 11, 136
Endotoxin, 10, 16, 29, 30, 49
Energy production, bacterial, 17
Engerix B, 110
Engineering controls, 93, 100-102, 247, 248
Enveloped virus, 19
Environmental Protection Agency (EPA), 92
  disinfectants and, 185
  waste definition and, 222, 223, 224, 228

Environmental surface
  cleaning and disinfection of, 82-188
  protecting with cover, 177-188
Enzyme
  collagenase, 29, 33
  extracellular, 14
  glucosyltransferase, 47, 48
  histolytic, 29, 30
  hyaluronidase, 27
  lactate dehydrogenase, 17
  lysozyme, 10, 31
  mechanism of action, 16-17
  protease, 14
  superoxide desmutase, 15
EPA; *see* Environmental Protection Agency
Epstein-Barr virus
  oral spread of, 71
  presence in mouth, 211
Equipment asepsis, 175-188
Equipment for infection control and safety, 169,
    241
Escherichia coli, 13, 14, 36, 39
Ethanol, 153, 262
Eyewash stations, 41, 270
Eyewear; *see* Protective eyewear
Eubacterium sp., 44
Exposure
  body fluids and, 98
  chemicals and, 248
  control plan, OSHA, 93-94, 242
  determination, OSHA, 94
  incident report, 308-309
  medical evaluation, 98-100

F

Faceshield, 129
Facultative anaerobe, 14, 15
FDA; *see* Food and Drug Administration
Federal Register, 275
Fermentation, 17-18, 48
Fever blisters, 70
Film, radiographic, 217-220
Fire extinguishers, 240, 241, 278
Fire prevention plans, 227-278
Flagellum, 8, 9, 11
Fimbriae, 8, 9, 11
Flash sterilization, 143,148, 152
Food and Drug Administration, 91-92
  resources and, 281
  sterilants and, 185
Formaldehyde, 153, 262
Fulminant hepatitis, 54
Fungus, 21
Fusobacterium, sp., 44, 50
Fusobacterium nucleatum, 29

G

Gamma globulin, 57
Genes, 9, 11
German measles; *see* Rubella
Giardiasis, 64
Gingivitis
    plaque and, 45-46
    types of, 49
Gingivostomatitis, primary herpetic, 70
Gloves, 115-124
    bloodborne pathogens standard and, 102-103
    chairside asepsis, 230-234
    instrument processing and, 137-138
    laboratory asepsis and, 210
    operatory clean-up and, 182
    placing and removing, 133-134
    radiographic asepsis and, 217-220
Glucans, 47, 48
Glucosyltransferase, 47, 48
Glutaraldehyde
    as a liquid sterilant, 171-172, 173, 31
    laboratory asepsis and, 212, 214
Glycoprotein, 7
Common cold, 71
Gonococcal pharyngitis, 71, 73
Gown, protective clothing, 129-133
Gram stain, 5
Gram-negative, 5, 10, 30, 44, 50
Gram-positive, 5, 10, 44
Grinding, laboratory, 215

H

Haemophilus influenzae type b,
    asymptomatic carrier, 71
    vaccine for, 107
Hairy leukoplakia, 64
Handpiece
    aerosols and, 127
    cleaning and sterilizing of, 171-172
    waterline contamination and, 190, 191, 195, 198
Handwashing, 124-136
Hand-foot-mouth disease
    discovery of cause, 36
    oral disease and, 71
    characteristics of, 74
Hayfever, 23, 34
Hazard communication standard (OSHA), 247
    compliance officer and, 240
    disposal of chemical and, 264
    "employee-right-to-know" and, 254
    engineering controls and, 93, 100-102, 247, 248
    hazard determination and, 254-256
    health hazard and, 249
    "HazCom" program and, 247, 249
    labeling chemicals and, 259-260

Hazard communication standard (OSHA)—cont'd
    MSDS and, 260-264
    NFPA 704 diamond labeling system and, 259
    OSHA problem solving and, 265-267
    personal protection devices and, 249
    purpose of, 251
    trade secrets and, 265
    training and, 236, 264-265
    warning signs and, 259-260
    work practices and, 247, 248
    written hazard communication program and,
        254-258
Hazard warning, 248
Hazardous chemical, 248, 267-274
Hazardous waste, 223
Health hazard, 249, 252
Heat-sensitive indicator, 161-163
Heat-resistant gloves, 118-119
Helicobacter pylori, 36
Hemophilia and HIV disease, 65
Hepatitis A,
    discovery of cause, 36
    characteristics of, 54, 56, 61
    serology of, 57
    vaccine for, 107
Hepatitis B, 54-60
    bloodborne disease, 54
    discovery of cause, 36
    OSHA and, 92-93
    risk for dental patient and, 59-60
    risk for dental team and, 59
    transmission of, 55-59
    vaccine for, 60, 97-98, 107, 109-113
Hepatitis B core antigen (HBcAg), 57
Hepatitis B e antigen (HBeAg), 57
Hepatitis B immune globulin (HBIG), 57
Hepatitis B surface Antigen (HBsAg), 57
    antibody to, 57
Hepatitis B vaccine
    antibodies to, 57
    doses of, 111
    employee refusal and, 113, 337
    OSHA and, 997-98, 112-113
    response to, 110-111
    safety and efficacy of, 110-111
    types of, 110
Hepatitis B virus
    characteristics of, 55
    resistance of, 55
    antigens from, 57
Hepatitis C
    bloodborne nature of, 54, 55
    characteristics of, 56, 60, 61
    discovery of cause, 36
    serology of, 57

Hepatitis D
    bloodborne nature of, 54, 55
    characteristics of, 56, 60-61
    discovery of cause, 36
    serology of, 57
Hepatitis E
    characteristics of, 54, 56, 61-62
    discovery of cause, 36
    serology of, 57
Hemophilia and HIV diseae, 65
Herpangina, 71, 74
Herpes simplex virus
    AIDS and, 63, 64
    asymptomatic infection from, 70
    oral diseases and, 63, 70
    pathogens in the mouth and, 211
    whitlow, 70
Herpes labialis, 70
Herpetic whitlow, 70
High volume evacuation, 101, 201, 205-206
Histolytic enzyme
    as a pathogenic property, 29, 30
    bacterial nutrition and, 14
    examples of, 29, 30
    in periodontal disease, 48, 49
    mesosomes and, 9
Histoplasmosis, 21, 64
HIV; see Human immunodeficiency virus, type 1
HIV disease, 62-68
    AIDS, 63
    HIV infection, 63
    HIV-testing, 63
    HIV periodontitis, 50
    oral manifestations of, 63
    prevention of, 68
    risk behaviors for, 65
    risk for dental patient and, 66-67
    risk for dental team and, 66
Holding solution, 136, 138-139
Homosexual men and HIV disease, 65
Hospital disinfectant, 183
Host defense, 30-34
Host-microorganism interaction, 27-34
Hot oil "sterilizer," 1173-174
Human herpes virus, 70, 72
Human immunodeficiency virus, type 1 (HIV)
    characteristics of, 62-63
    discovery of, 36
    pathogenic properties of, 62
Hyaluronidase, 27
Hydrocolloid impression material, 214
Hydrophilic virus, 185, 187

I

Immune serum globulin (ISG), 57

Immunization
    available vaccines and, 107
    hepatitis B and, 60, 97-98, 110-113
    influenza and, 108-109
    OSHA and, 97-98, 112-113
    tetanus and, 107-108
Immunity
    acquired type, 2
    antibody-mediated type, 32
    artificial type, 33, 106-114
    cell-mediated type, 32
    vaccines and, 106-114
Impression disinfection, 213-215
Incubation stage of disease, 24-25
Indirect contact, 26
Infection control
    goal of, 89-90
    in the laboratory, 210-217
    in radiology, 217-221
    clinical protocol for, 230-234
    rationale for, 83-90
    recommendations for, 90-91
    regulations for, 91-105
    procedures for, 84-86
Infectious disease
    bloodborne types, 54
    development of, 23-27
    endogenous types, 23
    exogenous types, 23
    host defense against, 30-34
    oral types, 44-52, 71
    opportunistic types, 23, 63, 64
    prevention of, 84-86
    respiratory types, 71, 72, 75-80
    stages of, 24-25
    systemic types, 71
    transmission of, 25-27, 80-89
Infectious mononucleosis, 71, 72, 74-75
Infectious waste, 223
Influenza, 71, 80, 107, 108-109
Injection drug use and HIV disease, 65
Instruments
    cassettes for, 140, 143, 144, 146
    cleaning of, 139-142, 160-168
    lubricating, 142
    packaging, 142-147, 166-168
    protection of, 170
    sharpening, 170
    storage of, 165-166, 168
    sterilizing, 147-156, 167-168
    unwrapped, 147
Innate host defense, 30-32
Interferon, 31
Iodophors, 185-186
    examples of 312-313
    hepatitis B and, 55

Iodophors—cont'd
  use on appliances, 211
  use on impressions, 214
  use on surfaces, 182

J

Jaundice in hepatitis, 59
Juvenile periodontitis, 04

K

Kaposi's sarcoma, 36, 71, 64
Kilopascals (kPa), 147
Koch, Robert, 2

L

Labels, warning
  for biohazard, 96
  for hazardous chemical, 249, 258, 259-260
  laundry and, 104-105
  OSHA and, 96, 259-260
Laboratory asepsis
  appliance disinfection and, 210-213
  blasting procedures and, 215
  grinding procedures and, 215
  impression disinfection and, 213-315
  intermediate cases and, 215-216
  laboratory office relations and, 210
  polishing procedures and, 215, 216
  protheses disinfection and, 210, 213
  pumice and, 215, 216
  stone casts and, 212
Lactate dehydrogenase, 17
Lactic acid
  fermentation and, 17, 18
  structure of, 17
  dental caries and, 47, 48
  Streptococcus mutans and, 48
Lactobacillus sp.
  caries and, 47
  in dental unit water, 192
  fermentation and, 17
  in the mouth, 44
  pathogenic properties of, 47
Lactobacillus acidophilus, 29, 47
Lathe, dental, 215, 216
Laundry, 104-105, 133
Leeuwenhoek, Antoni, 2
Legionella pneumophilia
  AIDS and, 64
  discovery of, 36
  pathogenic properties of, 29
  in waterlines, 192, 194
Legionnaire's disease, 36, 39-40, 192, 194
Lipid
  bacterial nutrition and, 16
  composition of, 7

Lipid—cont'd
  cytoplasm and, 7
  cytoplasmic membrane and, 9
  viral envelope and, 19
Lipopolysaccharide
  composition of, 7
  endotoxin and, 10
Lipoprotein, 7
Lockjaw; *see* Tetanus
Lyme disease, 36
Lymphocytes,
  role in immunity, 32
  HIV disease and, 62
Lymphokine, 32
Lymphoma, non-Hodgkin's, 64
Lysozyme, 10, 31

M

Macrophage, 32
Material safety data sheet (MSDS), 249, 258, 260-264, 274
Mask, 127-128
  bloodborne pathogens standard and, 102-103
  chairside asepsis and, 231
  instrument processing and, 138
  laboratory asepsis and, 210
  operatory clean-up and, 182, 233
  placing and removing, 133-134
  radiographic asepsis and, 217
Measles, rubeola; *see also* Rubella
  oral spread of, 72, 80
  vaccine for, 107
Medical records, 100
Medical waste, 223
Meningitis, 71
Mesophile, 13
Mesosome, 8, 9
Metabolism, bacterial, 16-18
Microaerophile, 14
Micrococcus sp., 44
Micrometer, 7
Miller, Willoby D., 3
Mitsuokella sp., 44
Modes, disease spread, 26-27, 83-89
Molds, 21
Monitoring; *see* Sterilization monitoring
Moraxella sp., 44
Mouthrinse, preprocedure, 207
MSDS; *see* Material safety data sheet
Multiple-drug-resistant TB, 40, 77-78
Mumps
  oral spread of, 71, 80
  vaccine for, 107
Mumps virus, 71, 211
Mutans streptococci, 46, 47
Mycobacterium sp., 136

Rothia sp., 44
Routes of entry, 27
Rubber dam, 206-207
Rubella
   oral spread of, 72, 80
   vaccine for, 107
Rubella virus, 72
Rubeola virus, 72
Rust, control, 142

S

Safety coordinator, 236
Saliva
   aerosols
      mask and, 127-128
      protective eyewear and, 129
      rubber dam and, 206-207
   as infected body fluid, 65, 94
   normal flora and, 43
Salmonella sp., 64
Salmonella choleraesuis
   resistance to chemicals and, 136
   hospital disinfectant and, 183
Scarlet fever, 11, 71, 183
Scoop technique, 225-226
Selenomonas sp., 44
Semmelweis, Ignaz, 23
Septicemia, 51
Sexually transmitted disease
   Chlamydia and, 16
   gonorrhea, 71
   hepatitis B, 55, 58
   hepatitis C, 60
   herpes infections, 73
   HIV disease, 63
   syphilis, 71
Sharps
   disease spread
      hepatitis B and, 58
      HIV disease and, 67
      mode of spread and, 83, 84
   handling and disposal of, 225-228
   instrument cleaning and, 141
   OSHA and, 101
   regulated waste and, 225-228
Shelf-life, 165-166, 173
Shigella flexneri, 64
Shingles, 72
Silicone impression material, 214
Skin flora, 125
Smoke alarm, 241, 279
Sodium hypochlorite, 185, 186
   hepatitis B and, 55
   use on appliances, 212
   use on impressions, 214
   use on surfaces, 182

Spatter, 101, 205
Spirochete, 73
Spore; *see* endospore
Spore strips; *see* Sterilization, monitoring, biological
Spore-testing; *see* Sterilization, monitoring, biological
State regulations, infection control, 91, 105, 158
Staphylococcus aureus
   asymptomatic carriers, 72
   cell morphology, 8
   hospital disinfectant and, 183
   pathogenic properties of, 29
   pathogens in the mouth and, 211
   resistance to chemicals and, 136
Sterilant, liquid; *see also* Glutaraldehyde
   heat-labile items and, 171-172
   proper use of, 173
Sterility assurance, 137
Sterilization
   failure of, 156, 157
   of instruments, 147-156
   importance of
      instrument processing and, 135-36
      killing pathogens and, 136
      sterility assurance and, 137
   monitoring
      biological, 156-161
      chemical, 161-163
      instrument processing and, 156-165
      physical, 163-164
      spore-testing, 148-149, 156-161
      sterilizers and, 148-149
   methods for, 147-156
   of sharps containers, 228
   regulations and, 105
   temperatures of, 148-149
   universal, 137
   wrap, 143
Sterilizer
   chemical vapor
      advantages of, 148
      precautions for, 148
      monitoring of, 148, 156
      use of, 153-154
   dry heat
      advantages of, 149
      precautions for, 149
      monitoring of, 149, 156
      use of, 154-156
   ethylene oxide, 172-173
   steam
      advantages of, 148
      precautions for, 148
      monitoring of, 148, 156
      use of, 147, 152
Stone cast disinfection, 212

Storage, instruments, 165–166

Streptococcal pharyngitis, 71, 75

bacterial attachment and, 11

exogenous disease and, 23

oral disease, 71

Streptococcus sp., 44

Streptococcus cricetus, 47

Streptococcus faecalis, 136

Streptococcus mutans

acidogenic nature and, 46, 47

aciduric nature and, 46, 47

fermentation and, 18, 48

nomenclature and, 5

normal flora and, 43

pathogenic properties of, 47

plaque formation by, 47, 48

Streptococcus pneumoniae

AIDS and, 64

asymptomatic carriers, 72

capsule and, 10

pathogenic properties of, 29

Streptococcus pyogenes

asymptomatic carriers, 72

pathogenic properties of, 29

pathogens in the mouth and, 211

streptococcal sore throat and, 71, 75

strep throat and, 71, 75

scarlet fever and, 71, 75

Streptococcus rattus, 47

Streptococcus sanguis, 29

Streptococcus sobrinus, 46, 47

"Strep throat"; *see* Streptococcal pharyngitis

Structure

bacterial, 7, 8

viral, 19

Subacute bacterial endocarditis, 51

Sucrose, 47, 48

Suction devices, 205, 206, 208

Supplies for infection control, 169, 241

Surface disinfection

bloodborne pathogens standard and, 103–104

disinfectants and, 182–188

laboratory asepsis and, 210–215

procedures for, 182

Surface covers

in radiology, 217–219

types of, 175–177

use of, 177–181

Symptoms, 24,

Synthetic phenolic disinfectants, 186, 187–189, 312–315

use on surfaces, 182

Syphilis, 71, 73, 74

T

Tetanus, 107–108

Thermophil, 13

T-lymphocytes; *see* Lymphocytes

Trachoma, 16

Trade secrets, 257, 258, 265

Training, OSHA

bloodborne pathogens, 94–96

hazard communication, 254–258

Treponema sp., 44

Treponema denticola, 8, 50

Treponema pallidum, 71, 211

Triclosan, 125

Toxic shock syndrome, 36

Toxic waste, 223

Toxin, 29, 30

Toxoplasmosis, 64

Transfusion

hepatitis C and, 60

HIV disease and, 65

Transient bacteremia, 51

Transient skin flora, 125

Tuberculosis, 71, 75–78

CDC and prevention of, 295–297

Typhoid fever, 107

U

Ultrasonic cleaning, 139–141

Unit dosing, 189

Universal precautions

asymptomatic carriers and, 24

basis for, 24

OSHA and, 100

Utility gloves

instrument handling and, 137, 138, 241

surface disinfection and, 182

types of, 117, 118

V

Vaccines; *see* Immunization

Varicella-zoster virus,

oral spread of, 71

presence in the mouth, 211

Veillonella sp., 44

Viral hepatitis, 54–62; *see also* Hepatitis

Virology, 2

Virus

bacterial, 3

control of, 21

life cycle of, 20–21

pathogenic properties of, 28, 29, 30

structure of, 19

Vitamins, bacterial, 16

Virulence, 89

W

Warts, 21
Waste management
    blood and, 224
    infectious waste and, 223-224
    medical waste and, 223
    OSHA and, 104
    pathogenic waste and, 224
    sharps and, 225-228
Waste products, bacterial, 16
Water-based phenolics, 186, 312-313
Waterborne disease agents, 80-82
Waterline, dental unit, 190-194
Wax rims and bites, 212
White blood cells, 10

Whooping cough, 107
Wolinella sp., 44
Wolinella recta, 50
Work practice control, 100-102, 247, 249
Wrap, sterilization, 143
Written opinions, OSHA
    hepatitis vaccination and, 97, 98
    post-exposure follow-up and, 99, 100

Y

Yeast, 21, 73
Yellow fever, 107

X

X-ray; *see* Radiographic asepsis

Learning
by Heart